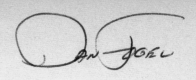

THE
PURSUIT OF
HAPPINESS

THE PURSUIT OF HAPPINESS

DISCOVERING
THE PATHWAY
TO FULFILLMENT,
WELL-BEING,
AND ENDURING
PERSONAL JOY

DAVID G. MYERS, PH.D.

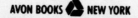
AVON BOOKS ▲ NEW YORK

Grateful acknowledgment is made for permission to reprint from the following:

Culture Shift in Advanced Industrial Society, copyright © 1990 by Ronald Inglehart, Princeton University Press.

Optimal Experience: Psychological Studies of Flow in Consciousness, copyright © 1988 by Mihaly and Isabella Csikszentmihalyi, Cambridge University Press.

Social Indicators of Well-being, copyright © 1976 by Frank Andrews and Stephen Withey, Plenum Press.

"National Estimates of Cohabitation," from *Demography*, copyright © 1989 by Larry Bumpass and James Sweet, University of Wisconsin.

AVON BOOKS
A division of
The Hearst Corporation
1350 Avenue of the Americas
New York, New York 10019

In gratitude for twenty-five happy, satisfying years
shared with students and colleagues
in a community of Hope

Everything should be made as simple as possible, but not simpler.

ALBERT EINSTEIN

Contents

THE
PURSUIT OF
HAPPINESS

Acknowledgments

My gratitude flows mostly to the researchers whose work inspired this book. Reading them persuaded me that their discoveries are humanly significant and deserving of a wide audience. This book therefore builds upon the efforts of an international community of scholars, including Ronald Inglehart, Frank Andrews, Randy Larsen, and the late Angus Campbell at the University of Michigan, Ed Diener and co-workers at the University of Illinois, George Gallup, Jr., at the Gallup Organization, Michael Argyle at Oxford University, Ruut Veenhoven at Erasmus University of Rotterdam, Andrew Greeley at the University of Arizona, Norval Glenn at the University of Texas, Alex Michalos at the University of Guelph, Robert Emmons at the

University of California, Davis, Norbert Schwarz and Fritz Strack at Mannheim University, Martin Seligman at the University of Pennsylvania, Shelley Taylor at UCLA, Bruce Headey at Melbourne University, William Stock and Morris Okun at Arizona State University, Jonathan Freedman at the University of Toronto, Mihaly Csikszentmihalyi and Tom Smith at the University of Chicago, Faye Crosby at Smith College, the late Richard Kammann at the University of Otago, and hundreds of others credited in the source notes. Because this book is also a personal essay, none of them will agree with everything I have written, nor should any of them be held responsible for it. Nevertheless, kudos to each. Without their pioneering explorations, this book would not exist.

I am additionally grateful to several friends for their kindness and criticism. Dennis Voskuil and Wallace Voskuil urged me to believe that others might share my fascination with the new research on well-being. Special thanks also to my wife, Carol, for her sage advice; to my daughter, Laura, who engaged me in a revealing oral reading of parts of the manuscript; to Les Beach, William Brownson, Max De-Pree, Jane Dickie, John Hesselink, Charles Huttar, Chris Kaiser, Tom Ludwig, Peter Schakel, John Stapert, and Merold Westphal for their ideas and encouragement; to Alison Husting and Suzanne Lipsett for helping me cast the material into a form suitable for a general audience; to Kim Bundy, Melissa Johnson, and Dawn Luchies for their help in tracking down information; to Phyllis Vandervelde for her painstaking revision of the notes and bibliography; and to my poet-colleague and friend, Jack Ridl, for once again guiding the voice that speaks through these pages.

I am further indebted to my agent, John Brockman, for his belief in this book, to my editor, Maria Guarnaschelli, for her careful, candid, and supportive guidance, and to Kathy Antrim, for her meticulous support in preparing the final manuscript for publication.

Finally, I pay tribute to the hundreds of thousands of people whose life experiences this book mirrors. By generously sharing with researchers the events and emotions of their lives, they have provided all of us with a clearer view of the things that do, and don't, make for enduring joy.

About This Book

Books, books, and more books have been written on psychology's analyses of misery, and how to relieve it. During psychology's first century, studies of negative emotions—depression, anxiety, stress—have greatly overshadowed studies of positive emotions. Thus, psychology's textbooks (as I know well, having written some) have far more to say about suffering than joy.

That is now changing. Thanks to a new generation of researchers, we have a fresh perspective on that age-old conundrum: What is happiness, and how can we attain it? In *Psychological Abstracts* (a sort of reader's guide to psychology) the number of articles pertaining to "happiness," "life satisfaction," or "well-being" mushroomed from 150 in 1979 to 780 in 1989. This book reports what we have learned so far, and although the new research offers no easy how-to-be-happy formula, the findings are enlightening. Looking over scientists' shoulders in their pursuit of happiness in human lives informs our personal pursuit of happiness.

The scientific study of emotional well-being is new, but theories about the secrets of happiness are ages old. The philosophers of ancient Greece pondered the happiness question intensely. Their answer: Happiness arises from a life of leisurely and intelligent reflection. "There is no fool who is happy, and no wise man who is not," echoed the Roman statesman Cicero (106–43 B.C.). For the Greeks, and for Cicero, the pleasures of life were therefore more of the mind and less of the body. To be happy was to live serenely, above the world's swings of passion and material fortune.

The Epicurean and Stoic philosophers offered variations on this song of happy contemplation. For Epicurus (342–270 B.C.), happiness flowed from life's simple, sustainable pleasures, such as tranquil peace of mind. He held that wise people remember the past with gratitude, take delight in present pleasures, and regard the eternal future without fear. To the Stoics, happiness was less the enjoyment of simple pleasures than the attainment of virtuous attitudes—the wisdom to know what is good and bad, what to fear and what not to fear, and how to control one's passions. Better to accept one's situation than to covet something different. Pretty cool, cerebral folks, those Greeks.

In the centuries since, other sages have offered radically different ideas about the roots of happiness. They've told us that happiness comes from living a virtuous life and that it comes from getting away with evil; that it comes from knowing the truth and from preserving illusions; that it comes from restraint and from purging ourselves of pent-up rage and misery. They also have told us that happiness comes from living for the present and living for the future; from making others happy and from enjoying our enemies' misery; from being with others and from living in solitude. The list goes on, but the implication is clear: To sift the true myths from the false, it's time for some careful investigation.

Enter the new science of well-being. We have long done a bang-up job of measuring our physical and material well-being, by monitoring people's diets, death rates, dollars, and dwellings. Without discounting these measures of "objective well-being," psychologists and sociologists in North America, Europe, and elsewhere now regularly assess people's "subjective well-being"—their feelings of happiness, their sense of satisfaction with life. The overriding question: What are the experiences, circumstances, traits, and attitudes that enable some people to experience well-being, others not? Simply put, who is happy—and why?

Like everyone who has written or read one of the scores of how-to-be-happy books, social scientists have their own hunches about the secrets of happiness. To test their hunches—to sift the true accompaniments of well-being from the merely plausible hunches—well-being researchers do two things. They survey representative samples of people. And they experiment.

To survey the experiences and emotions of a representative cross section of people, they gather a random sample—one in which everyone in the population under study has an equal chance of participating. Imagine a giant barrel containing 60 million white beans thoroughly mixed with 40 million green beans. A scoop that randomly sampled 1,500 of them would contain about 60 percent white and 40 percent green beans, give or take 2 or 3 percent. Sampling people is no different; 1,500 randomly sampled people provide a similarly accurate snapshot of 100 million people.

The popular alternative to representative random sampling is haphazard sampling. People who disbelieve the results of a careful survey typically do so based on their own hunches and their haphazard sampling of acquaintances. They're not so much doubting the survey findings as preferring their own informal survey to a more systematic one. From this it's only a short step to, say, Shere Hite's *Women and Love* survey, based on a 4.5 percent response rate from mailings to an unrepresentative sample of 100,000 American women. This was doubly unrepresentative, because not only did she have a modest, self-selected return, but the women initially contacted were members of women's organizations. Nonetheless, "It's 4,500 people. That's enough for me," reported Hite.

Apparently it was also enough for *Time*, which made a cover story of her findings—that 70 percent of women married five years or more were having affairs, and that 95 percent of women feel emotionally harassed by the men they love. Those who lapped this up seemingly cared little that on less publicized surveys, *representatively* sampled American women express much higher levels of satisfaction: Half or more report feeling "very happy" or "completely satisfied" with their marriages; only 3 percent say they are "not at all happy"; and only 10 percent report having had an affair during their current marriage.

You can forecast the weather by taking a haphazard sample—by looking at the clouds and holding your finger in the wind—or you can look at weather maps derived from comprehensive reporting. You can describe human experience using hunches, conventional wisdom, and haphazard samples. But for an accurate picture of the experiences and attitudes of a whole population there's only one game in town—the representative survey.

Aided by surveys, we can *describe* people's self-reported happiness. We can also answer many intriguing questions. If you wanted to predict someone's happiness, what would it help to know? Whether the person is young or old? female or male? outgoing or introverted? Is happiness linked with health? wealth? relationships? one's line of work? spirituality?

Answering these questions will *hint* at what causes happiness, and what you and I might do to put more joy in our lives. But to pin down cause and effect, social scientists *experiment*. To gauge the impact of some suspected factor, they give two equivalent groups an experience that differs only in that factor.

So, can listening to positive messages on subliminal tapes cause us to become happier (or to stop smoking, learn more easily, or warm up sexually)? To find out, an experimenter would randomly assign people to two groups, one that listens to a music tape with an embedded pertinent subliminal message, one to a music tape without the message. Because the subliminal message can't be consciously heard, neither group knows which tape it has. (For the results of such experiments, see Chapter 5.)

Or consider: Are people made happier by finding money? by having their expectations and points of comparison changed? by spending a leisurely day at the beach? by undergoing psychotherapy? Again, to answer such questions we experiment, by randomly assigning people either to experience or not experience the factor of interest.

Obviously, some possibilities don't lend themselves to experiments. To analyze whether marriage enhances happiness it might be nice to randomly assign people to lifelong marriage or single life, but there wouldn't be many volunteers. So we do the best we can, by ferreting out intricate links between marriage and well-being and drawing reasonable conclusions.

Before exploring this new science of well-being, let's clear the decks of some inevitable questions.

Is it selfish to focus on our own happiness? Should happiness really be our ultimate concern? John Stuart Mill thought not: ". . . better to be Socrates dissatisfied than a pig satisfied."

To help people evaluate the importance of happiness, Michael Fordyce, a Florida psychologist who teaches and studies happiness, suggests a mental exercise. Imagine that someone could grant you fame and fortune or happiness. You could have all the adulation and money you've ever dreamed of without knowing happiness. Or you could be joy-filled day after day but possess only life's necessities. Which would you choose?

John Stuart Mill may be right that being happy isn't, or shouldn't be, our ultimate purpose. But when we pit happiness against many things that we long for—robust health, social respect, large incomes—most of us choose happiness. Indeed, our search for happiness and for relief from misery motivates a host of behaviors, from success seeking to sex to suicide.

Aristotle (384–322 B.C.) supposed as much. He helped inspire the Greeks' philosophizing about happiness by arguing that happiness is the supreme good: It is so important that all else is merely a means to its attainment. So important that America rooted its Declaration of Independence in our human right to the pursuit of happiness. So important, believed the philosopher-psychologist William James, that "how to gain, how to keep, how to recover happiness is in fact for most men at all times the secret motive of all they do."

Still, does the quest for well-being seem unworthy? Does it smack of self-indulgence? Do satisfied people smirk contentedly while Rome burns?

Consider Dutch psychologist Ruut Veenhoven's distillation of research done on the accompaniments of happiness. When researchers study the self-reports, behaviors, and peer ratings of people who feel happy or unhappy, they find it's not happy people who are intensely self-focused, but those bereaved or depressed. People put in a sad mood (after imagining depressing situations) report twice as many current aches and pains as do less-self-focused people put in a happy mood. Depressed people tend to be lethargic, brooding, socially withdrawn, even hostile. In some respects, that's healthy. Like physical pain, psychological pain warns of dangers or threats of loss. There is sense in suffering, method in madness. A negative mood signals that all's not well, motivating people to ruminate and reassess rather than make snap judgments as carefree happier people do. But in presuming that other people are rejecting them, depressed people aren't entirely wrong; they are no joy to be around. Misery may love company, but company doesn't love misery. Although initially sympathetic and supportive, a depressed person's spouse and colleagues eventually tire of his hopeless attitude, the fatigue, the complaining.

Happy people, by contrast, are strikingly energetic, decisive, flexible, creative, and sociable. Compared to unhappy people, they are more trusting, more loving, more responsive. For example, as interviewers, they recall more of the positive behaviors of job applicants and rate them more highly than do unhappy interviewers. If made temporarily happy by receiving a small gift, people will report, a few moments later during a survey, that their cars and TV sets are working beautifully—better, if you took their word for it, than those belonging to folks who didn't receive a gift.

Happy people tolerate more frustration. They are less likely to be abusive and are more lenient. Whether temporarily or enduringly happy, they are more loving and forgiving and less likely to exaggerate or overinterpret slight criticism. They choose long-term rewards over immediate small pleasures. Given a chance to look at happy pictures (people laughing, playing) and sad pictures (funerals, disasters), they literally spend more time looking at the brighter side. Sad people look more at the gloomy side of life, and prefer less upbeat people, stories, movies, and music.

Moreover, in experiment after experiment, happy people are more willing to help those in need. It's the "feel-good, do-good phenomenon": Those made to feel successful are more likely to volunteer as a tutor. Those who have just found money in a phone booth are more likely to help somebody pick up dropped papers. Those whose mood has just been boosted by listening to a comedy album are more willing to lend someone else money. Robert Browning had the idea: "Oh, make us happy and you make us good!"

Evidence also accumulates that, as the writer of Proverbs said, "a cheerful heart is a good medicine, but a downcast spirit dries up the bones." Emotions are biological events. Our body's immune system fights disease more effectively when we are happy rather than depressed. When we are depressed, the number of certain disease-fighting cells declines. Stressed animals and distressed or depressed people are therefore more vulnerable to various illnesses.

So, human happiness is both an end—better to live fulfilled, with joy—and a means to a more caring and healthy society. As Helen Keller wrote, "Joy is the holy fire that keeps our purpose warm and our intelligence aglow." That being so, it is time we ponder not only our physical and material well-being, but also our inner well-being.

Our empirical sifting of competing ideas about happiness will affirm some of our culture's deeply held values while challenging others. This critical analysis can help us reassess our priorities. It may also assist our quest to recover a sense of shared values. In affirming certain values, my aim is less to make news than to report it. If it is "liberal" to report that wealth-accumulating materialism and self-focused individualism don't produce the hoped-for well-being, then the liberalism is in the human experiences that I report. If it is "conservative" to report that an active spirituality and close relationships such as marriage do enhance well-being, then the conservatism is less in my reporting than in the responses that I report.

Although we social scientists aim for objectivity, the truth of course is that pure, value-free objectivity does not exist. In questing for truth, we follow our hunches, our biases, our voices within. In deciding *what* to report and *how* to report it, our own sympathies subtly steer us, this way or that. This book was a pleasure to write precisely because it marries not only science with journalism, but facts with values.

My own sympathies lie first with psychology's empirical (scientific) tradition. As a research-oriented social psychologist—one who studies how people view, affect, and relate to one another—I'm not much persuaded by anecdotes, testimonials, inspirational pronouncements, or conventional wisdom. The pop psychology we've created from such sources is sometimes right, as we'll see. But representative surveys and careful experiments show that it's sometimes wrong, as we'll also see.

Rigorous research needn't be cold and dispassionate. Intellectual detective work can be conducted and reported both playfully and compassionately. Although this book's distinctiveness lies in its revelations based on research, I will connect its conclusions to the lives of real people. When discovering answers to the happiness question—who is happy, and why?—I will pause to ponder what the answers might mean for our everyday lives.

Although I identify with a profession not known for its piety, my sympathies also are colored by Christian values and spirituality. This may sound like an unusual combination—the skeptical bent of an empiricist blended with a biblical faith—but it's a stimulating mix. Religion without science shields itself from new understandings. Science without religion shields itself from deep understandings.

It's an old combination. Francis Bacon, Isaac Newton, and several other founders of modern science took seriously the biblical ideas that the created world was worth exploring, and that, owing no allegiance to any human authority, they should humbly submit their ideas to empirical testing and accept whatever truths nature revealed. It's also a combination that makes for a mind-expanding and purpose-filled approach to life. I don't feel dogmatic certainty about many things, but I am powered by (as the name of my institution suggests) a sense of Hope.

Knowing that I do not possess final answers to the mysteries of well-being—this being only an interim report on a fledgling science—I hope you will not feel pressed to agree with all that follows. Rather, I hope you will join me and the researchers in our unfinished search for joy. My aim for this book will be accomplished if their revelations, and my reflections on them, stimulate you to reflect on where you can find deeper meaning and satisfaction in your own life, and how all of us together can build a world that enhances human well-being.

1

What Is Well-being?

If one thinks that one is happy,
that is enough to be happy.

MME DE LA FAYETTE, LETTER TO GILLES MÉNAGE

We social scientists can count crimes. We can measure memories. We can assess intelligence. But how do we gauge happiness? Can we trust what people tell us? Oh, for a happiness thermometer.

If we considered well-being a thing—if it meant being well off, being successful, being healthy—we could measure that thing. However, like Madame de La Fayette, social scientists view well-being as a state of mind. Well-being, sometimes called "subjective well-being" to emphasize the point, is a pervasive sense that life is good. Well-being outlasts yesterday's moment of elation, today's buoyant mood, and tomorrow's hard time; it is an ongoing perception that this time of one's life, or even life as a whole, is fulfilling, meaningful, and pleasant.

It is what some people experience as joy—not an ephemeral euphoria, but a deep and abiding sense that, despite the day's woes, all is, or will be, well. Even when the surface waters churn, the deep currents run sure.

To probe people's sense of well-being, researchers have asked them to report their feelings of happiness or unhappiness along with their thoughts about how satisfying their lives are. Like tangerines and oranges, happiness and life satisfaction are subtly different yet share much in common. People who *feel* happy also tend to *think* their lives are satisfying.

Sometimes researchers probe with a simple, single question. Imagine yourself one of the tens of thousands of Americans approached by survey research teams from the University of Michigan and the University of Chicago and asked: "Taking all things together, how would you say things are these days—would you say you are very happy, pretty happy, or not too happy?"

And "How satisfied are you with your life as a whole these days? Are you very satisfied? satisfied? not very satisfied? not at all satisfied?"

Sometimes researchers probe with multi-item measures. For example, Chicago researcher Norman Bradburn wanted to assess people's positive and negative feelings separately. Imagine being asked about your positive emotions:

During the past few weeks have you ever felt . . .

> particularly excited or interested in something?
> proud because someone complimented you on something you did?
> pleased about having accomplished something?
> on top of the world?
> that things were going your way?

And about your negative emotions:

During the past few weeks have you ever felt . . .

> so restless that you couldn't sit long in a chair?
> very lonely or remote from other people?
> bored?

depressed or very unhappy?

upset because someone criticized you?

How many of the positive emotions have you been experiencing? How many of the negative emotions?

Alternatively, psychologists might define your happiness by summing your moment-to-moment positive feelings then subtracting your moment-to-moment negative feelings, or by computing the ratio of your positive to negative feelings. Bradburn's questions provide a quick self-estimate of what we would find.

How Happy Are People?

We are "not born for happiness," wrote Samuel Johnson, anticipating in 1776 a predominant opinion today. In his 1930 book, *The Conquest of Happiness,* philosopher Bertrand Russell echoed that most people are *un*happy, and recent warmhearted books for the would-be-happy, mostly written by people who spend their days counseling the unhappy, concur. Dennis Wholey (author of *Are You Happy?*) reports that experts he interviewed believe that perhaps 20 percent of Americans are happy. "I'm surprised!" responded psychologist Archibald Hart in his *15 Principles for Achieving Happiness.* "I would have thought the proportion was much lower!" In *Happiness Is an Inside Job,* Father John Powell agrees: "One-third of all Americans wake up depressed every day. Professionals estimate that only 10 to 15 percent of Americans think of themselves as truly happy." Even my esteemed fellow research psychologist, Mihaly Csikszentmihalyi, has written that "genuinely happy individuals are few and far between." And psychiatrist Thomas Szasz speaks for many in surmising, "Happiness is an imaginary condition, formerly attributed by the living to the dead, now usually attributed by adults to children, and by children to adults."

But when asked about their happiness, people across the world paint a much rosier picture. For example, in national surveys a third of Americans say they are *very* happy. Only one in ten say "not too happy." The remainder—the majority—describe themselves as "pretty happy."

Most people are similarly upbeat about their satisfaction with life. More than 80 percent rate themselves as more satisfied than dissatisfied. Fewer than one in ten rate themselves as more dissatisfied than satisfied. Likewise, some three fourths of people say, yes, they've felt excited, proud, or pleased at some point during the past few weeks; no more than a third say they've felt lonely, bored, or depressed.

To probe people's well-being in yet another way, University of Michigan researchers asked a national sample of Americans to express their feelings nonverbally: "Here are some faces expressing various feelings. Which face comes closest to expressing how you feel about your life as a whole?"

20%   46%   27%   4%   2%   1%   0%

Once again, we see that most people report feeling happy.

In Western Europe, well-being varies by country, from the Netherlands, where more than four in ten people say they are *very* happy, to Portugal, where fewer than one in ten say the same. Although Europeans, by and large, report a lower sense of well-being than North Americans, even they typically assess themselves positively. Four in five say they are "fairly" or "very" satisfied with their everyday lives.

Are People Lying?

Can we trust these generally bullish self-descriptions? Some would doubt it. Sigmund Freud believed that we delude ourselves by repressing painful feelings. Karl Marx believed we form a "false consciousness" that protects us from feeling the misery of injustice. Consider Martha, a devoted forty-three-year-old woman who learned her physician husband had been having affairs. She recalls "smiling and clutching my charge card on the way to the mall as I cheered myself by thinking he was just 'working late' today." Like Martha, might people not *say* they are happy while freely embracing the system that oppresses them?

To the happiness researchers, however, well-being is a state of mind. As we'll see in later chapters, our happiness depends less on our objective circumstances than on how we respond to them. "If you feel happy," writes research psychologist Jonathan Freedman, "you are happy—that's all we mean by the term." Moreover, if *you* can't tell someone whether you're happy or miserable, who can? Imagine that you felt, and told someone that you felt, very happy, deeply satisfied with how your life is going, and just plain grateful to be alive in this wonderful world. Would you not think it strange if someone said, "Sorry—you're deluding yourself; actually, you are miserable." Or imagine that you felt depressed, even distraught, but no one would believe you. Would you not think people arrogant to presume to report your own emotions more intimately and accurately than you can? Surely the people who participated in these studies would similarly feel bewildered at researchers' refusing to believe their experiences.

Still, even if people are the best judges of their own experiences, can we trust them to be candid? People's self-reports are susceptible to two biases that limit, but do not eliminate, their authenticity.

The first bias is their tendency to be agreeable, to put on a good face. People overreport good things. There is more reported voting (extrapolated from surveys) than actual voting, many fewer cigarettes smoked than actually sold, less tax evasion than known to occur. If people are uncertain about how to rate themselves, they shade the truth toward the positive, optimistic side. Given all that they hear about self-destructive negative thinking, my students are surprised to learn that most people exhibit what psychologists Margaret Matlin and David Stang call a "Pollyanna syndrome." Dozens of studies show that people more readily perceive, remember, and communicate pleasant than unpleasant information. Positive thinking predominates.

An example: Rutgers University researcher Neil Weinstein reports that college students consistently exhibit an "unrealistic optimism" about their future. They rate themselves as far more likely than their classmates to get a good job, draw a good salary, and own a house, and as far less likely to get divorced, have cancer, and be fired. As we will see in Chapter 6, this optimism is generally healthy. If we believe in our own possibilities and expect only good things to happen, we'll live more venturesome, upbeat lives (though perhaps failing to protect ourselves against such real risks as car accidents, AIDS, and heart attacks).

Another example: As they begin college, only 2 percent of students say there is a very good chance they will drop out, even temporarily. But we know the optimism of the other 98 percent is often unrealistic. For only about half of the students entering a four-year college or university graduate within five years. For one reason or another, the dream often dies.

So, when they answer survey questions Pollyannaish people—most people—probably do err on the bright side. This helps explain why, as we'll see in later chapters, certain other indicators (such as rates of depression and marital failure) paint a less rosy picture. But if people are all a bit Pollyannaish, this poses no real problem for research. If a hospital's thermometers all read 10 degrees too high, they would still allow us to compare people with relatively high versus low fevers. Likewise, we could downplay people's happiness reports by, say, 20 percent and still assume that our "happiness thermometers" are valid as relative scales. To discover who is happiest, and why, we need only assume that those who say they are "very happy" or "completely satisfied" do experience greater well-being than those who say they are unhappy or dissatisfied.

The second intriguing bias is people's momentary moods. If people are put in a buoyant mood—whether under hypnosis or just by a day's events (a World Cup soccer victory for the West German subjects of one study, for example)—they see the world through rose-colored glasses. They judge themselves competent and effective, other people well-intentioned, life in general wonderful. After rain, even a sunny day is enough to brighten people's reports of well-being. But let the emotional skies cloud over and suddenly they see everything negatively. Even memories change with moods.

Depressed adults are in one sense like children in a bad mood: They typically recall their parents as rejecting, punitive, and guilt-promoting. Inge, an occasionally depressed young woman, speaks for those who have known the plague of mood disorder. It's like viewing

28

life through dark-colored glasses: "My thoughts become negative and pessimistic. As I look into the past, I become convinced that everything that I've ever done is worthless. Any happy period seems like an illusion. My accomplishments appear as genuine as the false façade of a Western movie." *Formerly* depressed people describe their parents the same as do never-depressed people—positively. "In a blue mood even my favorite ice-cream cone tastes stale," says Ralph. "In an up mood, everything and everyone seems praiseworthy." Therapists beware: Patients' recollections of their terrible childhoods may say as much about their current moods as about their childhood experiences.

You and I may nod our heads knowingly. Yet, curiously, when in either a good or bad mood we persist in attributing our judgments to reality rather than to our temporary mood. When our mood changes, we perceive the world out there as actually different, and as having always been so. Passions exaggerate. Feeling elated, we think we'll ever be so. When the elation turns to gloom, we can hardly recall the jubilation. Elated again, we feel as if the elation never left.

By coloring people's assessments of the overall quality of their lives, temporary moods do reduce the reliability of their self-pronouncements. Their happiness thermometers are admittedly imperfect.

Though imperfect, they are nevertheless useful. We can acknowledge the biases of Pollyannaism and temporary mood and still assume, as I will, that people's reports of their own well-being are worth taking seriously. Why? First, when asked at various points in time to assess their happiness and life satisfaction, people's reports retain a respectable consistency. Those who today say their lives overflow with happiness and satisfaction are likely a year from now to say much the same.

Second, people who *say* they are happy give every indication of actually being so. They smile and laugh more during interviews. They have happier memories. They report more joy when their experience is sampled daily, sometimes over random moments (by using electronic pagers or watches with preset alarms that beep wearers to record their current activities and feelings). And their friends and family are more likely to see them as happy people.

Having people report their well-being is therefore like having them report the outdoor temperature. To get the most reliable and accurate reading, you're best off reading a thermometer. Lacking that, you can take the word of someone who just stepped outside to pick up the paper. But no! someone may object, that person's estimates will be biased by whether the person has just been exercising or inactive, whether the person is warmly dressed or not, whether the person has just been in a warm or a cool room. Yes, yes, and yes, you reply. Still, we can trust people's rough estimates of whether it is 70 or 60 degrees, and whether they are joy-filled or miserable.

So, most people experience a fair degree of well-being. But some experience more than others, and they can tell us as much.

We therefore wonder: What traits of personality, what circumstances of life, what states of mind correlate with well-being—with that enduring, joyful, and joy-spreading spirit that enables one to sense that being alive is the most wonderful of gifts? We shouldn't expect a single, simplistic answer, because complex human qualities such as intelligence, kindness, and happiness inevitably have many determinants. Breadstick-shaped explanations can't explain pretzel-shaped traits. Still, our question persists: Who is happy—and why? Let's begin by tackling head-on the American dream: Does happiness come by achieving wealth and success?

2

Wealth and Well-being

It's pretty hard to tell what does bring happiness.
Poverty an' wealth have both failed.

KIN HUBBARD, *ABE MARTIN'S BROADCAST*

Does well-being come with being well-off? More than ever, Americans of the 1980s *thought* so.

We may not have said it in so many words. But asked in a Roper survey how satisfied we were with thirteen different aspects of life, including our friends, our house, and our schooling, we expressed *least* satisfaction with "the amount of money you have to live on." When University of Michigan interviewers asked what hampers our search for the good life, our most frequent answer was, "We're short of money." Asked what would *improve* our quality of life, our first answer often was, "More money." Except for those with the highest incomes, most of us thought, and still think, that improved fiscal fitness—10 to 20 percent more money—would bring more happiness. And the more the better. According to a 1990 Gallup poll, one in two women, two in three men, and four in five people earning more than seventy-five thousand dollars a year would like to be rich.

These sentiments reflect a cultural shift toward greater materialism. What in a job is most important? From the early 1970s to the early 1980s, a "high income" rose to second in a series of rated criteria. It was surpassed only by "interesting and meaningful work."

This new "greening of America" was especially dramatic among collegians. In the American Council on Education's annual survey of over 200,000 entering college students, the proportion agreeing that an important reason for their going to college was "to make more money" rose from one in two in 1971 to nearly three in four by 1990. And the number who considered it very important or essential that they become "very well-off financially," rose from 39 percent in 1970 to 74 percent in 1990. These proportions flip-flopped with those who began college hoping to "develop a meaningful philosophy of life," whose numbers dropped from 76 to 43 percent. Similar percentages, but what a change in values!

During the six years in which he taught all the courses on corporate strategy at Duke University's School of Business, economist Thomas Naylor asked each of his students to write a personal strategic plan. "With few exceptions, what they wanted fell into three categories: money, power and things—very big things, including vacation homes, expensive foreign automobiles, yachts and even airplanes . . . Their request to the faculty was: Teach me how to be a moneymaking machine." All else was irrelevant, reported Naylor, including concerns for one's family, one's spirituality, one's workers, one's ethics and social responsibility. Alan Alda voiced the idea: "It isn't necessary to be rich and famous to be happy. It's only necessary to be rich." Thus as 1991 began Malcolm Forbes, Jr., marketed his magazine with a letter appealing to contemporary values: "I want to make one thing very clear about FORBES, namely—we are all about success and money. Period."

And why not? More money means more of the good things of life—a trip to Hawaii, a Colorado condo, a hot tub, flying business-class instead of coach, a large-screen video system, the best schools for one's

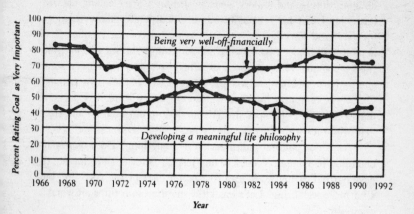

The materialism of the late 1970s and 1980s as seen in American college students' increasing desire for wealth
SOURCE: Eric L. Dey, Alexander W. Astin, and William S. Korn, *The American Freshman: Twenty-Five-Year Trends* (Los Angeles: Higher Education Research Institute, Graduate School of Education, UCLA, 1991); and Alexander W. Astin, Eric L. Dey, William S. Korn, and Ellyne Riggs, *The American Freshman: National Norms for Fall 1991* (Los Angeles: Higher Education Research Institute, Graduate School of Education UCLA 1991).

children, season tickets to the Philharmonic or the Lakers' games, eating out and eating well, stylish clothes, a retirement free from financial worry, and a touch of class in one's surroundings. Wouldn't you really rather have a Buick—or better a BMW or Mercedes? Wouldn't you rather have the power and respect that accompanies affluence? Knowing that money is one way we keep score in the game of life, wouldn't you rather win? And who wouldn't rather have ample security than be living on the edge?

The hunger for wealth and its accompaniments was evident not only in opinion surveys of the 1980s, but also in cultural symbols. *Dallas* and *Dynasty* were in. *The Waltons* and *Little House on the Prairie* were out. The Reagans, reaping two million dollars for a visit to Japan and with Nancy dressed in more than a million dollars' worth of designer dresses and jewelry, were in. Jimmy Carter nailing up wall-board for Habit for Humanity was out. Corporate takeovers, mega-mergers, and junk bonds were in. Savings accounts, certificates of deposit, and triple A bonds were out. Consumption was in. Contributions were out. (The Reagans preached voluntary generosity as an alternative to taxation and welfare, yet gave little of their own income.) On college campuses, business majors were, and still are, in. Education majors are out. A bumper sticker summed up our cultural affluenza: "He who dies with the most toys wins."

Are these cultural indicators on to something? Does money indeed buy happiness? Would having just 20 percent *more* money relieve our bill-paying woes, lead to a better taste of the good life, buy a bit more well-being? Let's break the question into three answerable questions.

Are People Living in Rich Countries Happier?

There *are* striking and consistent national differences in well-being. These country-to-country differences are most persuasively apparent from interviews conducted during the 1980s in what may well be the most extensive and important cross-national survey ever conducted—with representative samples of 170,000 people in sixteen nations, including ten Western European countries. In his 1990 book, *Culture Shift in Advanced Industrial Society,* University of Michigan political scientist Ronald Inglehart amasses the results. Result 1: Year after year, the Danes, Swiss, Irish, and Dutch feel happier and more satisfied with life than do the French, Greeks, Italians, and West Germans. These are genuine national differences, not mere differences in the connotations of the translated questions. For example, regardless of whether they are German-, French-, or Italian-speaking, the Swiss rank very high on life satisfaction—much higher than their German, French, and Italian neighbors.

The nations' well-being differences correlate modestly with national affluence: People in the Scandinavian countries generally are both prosperous and happy. But the link between national affluence and well-being isn't consistent. West Germans, for instance, averaged more than double the incomes of the Irish, but the Irish were happier.

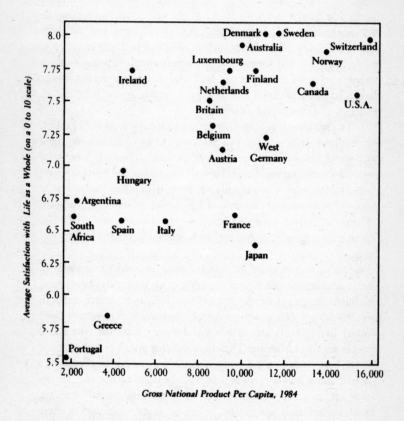

National wealth and well-being
SOURCE: Ronald Inglehart, *Culture Shift in Advanced Industrial Society* (Princeton: Princeton University Press, 1990).

And Belgians tend to be happier than their wealthier French neighbors.

Moreover, the surveyed nations differ in ways other than affluence, making it hard to disentangle cause and effect. For one thing, the most prosperous nations have enjoyed stable democratic governments, and there is a striking link between a history of stable democracy and national well-being. The thirteen nations that have maintained democratic institutions continuously since 1920 *all* enjoy higher life satisfaction levels than do the eleven nations whose democracies developed after World War II or have not yet fully emerged. Moreover, countries that in 1980 had both democracy and a free press also had happier people, report Dutch sociologists Ruut Veenhoven and Piet Ouweneel. So it may not be the wealth of the Scandinavians and Swiss that matters so much as the trust engendered by their history of freedom.

Recently, my family and I spent a sabbatical year in the beautiful historic town of St. Andrews in Scotland. As we compared life there with life in America, we were struck by the lack of connection between national wealth and well-being. To most Americans, Scottish life would seem Spartan. Incomes were markedly lower than in the United States. Among families in the Kingdom of Fife, which includes St. Andrews, 44 percent did not own a car, and we never met a two-car family. Though eight hundred miles north of Minneapolis, central heating was for many a luxury.

During that year we participated in or listened to hundreds of conversations—over daily morning coffee in my university department, in church groups, at needlework get-togethers, over dinner or tea in people's houses. It was our consistent observation that, despite their simpler living, Scots are no less joyful than Americans. We heard complaints about Margaret Thatcher's national priorities, but not once did we hear a whine about being underpaid or unable to afford one's "needs," as we hear so often in America. We heard no one say, "If only I could afford a car" (or eat out more or have a Continental vacation). There was certainly less money, but so far as we could discern there was no less satisfaction with life, no less warmth of spirit, no less pleasure in one another's company.

Within Any Country
Are the Richest the Happiest?

So, although national affluence and well-being correlate, the correlation is modest and entangled with a stronger link between democratic history and well-being. Let's therefore approach the money-happiness question from a second angle. Within any country, are the rich happier?

Here we again find a modest link between well-being and being well-off. Lest we romanticize poverty, hoping to convince ourselves that others' destitution is nothing for us to worry about, consider: Those who live amid affluence, yet themselves struggle to make ends meet on low incomes, typically live with less joy and more stress than do those who live with the comfort and security of incomes over forty-five thousand dollars. They less often report feeling "very happy" and more often suffer stress-related illness and emotional disorder. Poverty is not merely relief from the hassles of wealth, notes Jesse Jackson: "Most poor people . . . catch the early bus. . . . They raise other people's children. . . . They clean the streets." No, they're not carefree. Instead, they more likely work menial jobs, experience impoverished leisure time, feel things out of control, live with hopelessness.

No one denies that we genuinely *need* money enough to evade privation. We humans *need* food, rest, warmth, and social contact. For starving Sudanese and homeless Iraqis, more money *would* buy more happiness. In Britain, France, the Netherlands, and West Germany at the end of World War II, housing and food supplies were insufficient and self-reported happiness was similarly scarce. As the economies of these countries rebounded to provide for people's needs, happiness rebounded too.

But having more than enough provides little additional boost to well-being. To acknowledge that we "cannot live by bread alone" suggests that we do need bread, but that, when we have it, other needs—to belong, to feel esteemed, and so forth—come to the fore (as psychologist Abraham Maslow's famous "hierarchy of needs" recognizes). Once we're comfortable, more money therefore provides diminishing returns. The second helping never tastes as good as the first. The second fifty thousand dollars of income means much less than the first. Thus the correlation between income and happiness is modest, and in both the United States and Canada has now dropped to near zero.

In Europe, too, reports Ronald Inglehart, income "has a surprisingly weak (indeed, virtually negligible) effect on happiness." When we have basic human rights, secure food and shelter, meaningful activity, and enriching relationships, our happiness is unaffected by whether we drive a BMW or, like so many of the Scots, walk or ride a bus. We needn't adopt the asceticism of the Roman statesman-philosopher Seneca ("When we have provided against cold, hunger, and thirst, all the rest is but vanity and excess") to say that if little Athina Roussel were destined to inherit only $1 million of the Onassis fortune, rather than $1 billion, she would likely live no less happily. That being so, the other $999 million surely is excess.

Bringing the point down to my own world, I therefore wonder: Where is the point of diminishing returns beyond which more money does little to enrich our lives? How much money should we leave our own children? Should our financial goal be to leave these special people as wealthy as we can, or to benefit the rest of the world? How can we be generously loving and supportive, now and later, without demotivating their own achievements or needlessly diminishing what we can do for others?

Likewise, where is the point of diminishing returns in our consumption of material goods? Although it eluded me, I am sure there is a difference between the racks of eighteen-hundred-dollar Christian Lacroix dresses I saw at Chicago's Marshall Field the other day and the nearby racks of two-hundred-dollar Bonnie Marx dresses. But is the sixteen-hundred-dollar difference—money enough, UNICEF director James P. Grant tells me, to fund the survival of three ill or malnourished children at five hundred dollars per child—really going to affect the wearer's well-being? I don't mean to sound miserly, for I do enjoy the conveniences and pleasures of life in an affluent society. Still, for each of us there is a point of diminishing returns. With our needs comfortably met, more money can now buy things we don't need and hardly care about, or if unspent becomes blips on a bank computer or numbers on a stock report. Beyond this point of diminishing returns, why hoard more and more wealth and wares? What's the point?

This may be a surprise, but in the University of Michigan's national surveys what matters more than absolute wealth is perceived wealth. Money is two steps removed from happiness: Actual income doesn't much influence happiness; how *satisfied* we are with our income does. If we're content with our income, regardless of how much it is, we're likely to say we're happy. Strangely, however, there is only a slight tendency for people who make lots of money to be more satisfied with what they make. It's true: Satisfaction isn't so much getting what you want as wanting what you have.

This implies two ways to be rich: One is to have great wealth. The other is to have few wants. "Peace in a thatched hut—that is happiness," says a Chinese proverb. My friend Ruth, a former nurse in a Nigerian village, recalls "a group of five- to seven-year-old boys wearing rags for clothes and racing along our compound's driveway with a toy truck made of tin cans from my trash. They had spent the greater part of a morning engineering the toy—and were squealing with delight as they pushed it with a stick. My sons, with Tonka trucks parked under their beds, looked on with envy."

Moreover, our incomes don't noticeably influence our satisfactions with marriage, family, friendship, or ourselves—all of which, as we will see, *do* predict our sense of well-being. If not wracked by hunger or hurt, people at all income levels can enjoy one another and experience comparable joy. Third World theologian Gustavo Gutierrez observes that "the believing poor have never lost their capacity for having a good time and celebrating, despite the harsh conditions in which they live."

The overlapping joy-to-misery distributions among the rich and the poor imply that one can find pockets of joy among the poor that contrast with pockets of despair among the rich. After returning from a year spent living amid Peruvian peasants, theologian-priest Henri Nouwen was struck by the relative joylessness of North Americans. Over lunch with several of us here, he described the greater joy he observed among his impoverished Peruvian friends. At a party they could delight not only in one another's company, but also in tastes savored from a few divided cookies and shared sips of a Coke. Back home in North America, his more affluent friends displayed comparatively somber reflections, melancholic emotions, and pessimistic outlooks: "Often they suffered from strained relationships with their family, had difficulty in developing close relationships with their peers, and felt hostile toward people in authority. . . . Seeing and feeling this deep suffering in my ambitious, successful friends, I was increasingly overwhelmed by the immense spiritual crisis of the so-called First World."

Psychiatrist Robert Coles also was struck by the joy, as well as the misery, that he detected in his interviews with rich and poor. In both groups one finds defeat and despair, but also courage and hope. University of Illinois psychologist Ed Diener and his colleagues agree. They surveyed forty-nine of the wealthiest Americans, as listed by *Forbes*, and found them to be only slightly happier than average. Wealth, after all, brings prestige, more choice of activities such as travel, and opportunities to satisfy one's desires to help others and change the world. Still, four in five of these people, all with net worths well over $100 million, agreed that "money can increase *or* decrease happiness, depending on how it is used." And quite a few were, indeed, unhappy. One enormously wealthy man said he could never remember being happy. One woman reported that money could not undo the misery caused by her children's problems. A student of mine illustrates, writing of her misery after eight years living with her mother and a wealthy but emotionally abusive stepfather. "Needless to say this is not a very pleasant situation. But wait . . . He drives a BMW and just bought her a Mercedes. They gave me a Mazda 626. He shops at Bloomingdale's and bought her a Gucci watch. One year he gave me a sailboat. Then he later bought me my own Windsurfer. Our house has two VCRs and three Hitachi televisions! Do these things make me happy? Absolutely not. I would trade all my family's wealth for a peaceful and loving home." "Show me one couple unhappy merely on account of their limited circumstances," wrote Samuel Taylor Coleridge, "and I will show you ten who are wretched from other causes."

As examples of the latter, one thinks of Howard Hughes, Christina Onassis, or J. Paul Getty. Or Erno Rubik, whose puzzle cube transformed him overnight from a $150-a-month professor of design to Hungary's richest person. The toy he built in his room in his mother's apartment perplexed half a billion people, yet left its taciturn inventor unable to solve the greater puzzle of happiness. While he was showing interviewer John Tierney through his new house, with its pool and sauna and three-car garage and Mercedes, the never-smiling Rubik's emotions were as gray as the sky. Noting that Rubik eliminated the dining room when remodeling his house, Tierney wondered: "Do you plan to have many people over to dinner?" Puffing on a cigarette and gazing out a window, Rubik frowned. "I hope not."

Does Our Happiness Rise with Our Affluence?

We have scrutinized the American dream of wealth and well-being from two angles, by comparing, at given points in time, rich and unrich countries and rich and unrich people. This leaves the clincher question: Over time, does our happiness grow with our paychecks? Rubik's experience suggests not, but is he the exception that proves the rule?

In the United States as a whole, the answer is clearly no. Since the 1950s, our buying power has doubled. In 1957, the year John Galbraith was going to press with his famous book describing us as *The Affluent Society,* our per person income, expressed in today's dollars, was seventy-five hundred dollars. By 1990 it was over fifteen thousand, making us The Doubly Affluent Society—with double the goods that money buys. Compared to 1957, we now have twice as many cars per capita. We have color TVs, VCRs, home computers, air-conditioners, microwave ovens, garage door openers, answering machines, and $12 billion a year worth of brand-name athletic shoes. Indeed, most Americans now rate as "necessities" such things as frozen food, clothes dryers, car stereos, and aluminum foil. (Even as I write this our family's microwave oven is being repaired, and we are discovering that our onetime luxury has become a seeming necessity.)

With so much more of what money buys, are we happier?

In 1990, as in 1957, only one in three Americans told the University of Chicago's National Opinion Research Center they were "very happy." So: *We're twice as rich—not just 20 percent richer—yet we're no happier.*

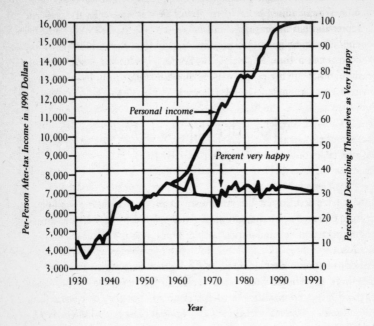

Year

Does more money buy more happiness? Thanks to rising incomes, more workers, and shrinking family size, buying power has doubled since the 1950s, but self-reported happiness is unchanged.

SOURCE: National Opinion Research Center happiness data from Richard Gene Niemi, John Mueller, and Tom W. Smith, *Trends in Public Opinion: A Compendium of Survey Data* (New York: Greenwood Press, 1989); and from Tom W. Smith (personal communication). Income data from *Historical Statistics of the U.S., Colonial Times to 1970*, pt. 1 (Washington, DC: Bureau of the Census, 1976), p. 225, and *Economic Indicators* (November 1980) : 6 and (November 1991) : 6, adjusted to 1990 dollars.

Between 1955 and 1971 the average income of Detroit families increased 40 percent in constant dollars. Yet compared to Detroit housewives in 1955, those interviewed in 1971 were no more satisfied with their "standard of living—the kind of house, clothes, car, and so forth." In fact, between 1956 and 1988, the percentage of Americans who reported they were "pretty well satisfied with your present financial situation" *dropped* from 42 to 30 percent.

If anything, to judge from a postwar rise in depression rates, we're more likely to be miserable. Among Americans born since World War II, depression has increased dramatically—*tenfold*, reports clinical researcher Martin Seligman. Twenty-five-year-olds today are much more likely to recall a time in their life when they were despondent and despairing than are their seventy-five-year-old grandparents, despite the grandparents having had many more years to suffer all kinds of disorder, from broken legs to the anguish of depression. Similar trends are evident in Canada, Sweden, Germany, and New Zealand, report psychiatric researchers Gerald Klerman and Myrna Weissman. Everywhere in the modern world, it seems, more younger adults than older adults report having ever been disabled by depression.

Do older adults simply forget long-ago depressive episodes? Apparently not, for the age difference persists when people report just their recent depressive symptoms. Well, then, do younger adults recall and report more depression merely because it's now more acceptable to admit such feelings? Or is it because young adults are less likely to consider temporary despair as part of the normal ups and downs of life, something to grin and bear? If so, then defining depression by other criteria—being hospitalized for depression, the duration of episodes, and so forth—should eliminate the depression age gap. But no matter how we define depression, the finding persists: Today's younger adults have grown up with more affluence, more depression, and (as Chapter 9 will show) more marital and family misery. They also know more of depression's consequences—suicide, alcoholism, and other forms of substance abuse.

The same story holds for the social well-being of adolescents. Between 1960 and the late 1980s America's teens enjoyed the benefits of declining family poverty, smaller families, increased parental education, doubled per-pupil school expenditures (in constant dollars), double the number of teachers with advanced degrees, and an 11 percent drop in class size. Simultaneously, their delinquency rate doubled, their suicide rate tripled, their homicide rate tripled, and the birthrate of the unmarried nearly quadrupled. While standing tall during the 1980s, believing a comfortable lie that all was well in a prosperous and militarily successful America, the uncomfortable truth was that social battles were being lost at home.

So, whether we base our conclusions on self-reported happiness, rates of depression, or teen problems, *our becoming much better-off over the last thirty years has not been accompanied by one iota of increased happiness and life satisfaction.* It's shocking, because it contradicts our society's materialistic assumptions, but how can we ignore the hard truth: *Once beyond poverty, further economic growth does not appreciably improve human morale.* Making more money—that aim of so many graduates and other American dreamers of the 1980s—does not breed bliss.

Shocking, but not original. Seneca observed nearly two thousand years ago that

> our forefathers . . . lived every jot as well as we, when they provided and dressed their own meat with their own hands, lodged upon the ground and were not as yet come to the vanity of gold and gems . . . which may serve to show us, that it is the mind, and not the sum, that makes any person rich. . . . No one can be poor that has enough, nor rich, that covets more than he has.

To be rich, Seneca would say, is less an ample bank balance than a state of mind. To be rich is to have wants that are simpler than our incomes can afford.

With my colleague Thomas Ludwig I first reflected on the money-happiness question in a 1978 piece in *Saturday Review.* We questioned middle-class "poortalk"—that grousing about how (despite the recreational vehicle in the driveway) one can't afford the rising price of milk and toothpaste. When our spending outstrips our income, we feel underpaid, defeated by inflation and taxes, unable to afford things we now define as necessities. And so we talk poor.

Such poortalk among the affluent is objectionable on two counts. First, it is insensitive to the truly impoverished, just as self-pitying "fat-talk" by a slightly overweight person is insensitive to the truly obese, or "dumb-talk" by an A student who just received a B is insensitive to the friend who longs for a B.

Second, poortalk sours our thinking. One of social psychology's maxims is that what we *say* influences what we think and feel. Positive talk promotes positive attitudes. Complaining magnifies discontent. Social psychologists call it the "saying becomes believing" effect.

When the subjects of countless experiments speak or write on behalf of some point of view, they come to believe it more strongly. Cognitive therapists harness the principle, by getting people to talk to themselves, and to others, in more positive, less self-defeating ways.

Thus one way for middle-class people to gain a healthier perspective on their situation is to cut the poortalk. "I need that" can become "I want that." "I am underpaid" can become "I spend more than I make." And that most familiar middle-class lament, "We can't afford it," can become, more truthfully, "We choose to spend our money on other things." For usually we *could* afford it—the snowmobile, the CD player, the Disney World vacation—*if* we made it our top priority; we just have other priorities on which we choose to spend our limited incomes. The choice is ours. "I can't afford it" denies our choices, reducing us to self-pitying victims.

When I first voiced these thoughts our family of five was living comfortably, but not luxuriously, on a twenty-two-thousand-dollar income. Having not entertained the idea of textbook writing, little did I expect that our income would multiply many times over. Given this sudden wealth—unbidden and beyond all expectations—my experience confirms the message of this chapter and the next: The river of happiness is fed far less by wealth than by the streams of ordinary pleasures. "What keeps our faith cheerful," says Garrison Keillor, "is everywhere in daily life, a sign that faith rules through ordinary things: through cooking and small talk, through storytelling, making love, fishing, tending animals and sweet corn and flowers, through sports, music, and books, raising kids—all the places where the gravy soaks in and grace shines through. Even in a time of elephantine vanity and greed, one never has to look far to see the campfires of gentle [and happy] people."

To be sure, I love the freedom that money buys, the empowerment to choose my circumstances and use of time. My wife and I also enjoy the freedom from financial stress, for which we gladly endure the smaller stresses of jointly deciding the disposition of money (and dealing with people who'd like to help us make those decisions). And we take pleasure in supporting things we care deeply about.

But the greater pleasures, the ones that sustain (or, at times, erode) my sense of joy, come, as Garrison Keillor predicted, through more ordinary, ongoing moments of cheer—through identifying with my children as they ride their adolescent roller coasters, through laughter and tears shared with friends, through work created and completed, through daily games of pickup basketball with friends, through happy recollections of Scottish tearooms, of family beach fires back home on Bainbridge Island, of falling in love.

Realizing that well-being is something other than being well-off is liberating. It liberates us from spending on eighteen-hundred-dollar dresses, on stockpiles of unplayed CDs, on luxury cars, on seagoing luxury homes—all purchased in a vain quest for an elusive joy. It liberates us from envying the life-styles of the rich and famous. It liberates us to invest ourselves in developing traits, attitudes, relationships, activities, environments, and spiritual resources that *will* promote our own, and others', well-being.

3

A Satisfied Mind

We are never happy for a thousand days,
a flower never blooms for a hundred.

CHINESE PROVERB

We have pondered a remarkable fact, one that impresses researchers and astonishes all of us who assume that inner well-being follows wealth or priviledge. As the late New Zealand researcher Richard Kammann put it, "Objective life circumstances have a negligible role to play in a theory of happiness." Having seen the negligible role of economic circumstance, let's consider other sorts of successes and setbacks, and then ask *why* the emotional dividends of wealth and success seldom endure.

To be sure, the events of our lives do influence our emotions, but only temporarily. Bad events—an argument, a rejection, a headache—put us in the dumps. Good events—a pay raise, winning a game, getting an A on a test, a first passionate kiss—increase happiness, for a while. But within a day or two, our moods usually return to normal, with ups and downs reflecting that day's events. Happiness, said Benjamin Franklin, "is produced not so much by great pieces of good fortune that seldom happen as by little advantages that occur every day." Happiness is less often found around the corner than right in front of us.

Surely you've noticed: Dejection and elation are *both* hard to sustain. We can usually count on rebounding from a funk. Stung by criticism or rejection, we wallow in relative gloom, but for only a day or two. Delighted by success or acclaim, we relish the joy, but not for long.

Incredibly, these emotional rebounds occur even for those who experience the extremes of tragedy or triumph. Given time, we humans have an enormous capacity to adapt to changed circumstance. The emotional well-being of cancer patients, and their satisfaction with different aspects of their lives, rivals that of healthy people. People who become blind or paralyzed will, after a period of adjustment, typically recover a near-normal level of day-to-day happiness. "The Lord lifts up those who are bowed down," observed the psalmist. "Weeping may linger for the night, but joy comes with the morning."

I know this sounds too easy, too unrealistic. But consider: One study of Michigan car accident victims found that three weeks after they suffered a paralyzing spinal cord injury, happiness was again the prevailing emotion. A University of Illinois study found that able-bodied students described themselves as 50 percent of the time happy, 22 percent of the time unhappy, and 29 percent of the time neutral. To within one percentage point, disabled students described their emotions identically. Another Illinois study revealed that students rate their disabled friends as equally happy as their nondisabled friends.

Without minimizing catastrophe, the consistent and astonishing result is that the worst emotional consequences of bad events are usually temporary. With major setbacks or injuries, the emotional after-effects may linger a year or more. Yet within a matter of weeks, one's current mood is more affected by the day's events—an argument with one's spouse, a failure at work, a rewarding call or a gratifying letter from a dear friend or child—than by whether one is paralyzed or mobile, blind or sighted.

W Mitchell was a modern-day Job. In 1971 he was horribly burned, nearly killed, and left fingerless from a freak motorcycle accident. Four years later tragedy struck again. This time he was paralyzed from the waist down in a small plane crash. Though terribly disfigured, he chose not to buy the idea that happiness requires handsomeness. "I am in charge of my own spaceship. It is my up, my down. I could choose to see this situation as a setback or a starting point." Mitchell today is a successful investor, an environmental activist, and a speaker who encourages people to step back from their own misfortunes: "Take a wider view and say, 'Maybe that isn't such a big thing after all.' "

Many victims report that their tragedy entails a mix of negative and positive consequences. Lucio, one of many such people interviewed by University of Milan psychologist Fausto Massimini, was a happy-go-lucky but purposeless twenty-year-old gas station attendant when paralyzed below the waist in a motorcycle accident. The tragedy somehow awakened a new resolve, challenging him to enroll in and complete college, and to become a successful tax consultant and regional archery champion. "When I became a paraplegic, it was like being born again. I had to learn from scratch everything I used to know . . . it took commitment, willpower, and patience. As far as the future is concerned, I hope to keep improving, to keep breaking through the limitations of my handicap."

In their interviews with many dozens of breast cancer patients, UCLA health psychologists Shelley Taylor and Rebecca Collins were surprised to discover that many claimed to have benefited from their experience. Victims of cancer (and other life-threatening events) often reappraise their lives, reorder their values and priorities, and renew their close relationships. Things they formerly took for granted, even the opportunities of each new day, they now pause to appreciate. As a result, many think they are better adjusted than before suffering cancer. Said one woman, "I have much more enjoyment of each day, each moment. I am not so worried about what is or isn't or what I wish I had. All those things you get entangled with don't seem to be part of my life right now." Another patient reflected that

> you take a long look at your life and realize that many things that you thought were important before are totally insignificant. That's

probably been the major change in my life. What you do is put things into perspective. You find out that things like relationships are really the most important things you have—the people you know and your family—everything else is just way down the line. It's very strange that it takes something so serious to make you realize that.

This has been my brother's experience. Jim is a victim of one of nature's horrible afflictions, motor neuron disease. For most people, the disease progressively erodes the capacity to control their limbs and, in the end, even to speak or breathe—all the while leaving their senses and minds fully alert and aware of this degeneration. ALS—Lou Gehrig's disease—is its best-known form. Now in an early stage, Jim has difficulty tying his shoes, buttoning his shirts, typing at his job as a network TV station promotions director. Nevertheless, what continually amazes me is the resilience of his spirit, the joy he takes in being with his young daughters, the enthusiasm he feels for his volunteer church work, the happiness he finds in knowing that his initial prognosis was too grim and that an experimental new drug may be slowing the course of his disease and giving him the great gift of seeing his daughters grow to maturity. After staring death in the face, he knows what matters. "Life itself seems more precious and real," he says. As a fellow motor neuron disease survivor, Cambridge physicist Stephen Hawking put it, "When one's expectations are reduced to zero, one really appreciates everything that one does have."

Surely, none of these victims of tragedy would wish their disease upon anyone else. Few would say that these bad things are, on balance, good. Yet most discover that even bad things can work for good. Indeed, just being close to such a person can give each of us pause to wonder: If I knew I had a month to live, what would I care most about? On my deathbed, what will I wish I had spent more time doing? Am I living out my real priorities?

If the emotional impact of most bad events is temporary, the impact of dramatically positive events is similarly temporary. Looking back, Illinois state lottery winners and British pool winners tell researchers they were delighted to have won. But the rush of euphoria didn't last. In fact, ordinary activities they previously enjoyed, such as reading or eating a good breakfast, actually became less pleasurable. Winning the lottery was such an emotional high that, by comparison, their ordinary pleasures paled.

On a smaller scale, a jump in income can buy a temporary jolt of happiness. We notice with pleasure the effect of the raise on our next few paychecks. "But in the long run," notes Ronald Inglehart, "neither an ice cream cone nor a new car nor becoming rich and famous produces the same feelings of delight that it initially did. . . . Happiness is not the result of being rich, but a temporary consequence of having recently become richer."

Why? Why could Seneca notice that "no happiness lasts for long"? Why does happiness not follow economic success on its upward climb? Why do most families in the industrialized world—living with comforts unknown to *wealthy* families two centuries ago—not consider themselves wealthy? Why do yesterday's luxuries become today's necessities? Why are the satisfactions of success so short-lived?

Two psychological principles solve this enigma, each by suggesting that happiness is relative.

Adaptation Level:
Happiness is Relative to Our Prior Experience

This first principle reaches from ancient philosophy to contemporary experiments, which show that we judge various experiences relative to our previous experiences. From our recent experience we calibrate "adaptation levels"—neutral points at which sounds seem neither loud nor soft, lights neither bright nor dim, experiences neither pleasant nor unpleasant. We then notice and react to variations up or down from these levels. A marching band seems "loud" to a chamber musician but not to a rock musician. Here in Michigan, a 60-degree day in July feels cold, but the 60-degree Christmas day we had several years ago felt distinctly warm.

What matters, then, is whether things have just changed—for better or for worse. Better than a high income is a rising income. If we get a pay raise, receive an improved test grade, bring home a promotion, or get asked out, we feel an initial surge of pleasure. But if these new realities continue, we adapt. Black-and-white television, once a thrill, began to seem ordinary until we got that exciting nineteen-inch color set, which itself will be replaced by a bigger fix—a twenty-seven-inch set or maybe even high-definition television. So it happens that luxuries become necessities.

Indeed, as our experience changes, relative luxury may even begin to feel like poverty. Thus in 1990 psychiatrist Lewis Judd resigned as director of the National Institute of Mental Health because "simply put, I found that . . . my family and I can no longer afford to remain in government service"—on a mere $103,600-per-year salary. William Bennett must have sympathized. In spurning a $125,000 offer to become chair of the Republican National Committee he remarked, "I didn't take a vow of poverty"—which apparently is what $125,000 feels like after making a reported $240,000 in speaking fees during the preceeding four months. But even double $240,000 doesn't feel like wealth to some professional athletes. "People think we make $3 million or $4 million a year," explained Texas Ranger outfielder Pete Incaviglia. "They don't realize that most of us only make $500,000."*

I roll my eyes at such insensitivity to those hungry or homeless. But are any of us immune to adaptation? As married students in the 1960s, my wife and I lived in a drafty $62.50-per-month war-surplus Quonset hut, with enough money from a National Science Foundation fellowship to cover expenses and occasionally splurge on take-out chicken. When I became an assistant professor our income nearly doubled, we rented a $100-a-month house, and again, we met expenses with a little left over for an occasional meal in a restaurant. Over the next twenty years our real income doubled again; we moved to a nicer house, traveled a bit more, ate better, even gave more away—yet still seemed to have just enough to cover our needs. We were no more or less happy than when snuggled in our Quonset hut, but we wouldn't have happily traded our Victorian house for the hut. No, with each

---

*If Boston Red Sox pitcher Roger Clemens throws thirty-five 100-pitch games for his $5.2 million annual salary, he can imagine another $150,000 in the bank every time he shows up to pitch, or $1,500 after every throw. But then Clemens can point to H. J. Heinz CEO Anthony O'Reilly, whose reported $38.5 million in 1990 compensation came to $150,000 a day for 250 days a year or, assuming a ten-hour day, a cool $15,000 per hour.

raise the extra money soon ceased to be extra, the new luxuries soon lost their luxurious feeling. So it goes as the treadmill elevates to incomes of over a hundred thousand dollars. At lower incomes people *think* that with more money they'd be happier and more generous. But seldom is this so. Indeed, a recent Gallup poll offered the astonishing result that people with incomes of under ten thousand dollars give 5.5 percent to charity, and those earning fifty to sixty thousand give a stingier 1.7 percent. Even those earning over a hundred thousand dollars are proportionately less charitable than the poor, giving 2.9 percent of their household income. Moreover, as family affluence has multiplied since the 1930s giving as a percentage of income has not changed.

We can thank the adaptation-level phenomenon for fueling our ambition and achievements. Without it we'd dwell contentedly on our first plateau of success, feeling no drive to accomplish more. As we instead pursue expectations bred by our rising achievements, staying even just won't do. As Dutch emotion researcher Nico Frijda says, "Continued pleasures wear off. . . . Pleasure is always contingent upon change and disappears with continuous satisfaction."

The point cannot be overstated: *Every* desirable experience— passionate love, a spiritual high, the pleasure of a new possession, the exhilaration of success—is transitory. True, some individuals are characteristically happier than others—or more in love, or more spiritually alive, or more delighted with their success. Still, life could be an unending pleasure cruise only if happiness were continually rejuiced by new upward surges—highs followed by higher highs. If you're headed for the top, the pleasure of going by stairway will outlast that of a fast elevator ride.

At the end of his Narnia tales, C. S. Lewis offers such a vision of paradise. Having survived the last battle, with their world collapsing behind them, its creatures step into a joyous never-ending story. "All their life in this world and all their adventures in Narnia had only been the cover and the title page: now at last they were beginning Chapter One of the Great Story which no one on earth has read: which goes on forever: in which every chapter is better than the one before."

This side of heaven, we can never create a paradise of endless joy. What would your utopia involve: morning golf with scores in the seventies? sumptuous poolside lunches with friends? sexual ecstasy every evening? no bills, no ills? Even if we found a home in our utopia we would eventually adapt, leaving us, once again, sometimes feeling gratified (when what we got surpassed what we've come to expect), sometimes deprived (when our attainments didn't reach our expectations), and much of the time, well, we'd just mellow out.

Our very human tendency to adapt to new circumstances explains why, despite the elation of triumph and the anguish of tragedy, even million-dollar lottery winners and paraplegics eventually return to variations on moment-to-moment happiness. And it also explains why material wants can be insatiable—why Imelda Marcos, living in splendor insulated from Philippine poverty, would buy 1,060 pairs of shoes; why, having achieved the economic miracle of a chicken in every pot, a steak-hungry but recession-plagued Long Island teacher could complain that "if I see chicken or hamburger once more I'll scream"; and why many a child "needs" just one more Barbie outfit, one more Nintendo game, one more CD. When the victor belongs to the spoils, when the possessor is possessed by possessions, adaptation level has run amuck.

Even in the short run, emotions seem attached to elastic bands that snap us back from highs or lows. For many pleasures we pay a price, and for much suffering we receive a reward. For the pleasure or euphoria of a drug high, we pay the price of craving and increased depression when the drug wears off. For suffering through hard exercise, we afterward enjoy the dividend of a pleasing glow. With support from studies of both animal and human emotions, University of Pennsylvania psychologist Richard Solomon formalized an "opponent-process" principle: Emotions trigger opposing emotions. After a terrifying parachute jump, parchutists typically feel elated. After the pain of labor and childbirth, a woman experiences happy relief or even euphoria. After a holiday, we may get the blues.

As with all psychological phenomena, there are corresponding biological events. Take the drug high. Cocaine, for instance, produces a "rush" by flooding the brain with excitatory neurotransmitters (the nervous system's chemical messengers). But this reduces the brain's own supplies of these neurotransmitters, producing a crash of depression when the drug wears off. For suppressing the body's own neurotransmitter production, nature charges a price.

This emotions-trigger-opposing-emotions principle has a corollary: With repetition, the lingering opposing emotion gains strength. Thus the rush of a drug high becomes more and more swiftly knocked down by an opposing reaction. This leads the user to use more of the drug to re-create the high (a phenomenon known as drug tolerance). Moreover, the user may experience hangovers (the opponent feelings that linger after knocking down the pleasure) and addiction (the craving for more of the drug to switch off the pain of withdrawal). "The more I drank the worse I felt when sober," says the recovering alcoholic, "so I found myself drinking more each day to restore my level of comfort."

Plato anticipated opponent emotions: "How strange would appear to be this thing that men call pleasure! And how curiously it is related to what is thought to be its opposite, pain! . . . Wherever the one is found, the other follows up behind."

As Solomon wisely notes, the opponent-process principle is bad news for hedonists: Those who seek artificial pleasures will pay for them later, and repetition will diminish much of the pleasure's intensity. There is no free lunch. With every kick comes a kickback. An old Spanish saying anticipated the phenomenon: " 'Take what you want,' said God. 'Take it, and pay for it.' "

But there is corresponding good news for ascetics: Long-term adaptations and short-term opponent processes reassure us that those who suffer will be recompensed. We needn't minimize evil or justify suffering to acknowledge some payback. Suffering lowers our adaptation level and triggers an emotional rebound.

There of course are exceptions. The trauma of rape, child abuse, combat, or a concentration camp can forever color one's view of the world. For nearly half of the Vietnam veterans who experienced heavy combat, often with friends dying beside them, the psychological wounds of war linger, as haunting flashbacks and nightmares. Many of these "post-traumatic stress disorder" victims have trouble sleeping and concentrating. When the Centers for Disease Control compared seven thousand combat veterans with seven thousand noncombat veterans, they discovered that combat stress doubled a Vietnam vet's risk of suffering bouts of depression, anxiety, or drinking.

One such soldier, Jack, served in a platoon that was repeatedly under fire. In one ambush, his closest friend was killed while standing a few feet away. Jack himself killed a boy Vietcong soldier by bludgeoning him with a rifle butt. Years later, images of these events keep intruding in Jack's mind. He still jumps at the sound of a cap gun or the backfire of a car. When annoyed by family or friends, he lashes out in ways he seldom did before Vietnam. To calm his continuing anxiety, he drinks more than he should.

So, in extreme cases—for survivors of vicious combat, abuse, or sexual assault—past traumas may still torment.

But for most of us, sorrows undone bring greater joy than had we never sorrowed. Parents of the child who matures after a troubled adolescence enjoy a gladness unknown to parents who never suffered. T. S. Eliot reported that the contrast with his long and miserable first marriage contributed to the rejuvenating happiness of his second marriage. Even Russians who survived the starvation of the Nazi's thousand-day siege of Leningrad reportedly felt well-off for a generation afterward, despite periodic food shortages. "Blessed are those who mourn, for they shall be comforted." For pain endured and remembered, we gain a sweeter joy.

Social Comparison:
Happiness Is Relative to Others' Attainment

Happiness is relative not only to our personal past experience, but also to our social experience. We are always comparing ourselves to others. And we feel good or bad depending on whom we compare ourselves to.

This simple fact explains why if you escape poverty your happiness increases, yet, paradoxically, societies do not become happier as they progress from relative poverty to affluence. Because what we perceive as a "need" is socially determined, those who live in richer places and times have a higher standard of comparison. Today's ghettos have more cars and TV sets than yesterday's suburbs, yet the continuing inequalities leave those with small pieces of the growing pie no more satisfied. Today's middle class has double the spending power of three decades ago, yet, because the rising tide lifts all boats, feels relatively deprived compared to their better-off neighbors.

Even the rich seldom *feel* rich. In a 1990 Gallup poll, Americans readily applied the label "rich" to others. The average person judged that 21 percent of Americans were rich. But virtually none—fewer than ½ of 1 percent—perceived *themselves* as rich. To those earning $10,-000 a year, it takes a $50,000 income to be rich. To those making $500,000, rich may be a $1 million income. When the Oakland Athletics signed outfielder Jose Canseco to a $4.7 million annual salary, his fellow outfielder Rickey Henderson became openly dissatisfied with his $3 million salary. Refusing to show up on time to spring training, he complained "I don't think my contract is fair." Other teammates, smirking, took up a collection for him. When Pittsburgh Pirate outfielder Barry Bonds's salary was raised from $850,000 in 1990 to $2.3 million in 1991, instead of the $3.25 million he had requested, Bonds sulked, "There's nothing Barry Bonds can do to satisfy Pittsburgh. I'm so sad all the time."

These "bawl players," as *Sports Illustrated* called them, illustrate a well-confirmed principle: How frustrated or contented we feel, personally, depends on who we compare ourselves to. How well a group as a whole is doing will influence its readiness to protest, to demonstrate, to strike. But our personal feelings of well-being hinge more on how we're doing compared to our peers—our fellow workers, our friends, our extended family. Such comparisons influence our expectations. And as University of Guelph researcher Alex Michalos has shown, happiness shrivels with the gap between what we have and what we want, what we have and what we expected to have by now, what we have and what our neighbors have.

Our social comparisons concern not only money, but also looks, smarts, and various forms of success. Researchers have found that moderately able students usually have a higher academic self-esteem if they attend a school where their peers are *not* exceptionally capable. If your classmates are brilliant, you may feel stupid in comparison. Able students' academic self-confidence may therefore fare best when they are *not* in public schools that separate "gifted" students or when not attending Ivy League universities. As measured by the further educational successes of their graduates—one crude index to a college's influence—some surprising success stories come from unheralded places. My own institution provides an example: During the half century from the 1920s through the 1960s (excepting the war years), Hope College tied Harvard University for twentieth place among America's colleges in the percentage of male graduates who went on to get Ph.D.s. Historically, black colleges provide a similar success story. They enroll only one in five African-American students, yet their graduates represent one third of new African-American Ph.D.s in science, math, and engineering. One stretches to imagine how this could be—how modestly endowed colleges unrecognized by much of the populace could rival rich, renowned universities with elite student bodies. The answer lies partly in the greater ease with which cream rises to the top in the less-competitive setting, enabling relatively capable students to develop intellectual self-confidence and ambition. How big the fish feels depends less on the pond than on who else is in the school. Social comparisons matter.

Henderson's and Bond's discontent illustrates another repeated finding: As we climb the success ladder we mostly look upward. Seldom do we compare ourselves with those below us. More often we compare ourselves with those a rung or two above, those whose level we now aspire to join. The philosopher Bertrand Russell saw no end to the upward comparison: "Napoleon envied Caesar, Caesar envied Alexander, and Alexander, I daresay, envied Hercules, who never existed. You cannot, therefore, get away from envy by means of success alone, for there will always be in history or legend some person even more successful than you are."

Advertisers exploit our eagerness to compare upward by bombarding us with images of people whose elegant possessions awaken our envy. Many television programs similarly enlarge our circle of comparisons, whetting our appetites for what some others have. In thirty-four American cities where television ownership became widespread in 1951, the 1951 larceny theft rate (for crimes such as shoplifting and bicycle stealing) jumped. In thirty-four other cities, where a government freeze delayed the introduction of television until 1955, a similar jump in the theft rate occurred—in 1955. Researcher Karen Hennigan and her colleagues attribute the jumps to resentments aroused when younger, poorer people compared their possessions "with (a) those of wealthy television characters and (b) those portrayed in advertisements."

Comparing "upward" also affects our satisfaction with our relationships, sometimes causing us to devalue our partners. In experiments, watching X-rated movies simulating easy and endless sexual ecstasy tends, back in the real world, to diminish satisfaction with one's own, comparatively less exciting, partner. Even viewing sexually attractive women on TV or in magazines leads men to devalue their own companions. After gazing at a perfect "10" in a centerfold, one's own partner seems less appealing—more like a "6" than an "8."

So, satisfaction and dissatisfaction are relative both to our past experience and to expectations influenced by our comparisons with others—typically those who swim in the same pond we do, and quite likely those who swim a little ahead than those who swim behind us.

When demoralized or feeling threatened, however, we more often than not compare ourselves with those less fortunate. Consider some uplifting effects of comparing downward:

- Following natural disasters, victims commonly feel lucky compared to those more severely victimized. Many who suffered broken dishes and windows in the 1989 San Francisco earthquake felt blessed—blessed not to have lived in the devastated Marina district. "Replacing these things sure beats being homeless."
- Anxious or depressed people feel better after considering people whose troubles are worse than their own. When agonizing over a child who is failing in school, knowing others who struggle with a child whose problems are more serious helps us keep our sense of perspective. "It could be worse, you know."
- If you fear you just bombed an exam, it secretly feels good to hear someone—even a friend—lament that she left half the questions blank. "At least I wasn't alone."
- Shelley Taylor reports that women who have had lumpectomies for breast cancer tend to compare themselves with those who've had mastectomies, who tend to compare with those who've lost more to cancer. Helga, a lumpectomy patient explains: "I had a comparatively small amount of surgery. How awful it must be

for women who have had a mastectomy. I just can't imagine. It would seem to be so difficult." But Maria, a mastectomy patient doesn't feel so awful: "It was not tragic. It worked out okay. Now, if the thing had spread all over, I would have had a whole different story for you." Dorothy, an older women with breast cancer maintains her morale by feeling sorry for "these young gals. To lose a breast when you're so young must be awful. I'm seventy-three. What do I need a breast for?"

Comparing downward can have its darker side, though, sometimes causing us to relish another's downfall. In experiments, people who have just experienced failure or been made to feel insecure will often alleviate their self-doubts by disparaging a rival group or person. It helps to have others to look down on, a fact that helps explain the persistence of prejudice. In *The Devil's Dictionary*, Ambrose Bierce defined happiness as "an agreeable sensation arising from contemplating the misery of another." For an ardent Chicago White Sox fan happiness is the White Sox winning *and* the Cubs losing. As Gore Vidal remarked, "It is not enough to succeed; others must fail."

But let's look on the brighter side. The processes of adaptation and social comparison reassure us that if forced to adjust our living standards downward, we could regain our sense of well-being. Imagine ecology's prophets are right—that the world's bulging population is stretching the earth's carrying capacity by depleting the remaining oil reserves, threatening the atmosphere, and requiring us to restrain our use of forests and fossil fuels. If the modern ideology of unending progress, of continuing improvement, of ever-more luxury were to crash against a wall of ecological limits, what then?

Simplifying our living would indeed cause some initial pain. (Even Donald Trump probably felt gloomy when financial troubles in 1990 necessitated trimming his daily expenses on food, shelter, and other living expenses from $19,200 to $14,800.) But, especially if we shared our sacrifices, we would adapt. And in time we would recover our normal mix of joy, discontent, and neutrality. During the energy crisis of the 1970s, many North Americans managed to curb their "need" for gas-slurping cars and, with only temporary feelings of deprivation, to adapt to smaller cars. Maybe improving technology and productivity will solve global problems and insulate us from sacrifice. Maybe not. If, that all might live, we must live more simply, returning to a standard of living that a century ago would still have been deemed luxurious, well, we'll manage, perhaps with thankfulness for the gift of life.

I take personal comfort in the resilience of well-being in the face of downward, as well as upward, adaptation. At age forty-nine, I find my hearing declining on a trajectory directly toward my eighty-two-year-old mother's utter deafness. Although it's not yet disabling—I still teach and carry on conversations with only occasional difficulty—I do find myself sitting front and center at plays and meetings, seeking quiet corners in restaurants, wearing an aid, using amplification devices for TV and telephone. And it can be frustrating to miss the punch line in a joke that everyone else is guffawing over, or to make what you later learn is an inappropriate reply to a soft-spoken person whose words you thought you heard.

But how will I cope, and what will happen to my emotional well-being, as the impairment becomes more serious? Will I gladly suffer being unable to talk to friends on the phone? to explain to friendly strangers that I cannot hear them? to lose the pleasure of listening to music? to end my teaching career prematurely? to struggle to communicate even with my wife and children?

Surely I will regret the loss and will remember wistfully the symphony of sound I once knew. Perhaps I will better appreciate why Helen Keller could say that she "found deafness to be a much greater handicap than blindness." But if I take seriously the findings and the human experiences that I have just reported—and I take them very seriously—then, I reassure myself, I will adapt. I will discover new joys, and maybe even find some good within the bad. How fortunate I am that I love to read, think, and write, activities that may even be enhanced by deafness. How even more fortunate if I can acquire the attitude that another scholar-writer, Scotland's William Barclay, expressed in his later years: "I am almost completely deaf. But this means I can sleep without trouble in a noisy hotel by a railway station! And I can concentrate far better on work and study for I have no distractions. . . . A handicap has its compensations."

Although I wish my hearing were acute, the prospect of deafness neither frightens nor depresses me. Without deluding myself that the compensations will pay the considerable price of a sensory disability, I am optimistic that I will adapt, that I will develop new sensitivities, that I will drink from other sources of continuing joy, and that goodness and mercy shall therefore follow me all the days of my life.

Managing Our Expectations and Comparisons

Knowing these things also makes me wonder: Can we find comfort if we restrain our impossible expectations? Shakespeare's Hamlet may have overstated the power of perception in saying, "There is nothing either good or bad but thinking makes it so." But it's true: Happiness depends less on having things than on our attitude toward the things we have. If our upward strivings and our social comparisons lead us to want and expect more than we have, we feel frustrated. Several years ago an anonymous *New York Times* editor complained that, although his yearly income was sixty-thousand dollars (in 1991 dollars), he was irritated. Rising "fixed" monthly expenses, for such things as newspapers, dry cleaning, and credit card payments, meant he could no longer afford lamb chops and exciting vacations. Though his life-style would be the envy of billions, he felt frustrated, cheated, and his enjoyment soured: "I have earned the right to have more for myself and my family, to have what I earn get us more of what this city and country have to offer."

Without turning a blind eye to economic injustice, how might we gain for ourselves an attitude of gratitude? Should we dwell on our happiest times from the past? One old chestnut counsels, we "are always happier for having been happy." Despite our enjoyment of happy memories, there is both theory and evidence to suggest that dwelling on the Camelot moments from our past makes the present seem pretty pedestrian.

In one experiment, German adults asked to recall and write down a significant low moment in their lives reported feeling better about their present life than if they recalled a high. Dwelling wistfully on the passionate peaks in the early years of my relationship with my wife renders our current emotions unremarkable. If we use our happiest memories as our yardstick for assessing the present, we doom ourselves to disappointment. Although the memories themselves are pleasant, nostalgia breeds discontent.

Indeed, ecstasies remembered exact a price: They dull our ordinary pleasures. UCLA psychologist Allen Parducci explains why. Like our perceptual judgments, our assessments of current happiness are relative to the *range* of our prior experiences. If our current experience is near the top of our best-to-worst range of experience, we feel happy. Raise the top end of your range (by taking an idyllic vacation, earning twice the commission you've ever earned before, sharing sexual passion such as you've never experienced, receiving a Christmas basket break from grinding poverty) and what happens? You now find your everyday experience—your weekends, your regular commission, your normal lovemaking, your everyday macaroni—less enjoyable. Ergo, *if superhigh points are rare, we're better off without them.* Better *not* to expose ourselves to luxury and excess, if their rarity only serves to diminish our daily quiet joys. Better to have our best experiences be something we experience fairly often.

It's also better to experience an occasional reminder of how bad things can be—to provide a point of contrast with one's comfortable daily experience. Given time to fully recover, people report greater happiness if they experienced a health problem requiring hospitalization. Indeed, contrasts define many of life's pleasures. The pangs of hunger make food delicious. Tiredness makes the bed feel heavenly. Loneliness makes a friendship cherished.

In 1943, University of Chicago theologian-to-be Langdon Gilkey was herded with eighteen hundred other foreigners into a Japanese internment camp in North China. In *The Shantung Compound: The Story of Men and Women Under Pressure,* Gilkey recalls the effects of two and a half years of crowding, privation, and malnutrition. After liberation he and his American and British comrades were unprepared for the luxury awaiting them at a hotel commandeered for them by the U.S. Army:

The hotel was out of this world, a galaxy of wonders to our unaccustomed senses. I stopped short after I had gone through the revolving doors—what *was* I standing on? I laughed at myself when I looked down and saw a thick carpet under my feet. A large room for two was stranger still. There was space to move about in, a dresser for clothes, and hot water that came out of the faucet when one turned it on! These elements of civilized life greeted us from every side; we said "Hello" to them with a most intense delight.

When he arrived home, America seemed a dreamworld.

I went with my mother to the grocery on the corner of 55th Street and Woodlawn Avenue in Chicago. It was by no means a supermarket—only an ordinary corner grocery. And yet it completely overwhelmed me. I stood in the middle staring at those shelves piled high with food, cereals, breads, canned vegetables, fruit, and meats, layer on layer of food, spilling over, piles of it in corners, and beyond the butcher's counter, there was more piled high in unopened crates and boxes.

I felt engulfed in food, drowned in immense and inexhaustible wealth, stuffed and bloated with so many fats, calories, and vitamins that I wanted to run outside. Meanwhile, people in the store were talking of their relief that the rigors of rationing were over. I understood then what real affluence meant.

In lesser ways we, too, can *experience reminders of our blessings.* The tent floor underneath the sleeping bag makes the bed back home feel softer. The sacrificial bowls of rice during Lent make the roast chicken tastier. The temporary separation from a loved one makes the reunion sweeter, the person less taken for granted. In such ways we can reframe our thinking, our attitude, our gratitude.

Reuben Bulka explains a related notion of "denial for the sake of pleasure" found within Jewish tradition. Pleasures routinized lose their pleasure-giving power. Thus in Jewish law, husband and wife experience abstinence during and for a week following menstruation. The Talmud's explanation: so that in coming together after separation they might eagerly anticipate and enjoy a warmth and emotional pitch reminiscent of the day they married. Likewise, the Islamic tradition of Ramadan—a month-long fast during daylight hours—whets each evening's appetite and renews appreciation for daytime eating.

Shelley Taylor further illustrates with a Jewish fable about a farmer who seeks a rabbi's counsel because his wife nags him, his children fight, and his surroundings are in chaos. The good rabbi tells him to go home and move the chickens into the house. "Into the house!" cries the farmer. "But what good will that do?" Nevertheless, he complies and two days later returns, more frantic than before. "Now my wife nags me, the children fight, and the chickens are everywhere, laying eggs, dropping feathers, and eating our food. What am I to do?" The rabbi tells him to go home and bring the cow into the house. "The cow!" cries the distraught man. "That can only worsen things!" Again, the rabbi insists, the man complies, and then returns a few days later more harried than ever. "Nothing is helping. The chickens are into everything and the cow is knocking over the furniture. Rabbi, you have made things worse." The rabbi sends the frantic man home to bring in the horse as well. The next day the man returns in despair. "Everything is knocked over. There is no room for my family. Our lives are in shambles. What shall we do?" Now the rabbi instructs, "Go home and take out the horse and cow and chickens." The man does so and returns the next day smiling. "Rabbi, our lives are now so calm and peaceful. With the animals gone, we are a family again. How can I thank you?" The rabbi smiles.

Recognizing that ever-rising desires mean never-ending dissatisfaction, we can also strive to *make our goals short-term and sensible.* Life's greatest disappointments, as well as its greatest attainments, are born of the highest expectations. Lyndon Johnson's announced goal of a Great Society—a new America where poverty and prejudice would be eradicated—was followed by explosions in America's cities when "the revolution of rising expectations" was unfulfilled. We need visionary dreams. But to constrain the frustrating gap between what you want and what you have, work toward them in realistic steps. Better to fulfill a succession of modest goals, and to enjoy the sense of competence such achievements provide, than to believe the promises of pop psychology book jackets and be ever reaching for the moon and failing. Better to face the fact that your organization is a pyramid, with fewer and fewer people reaching higher and higher levels, peaking in one CEO. Better to define success not as the world does—as surpassing other people (a never-ending quest)—but as fulfilling one's own potential. Better to let go of impossible expectations for success, for our children, for our marriages, writes Judith Viorst, than to clutch at "the dearest megalomaniacal dreams of our childhood. Growing up means knowing they can't be fulfilled. Growing up means gaining the wisdom and skills to get what we want within the limitations imposed by reality—a reality which consists of diminished powers, restricted freedoms, and, with the people we love, imperfect connections."

Finally, we can *choose our comparisons intentionally.* Vacationing amid the luxuries of Rancho Mirage, California, outside Palm Springs, my parents write of feeling relatively poor. We receive their letter in Scotland where, though living with somewhat less, our comparison with friends and neighbors makes us acutely sensitive to our relative wealth. It all depends on whom we compare ourselves with. As the psychologist Abraham Maslow noted, "All you have to do is to go to a hospital and hear all the simple blessings that people never before realized *were* blessings—being able to urinate, to sleep on your side, to be able to swallow, to scratch an itch, etc. Could *exercises* in deprivation educate us faster about all our blessings?"

Short of visiting the sick, befriending the bereaved, or hearing the voices and seeing the faces of the desperately poor, even imagining others' misfortunes can trigger renewed life satisfaction. A research team led by Marshall Dermer put University of Wisconsin–Milwaukee women through some imaginative exercises in deprivation. After viewing vivid depictions of how grim life was in Milwaukee in 1900, or after imagining and then writing about various personal tragedies such as being burned and disfigured, the women expressed a greater sense of satisfaction with the quality of their own lives. Today suddenly seemed not so bad after being made keenly aware, through slides and narrative, that "the good old days" were times of sickening hygiene, hungry unemployment, and crime, corruption, and despair.

In another experiment, State University of New York at Buffalo psychologists Jennifer Crocker and Lisa Gallo tested the wisdom of that old song "Count your blessings, name them one by one." After five times completing the sentence "I'm glad I'm not a . . ." people felt relatively happy and satisfied with their lives. By contrast, those who counted their unfulfilled desires, by completing sentences beginning with "I wish I were a . . ." came away feeling worse.

To repeat, if we seek greater serenity we can strive to restrain our unrealistic expectations, to go out of our way to experience reminders of our blessings, to make our goals short-term and sensible, to choose comparisons that will breed gratitude rather than envy.

4

The Demography of Happiness

Youth is pert and positive, Age modest and doubting:
So Ears of Corn when young and light, stand bold upright,
but hang their heads when weighty, full and ripe.

BENJAMIN FRANKLIN, *POOR RICHARD'S ALMANAC*

We have seen that, once beyond poverty, new levels of wealth and success bring but temporary pleasure. After adapting to the new circumstances, and raising one's standard of comparison, life settles back to its normal mix of emotions. Ergo, we needn't be so envious of the wealthy.

But what about other population groups? Who are the happiest? Are they mostly young? middle-aged? retired? Are they mostly women or men? One race or another? City folks or rural dwellers? Seems like a labyrinth of possibilities, doesn't it. Let's look for our own experiences within these demographic groups, beginning by considering well-being across the seasons of life.

Well-being Across the Life Span

It's a given—to live is to grow older. And that means all of us will likely look backward with either satisfaction or sorrow, and look forward with hope or dread. But actually, which periods of life should we most dread? Marguerite, her family's matriarch and a former world traveler and French professor at my college, still exudes mental vitality at age ninety-six. She challenges her retirement home neighbors to consider: "Is old age a reward or a punishment?"

When asked which periods of life are least rewarding, people often say that adolescents and the elderly are the unhappiest. In adolescence we are assailed by mood swings and insecurity, parental power and peer pressures, social anxieties and career worries. As one thirteen-year-old moaned, "Being this age isn't easy, you know. I feel like an adult trapped in a child's body." Being old doesn't look like much more fun. In later life, our income shrinks, our occupation is snatched away, our body deteriorates, our recall fades, our energy wanes, our family members and friends may die or move away, and the great enemy, the Grim Reaper, looms ever closer. Small wonder that we presume the teen and over-sixty-five years are the worst of times.

But there goes another myth, for they are not. Actually, people of all ages report similar feelings of well-being. Arizona State University psychologists William Stock, Morris Okun, and their colleagues boiled down the results of more than a hundred studies and discovered that less than 1 percent of the variation in well-being was related to age. Ronald Inglehart found the same in his amassing of the 170,000 interviews in sixteen nations. As the figure on the next page illustrates, age differences in well-being were trivial.

Does happiness, then, align itself more with any particular age? Do young adults have more fun? Surprisingly, and definitely, not.

But aren't there times when our well-being takes a predictable nosedive? Popular psychology tells us that despair may strike women during and after menopause, or when their children leave home (the

Percent "Satisfied with Life"

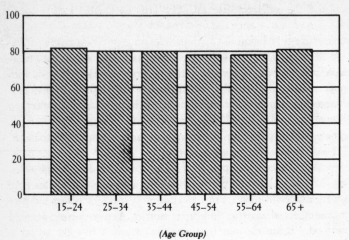

(Age Group)

Age and well-being in sixteen nations
SOURCE: Data from 169,776 people reported by Ronald Inglehart, *Culture Shift in Advanced Industrial Society* (Princeton: Princeton University Press, 1990).

"empty nest syndrome"). Actually, life's ups and downs are not so predictable. One survey of 2,500 middle-aged Massachusetts women found them no more or less depressed if experiencing menopause.

What determines the emotional impact of menopause is the woman's attitude toward it. Does she see menopause as a sign that she is losing her femininity and sexual attractiveness and beginning to grow old? Or does she look on it as liberation from contraceptives, menstrual periods, fears of pregnancy, and the demands of children? To learn women's attitudes toward menopause, University of Chicago developmental psychologist Bernice Neugarten and her colleagues did what, before the 1960s, no one had bothered to do: They asked questions of women whose experience of menopause had not led them to seek treatment. When asked whether it is true that after menopause "women generally feel better than they have for years," only one fourth of the premenopausal women under age forty-five guessed yes. Of the older women who had experienced menopause, two thirds said yes. As one woman said, "I can remember my mother saying that after her menopause she really got her vigor, and I can say the same thing for myself." And are women "generally calmer and happier after the change of life than before"? Of those under forty-five, 38 percent said yes; of those over fifty-five, 80 percent said yes. Social psychologist Jacqueline Goodchilds quips: "If the truth were known, we'd have to diagnose [older women] as having PMF—Post-Menstrual Freedom."

Moreover, says Neugarten, "Just as the major problem of middle-aged women is not the menopause, it is also not the empty nest. Most women are glad to see their children grow up, leave home, marry, and have their careers. The notion that they mourn the loss of their reproductive ability and their mother role does not seem to fit modern reality. No matter what the stereotypes tell us, it is not the way women talk when you listen."

Seven national surveys confirm that the empty nest is generally a happy place. Compared to middle-aged women who still have children at home, those whose nest has emptied report greater happiness and greater enjoyment of their marriage. Those whose nest refills with adult children returning home (an increasing tendency during divorce or financial woe) often suffer from the stress. Insanity is hereditary, says an old joke, you get it from your kids. Many parents whose nest has just emptied therefore experience what sociologists Lynn White and John Edwards call a "post-launch honeymoon," especially if they maintain close relationships with their children.

My friend Phoebe, a warm and energetic fifty-year-old, explains: "Our family is very close. When my two sons come home I can't wait till they get here, I stay excited throughout their stay, and I'm in tears after they leave. Yet within a day or two we're back to enjoying our freedom. My husband and I now worry less about them. We experience fewer of the aggravations that accompany raising teenagers. And we can spontaneously go out with friends—our time is ours!"

As for men, part of their "passage" to middle adulthood is supposedly an early-forties midlife crisis: They realize they will never be the company president, that the passion is long gone from their marriage, that their bodies are aging. Thus they are said to suffer an agonizing period of turmoil and despair that may trigger a search for new life meanings and relationships, perhaps even an ego-building affair. "While Diana puts on a brave face," proclaimed a 1991 *People* magazine cover, "a brooding [forty-two-year-old] Prince Charles grapples with a midlife crisis and retreats to his old girlfriends."

Or take Jim Tracy. At age forty-one he had risen to corporate vice president with thousands of people under him, and a six-figure salary. Yet he began to feel trapped. He started to question the social impact of his company's products and personnel policies. He began an affair, which led to his divorcing his wife and remarrying. And he felt guilt over so often being unavailable during his children's troubled transitions to adulthood. After remarrying, Tracy's illusions about his new marriage and family life slowly crumbled. All this plus his wife's allergies led him finally to resign his executive position and move with his new family to Denver, to enjoy not only the drier climate but also a new way of relating to work and family.

For Jim Tracy and others of the upscale, career-oriented American males sampled in two famous studies, a crisis at midlife appears to be a real event. Nevertheless, research with large, representative samples of adults tells us that such cases are not the norm. The fact is that most men in their early forties exhibit *no* dip in their sense of well-being. What's more, there is *no* upswing in job and marital dissatisfaction, career change, divorce, anxiety, depression, or suicide. Divorce, for example, is most common among those in their twenties, suicide among those in their seventies and eighties. The relatively unusual instances of middle-age divorce may, however, snare our attention—confirming our stereotype of midlife dissatisfactions.

Are these markers of crisis too crude to detect a more subtle midlife turmoil? National Institute of Aging researchers Robert McCrae and Paul Costa gave a "Midlife Crisis Scale" assessing the sense of meaninglessness and mortality, job and family dissatisfaction, and inner turmoil and confusion to 350 thirty- to sixty-year-old men. Still, they could find "no evidence at all" that such concerns peak at midlife. Surprised, they gave their scale to a new group of 300 men, and a measure of emotional instability to nearly 10,000 men and women. "The results were an exact reconfirmation: There was not the slightest evidence" that distress peaks anywhere in the midlife age range.

Other researchers have reached the same definitive conclusion:

Those tendencies that should be discernible, given a midlife crisis, are just not to be found—not even a midlife blip on the trend lines.* Contrary to the empty nest and midlife myths, it is not age that marks the transitions from one life stage to another, but significant life events. Whenever they occur, childbearing, child leaving, relocation, occupational shifts, divorce, illness, retirement, and widowhood can recast our lives.

The stability of well-being across the life span, even across the midlife years, does, however, obscure some interesting age-related emotional differences. As our years go by, our feelings mellow. Our highs are less high, our lows less low. So, while with age our *average* feeling level may remain stable, we find ourselves less often feeling excited, or intensely proud, or elated. But we also less often feel depressed. Compliments provoke less elation and criticisms less despair. Both become iotas of additional feedback atop a pile of accumulated praise and reproach.

University of Chicago psychologist Mihaly Csikszentmihalyi and his colleagues use the electronic pagers to map people's emotional terrain by beeping people at random intervals to stop and note their current activities and feelings. One finding: Young teenagers typically descend from elation or ascend from gloom in less than an hour. A snub from a friend and it seems the world is about to end. But then comes a phone call and all's forgotten. No wonder Gettysburg College researchers report that today's ratings of parental warmth by late adolescents living at home bear no relation to ratings made by the same adolescents six weeks before. When teenagers are down, their world, including their parents, seems inhuman; when their mood brightens, their parents' traits become admirable. Adult moods are less extreme but more enduring. Having survived past sufferings and enjoyed past thrills, mature people look beyond the moment.

The dean of well-being researchers, the late Angus Campbell at the University of Michigan, reported similarly. Age irons out the highs

---

*One wonders why such pop psychology myths do not die when countered by consistent, conclusive evidence. Is it because people find Jim Tracy-like anecdotes more memorable than population statistics? One of my underlying messages in this book is that intensive case studies of a few people can be suggestive; but we had best verify our conclusions with larger, more representative samples of people. I offer examples, such as Phoebe, not as evidence but as representative, real-life illustrations.

and lows. Old age therefore does offer less joy. But the compensation is contentment. Those things that used to irritate—poor service at a restaurant, slow traffic, rain on a picnic—no longer seem like that big a deal. "At seventy, I would say the advantage is that you take life more calmly," said Eleanor Roosevelt. "You know that 'this, too, shall pass!'"

At the outset of my career, having my research accepted by a leading journal led me to fantasize about becoming one of the world's most creative social psychologists; having the next submission rejected made me wonder if I had the smarts even to function in the profession. Now, two decades later, praise, though still welcome, is merely pleasant. And being criticized? Well, it's no longer a trauma. As we age, average well-being may be unchanged, but we ride a smoother roller coaster.

The stability of well-being across the life span also obscures changed feelings concerning specific domains of our lives. Compared with younger adults, older people report feeling slightly more satisfied with their work, their marriage, their standard of living, their housing, and their community. "There's an acceptance that comes with age," said Ted. "I feel less need to try to change my wife's behavior, to gain a better job, to have a better house. She, and they, are what they are. They're comfortable and familiar, so why not enjoy them?"

Offsetting these satisfactions of aging is a sadder side. Surveys reveal that older people often do feel lonelier and *less* satisfied with their health and attractiveness. Mary, an unhappy Arizona woman, was pleased to be so healthy at age eighty-four. Yet, she reported, "I don't see the sense of it. My husband of forty years is gone; my two sisters and brother are gone; two of my children are gone; everyone I cared about except only my youngest daughter is gone and she lives in Ohio."

So, satisfaction with life remains pretty stable because the up and down sides of aging roughly balance. Still, given all the reasons why people suppose the elderly must be finding life less satisfying, do the positive satisfactions really balance the sadder side? Is old age really as much a reward as a punishment? Usually, yes, for several reasons.

With age, stress declines. The upheavals and traumas of dating, child rearing, and vocation are behind. Even daily hassles diminish as demands lessen. University of Michigan researchers Regula Herzog and Willard Rodgers report that older adults more often describe their lives as "free" and "easy" rather than as "tied down" and "hard." True, those over sixty-five are more often plagued with chronic illnesses. But they are *less* susceptible to the discomforts of flu and other short-term illnesses. My seventy-five-year-old friend Chuck is typical: "I rarely get sick. The last cold I had was a year ago. I've got a lifetime full of antibodies protecting me."

Another reason: Older people better align their aspirations with their attainments. As we age we relinquish some of our earlier yearnings, dream fewer impossible dreams, and therefore reduce the frustrating gap between our aspirations and actualities. Our aspirations become colored by what we perceive as normal for our sort of folks. One survey for the National Council on Aging revealed that most elderly people think that others their age have some sort of serious health problem; but when asked about their own health, fewer than one in four report that *they* have such a problem. Perceiving themselves better off than others, most elderly people can reason, "I have a lot to be grateful for."

The stability of well-being across our life span does not contradict what we all plainly observe: Everyone's morale fluctuates, and individuals do indeed differ. People at ages fifteen, fifty, and seventy-five express similar average levels of well-being; yet at any age they vary from the depressed to the buoyant. That raises a question that has occupied dozens of researchers: What makes for well-being in later life? Are the things that predict satisfaction and happiness the same for the elderly as for the young?

Here we find fewer surprises. At any age, whatever aspects of our lives most preoccupy us are those that best predict our well-being. Older people are less occupied with work, more involved in leisure activities and social relations. And sure enough, compared with younger adults, their work satisfaction is a less important predictor of their well-being, while satisfaction with leisure activities and social relationships become more important. The happiest of senior citizens are those who are actively religious, who enjoy close relationships with friends and family, who have sufficient health, income, and motivation to enjoy a variety of activities. Anthropologist Ashley Montagu, who has studied aging both professionally and first hand, observes that the later years can be the happiest of one's life. Many of those who have achieved what others call old age have confessed to feeling embarrassingly young, as if such feeling were something anachronistic, an unexpected freshness. It is the kind of freshness that the long-distance runner experiences when at the peak of fatigue he experiences a second wind that takes him on to the finish line. This kind of freshness [is] that feeling of unadulterated joy in being alive that the romping child so gloriously feels—perhaps without the physical romping, but with that gaiety of spirit that has enabled one to grow young more effectively and more happily than was ever before possible—the last of life, for which the first was made.

Whatever the explanation—reduced stress, lowered aspirations, newfound sources of pleasure, acceptance of life and death—the bottom line from hundreds of thousands of interviews with people of all ages in many countries remains: Older people report just as much happiness and satisfaction with life as do younger people. Given that growing older is one sure consequence of living, an outcome that most of us prefer to its alternative, we can surely find comfort in this truth.

More than a hundred studies confirm that for adults of all ages, and certainly for older adults, one predictor of happiness is health and physical fitness. More exactly, ill health—chronic pain, depleted energy, or threat of death—can undermine our well-being. Listen to Frank, a terminal cancer patient: "It is hard to be twenty-two and wondering and questioning why you can't be happy and why you have to die. People teach us many things but not how to cope with dying. It's scary and so lonely."

Despite their illness, some people manage to maintain a joie de vivre. But usually we are more upset by illness than delighted by health. Health is like wealth. Although its utter absence can breed misery, having it is no guarantee of happiness.

More than we realized a decade and more ago, our behaviors and emotions affect our health and vitality. The three leading causes of serious illness and death—heart disease, cancer, and strokes—are influenced by our smoking and drinking habits, by how we react to stress, by our nutrition, by our willingness to exercise. Behavior kills. To learn why, and what to do about it, psychologists and physicians have created the profession of behavioral medicine.

Two lines of research in this new field provide clues to good health *and* to happiness for both young and old. One explores the effects of modifying the life-styles of intense, anger-prone Type A people. In one experiment, cardiologist Meyer Friedman and Diane Ulmer assigned hundreds of middle-aged San Francisco area heart attack survivors to one of two groups. The first group received standard advice concerning medications, diet, and exercise. The second group received similar advice plus counseling on how to slow down and relax—by walking, talking, and eating more slowly; smiling at others and laughing at themselves; admitting mistakes; taking time to enjoy life; and renewing their religious faith. Over the ensuing three years, the second group experienced half as many repeat heart attacks as the first group.

These spectacular results demand confirmation. In the meantime, studies have documented the therapeutic value of laughter. People who laugh readily and view life with a sense of humor find stressful events less disturbing. "Hearty" laughter tones the cardiovascular system, exercises the lungs, and releases muscle tension. Although it's probably an overstatement to say that "laughter is the best medicine," there is reason to suspect that, indeed, he who laughs, lasts.

Laughter works by first arousing us and then leaving us feeling more relaxed. So also does aerobic exercise (sustained exercise, such as jogging, that increases lung and heart fitness). Here the evidence is even stronger and the implications more practical: Aerobic exercise strengthens the spirit as well as the body. First, exercise boosts our well-being indirectly, by enhancing our energy and health. One sixteen-year study of 17,000 middle-aged Harvard alumni found that those who exercised regularly were likely to live longer. Another study of 15,000 Control Data Corporation employees found that those who exercised had 25 percent fewer hospital days than those who didn't. And a digest of data from forty-three studies revealed that, compared to inactive adults, people who exercise vigorously suffer half as many heart attacks.

Second, regular exercise lessens the odds of our becoming depressed or overwhelmed by stress. Repeated surveys, some by government health agencies, reveal that Canadians and Americans are more self-confident, self-disciplined, and psychologically resilient, and less anxious and depressed, if physically fit. More often than not, joyful spirits accompany strong, fit bodies.

But might cause and effect run in the other direction (maybe stressed or depressed people lack the energy to exercise)? To find out, psychologists have randomly assigned unhappy people either to aerobic exercise programs or to other treatments. In one such experiment, Lisa McCann and David Holmes assigned one third of a group of mildly depressed University of Kansas women students to a program of aerobic dancing and running, and another third to a treatment of relaxation exercises. For comparison purposes, the remaining third received no treatment. Ten weeks later, those in the untreated group were unchanged, those in the relaxation group were feeling better, and those in the aerobic exercise group were dramatically improved.

Exercise also provides a short-term boost. When I find myself feeling nervous, groggy, or depressed, nothing so effectively calms the jitters and clears the fog as a half-hour jog. Research reveals that even a ten-minute walk simulates a two-hour hike in well-being by raising energy levels and lowering tension.

Researchers are now debating *why* aerobic exercise enhances positive emotions. Is it because those who exercise evaluate themselves as looking and feeling younger (which they do compared to nonexercisers)? Is it because exercise lowers both blood pressure and the blood pressure reaction to stress (which it does)? Is it because exercise increases production of mood-boosting brain chemicals, such as the endorphins (which it does)? Are the emotional benefits a side effect of the increased body warmth or the muscle relaxation and sounder sleep that follow?

Regardless, the new research on moderate aerobic exercise is producing such consistent and encouraging results—and with such minimal cost and desirable side effects—that virtually anyone of any age seeking to boost health and well-being is well advised to join the movement movement. As one ninety-four-year-old man who worked up to walking three miles a day reported, "I sleep better, feel better." Chuck, my seventy-five-year-old friend, plays basketball daily with men half his age and younger. "If I don't exercise five times a week," he explained, "I begin to get the blahs. The stamina I get from exercising helps keep me optimistic about living."

"Mens sana in corpore sano," goes the ancient Latin wisdom. Sound mind in a sound body—for people at every age.

Gender and Joy

Another much-studied demographic predictor of well-being is gender. What do you know about the happiness of women and men? A little quiz can help you find out. True or false:

1. Men report higher levels of well-being than do women.
2. Women report more happiness and fulfillment if their lives feel rushed rather than free and easy.
3. Full-time homemakers have happier husbands.
4. Women are more likely than men both to become depressed *and* to express joy.
5. Men are more likely than women to attempt suicide.
6. Women tend to feel somewhat tense, irritable, or depressed during the two or three days before the onset of menstruation.*

In Western societies, which sex enjoys greater well-being? Is it men, because of their greater social power and higher incomes? Is it women, because of their greater capacity for empathy and intimacy? The answers are reminiscent of research on age and well-being: Knowing that someone is a man or a woman gives us little clue to the person's self-reported well-being. One statistical digest of 146 studies found that gender accounted for less than 1 percent of people's differing well-being; another review of research reported that women expressed only slightly greater happiness. Data amassed from the 1980s sixteen-nation surveys illustrate: Men and women are equally likely to report being "very happy" and "satisfied or very satisfied" with life. The same finding appears in a new study of 18,032 university students surveyed by sixty-eight researchers in thirty-nine countries around the globe.

*Statements 1, 3, 5, and 6 are false; 2 and 4 are true. For pertinent evidence, read on.

Given past inequities in the status of men and women, the finding is impressive. In well-being, if not in social power, the sexes are equal.

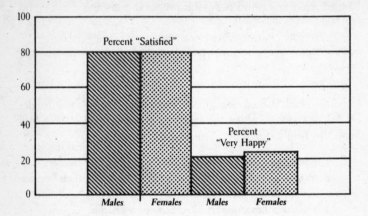

Gender and well-being in sixteen nations
SOURCE: Data from 169,776 people reported by Ronald Inglehart, *Culture Shift in Advanced Industrial Society* (Princeton: Princeton University Press, 1990).

But does this overall result obscure any important differences? Consider one obvious possibility: that employed women are more (or less) happy than those who don't work for pay. Does the flow of married women into the workplace—from 1890 when one in seven married women were in the work force, to 1940 when one in four were, to 1990 when nearly six in ten were—suggest that the alternatives to employment are less rewarding?

In fact, employed married women are only slightly more likely than those not employed to say they are very happy and fully satisfied with their lives. This rough equivalence has persisted even as women's attitudes and employment rates have changed dramatically.

One explanation is that the psychic costs and benefits of each role are roughly equal. On the negative side, housework can be repetitive, boring, and socially isolated. But let's not romanticize punching a cash register; employed women often have low-paying, unrewarding jobs, from which they come home to shoulder most of the housework and child care. (For most women, work is never done. Today's average husband does but one third of the household tasks, though that's up from 15 percent in 1965.) On the positive side, should one prefer the freer life and avocations enjoyed by those not employed? Or the identity enjoyed by those with careers?

Actually, middle-class housewives who feel *less* free—whose lives feel full and rushed rather than free and easy—express greater feelings of happiness and fulfillment. For these women, reports sociologist Myra Ferree, too little to do can be more of a problem than too much. Carol, a vigorous forty-six-year-old, paused to reflect: "I don't buy our culture's materialistic idea that work is meaningful only if compensated. My life is filled with challenge—nurturing a family, yes, but also giving volunteer leadership to church and community organizations. It adds time pressure, but my life is richer—both more interesting and more meaningful—than if I were either playing bridge or working only for money."

Although women's employment and divorce rates have risen together, employed women are not less satisfied with their marriage and family life. National surveys reveal that the combined stresses of motherhood and employment do erode some women's well-being by overloading their circuits. This is especially true for thirtysomething working mothers, who often feel most keenly the pressures of competing demands. But compared with married women who do not work for pay, those who do are no more or less likely to say they understand and are understood by their husbands. Moreover, their husbands are no more or less happy with their marriages.

Obviously, some husbands aren't happy about their wives working. "It's okay for both husband and wife to work, but only until one or the other gets pregnant," lampooned Sam Levenson. Still, when both spouses have jobs, the average marriage doesn't suffer. Typically, if married women feel supported in their endeavors, both by colleagues at work and by their husbands' attitudes and participation in child care and housework, they thrive. They enjoy good health and self-esteem, and feel positive about their spouses and their lives. Take my friend and colleague Jane, a spirited college professor: "Some say, 'You can't have it all.' And there surely are hectic times with meeting the demands of my job and wanting to enjoy our children and home life, too. But I'd have to say, I have felt real richness in my life having both a loving, challenging family and a meaningful career. I wouldn't have it any other way."

From their studies at the Wellesley College Center for Research on Women, Grace Baruch and Rosaline Barnett conclude that what matters is therefore not which roles a woman occupies—as paid worker, wife, mother—but the quality of her experience in those roles. Happiness is having work that fits your interests and provides a sense of competence and accomplishment. It's having a partner who is a close, supportive companion and who sees you as special. It's having loving children whom you like and take pride in.

Furthermore, reports Smith College researcher Faye Crosby, satisfaction in love and work feed each other: "Having important roles to play away from work (as, say, a wife, mother, or volunteer worker) enhances job satisfaction. Working outside the family—either for pay or in major volunteer work—enhances satisfaction with home life."

Freud would not have been surprised. The healthiest adult, he said, enjoys both love and work. For most people, *love* is centered on family relationships. *Work* is any activity, whether for pay or not, that enables one to feel productive and competent. Having both, as do Carol and Jane in their differing ways, is a big step toward well-being.

If women and men are surprisingly similar in their average well-being, they are as surprisingly different in their experiences of misery. In the United States and Europe, women are twice as likely as men to suffer the hopelessness and lethargy of a prolonged bout of depression. To be depressed, as women more often know, is to feel discouraged, dissatisfied, isolated, sad, lacking energy and appetite, unable to concentrate, even wishing one was dead.

Why are women more vulnerable to depression? Is it because society provides women with less independent control over their lives than men have? Consistent with this explanation, depression does tend to accompany the self-defeating beliefs that often arise when people feel powerless and helpless. Moreover, housewives and unassertive women are more vulnerable to depression.

But there is an additional explanation: Yale psychologist Patricia Linville reports that people who occupy several roles and therefore have multiple identities—as parent, spouse, worker, amateur athlete, community leader, or whatever—have their whole sense of self less threatened by problems in any given area. For both women and men, a sense of pride and satisfaction in one's roles at home can lessen the sting of disappointment at work. Likewise, a broken marriage will be less devastating to the one who can think "despite my marital problems, I am a good parent" (or a skilled and appreciated worker). As one woman said, "My job was my refuge from my husband's constant criticism. My success at work helped me know that I wasn't as incompetent as he made me out to be." For a short time, the stress of divorce may disrupt work. But thereafter, reports Faye Crosby, "Professional life proves enormously helpful to the typical woman as she goes through a divorce." Work structures the day, offers a focus, and provides self-esteem and pleasant interactions.

Which sex do you suppose most often feels worried or frightened? Again, the answer is women, who more often experience (or at least more often acknowledge) strong feelings, both negative (depression, anxiety, fear) and positive (joy). Texas A&M researchers Wendy Wood, Nancy Rhodes, and Melanie Whelan conclude that "women are more likely than men to be sensitive to and expressive of emotional experiences, and this is particularly the case with emotional aspects of intimate relationships." After studying hundreds of adults and university students, University of Illinois researchers Frank Fujita, Ed Diener, and Ed Sandvik concur. Under good circumstances, women more often than men report intense joy, but under bad circumstances they report more intense sadness. This helps explain why women's average happiness is equal to men's, yet women are twice as vulnerable to depression.

Women's greater empathy seems related to their skill at reading others' emotions. Studies consistently reveal women's greater sensitivity to nonverbal cues. For example, when shown a two-second silent film clip of the face of an upset woman, women are better than men at guessing whether she is angry or discussing a divorce. This helps explain why both men and women report their friendships with women to be more intimate, enjoyable, and nurturing. When wanting intimacy and understanding, both men and women turn to women. Don speaks for many men (and women): "I've got some close men friends who are great fun to be with, but sharing my worries and hurts somehow comes easier with my women friends." Such may also explain why men are more likely than women to say that their best friend is their spouse, and why four in five women say their best friend is another woman.

Time and again I am struck by how the findings I report in this book ring true in my own life. My department offers me five male and three female colleague-friends, each of whom I cherish for different reasons. But when I'm brooding over a sensitive matter or deeply concerned about one of my children, to which colleague am I most likely to disclose my concerns? Jane.

Given women's sensitivity and empathy, and their vulnerability to depression, we might expect them to commit more suicide. Women do, indeed, more often *attempt* suicide. But, depending on the country, men are two to three times more likely to succeed.* (Men more often use methods that are sure to succeed, like putting a bullet into the brain.) Men also are five times more likely to become alcoholic and eight times more likely to commit violent crime. So, though it's an oversimplification to say that either women or men are more prone to disorder, there are strong connections between gender and *type* of psychological disorder.

The newest gender myth proposes that women's well-being varies with their menstrual phase. Many women believe that their two or three premenstrual days, and perhaps the two or three days following the onset of menstruation, are the blahs—a time of increased irritability, tension, or depression. Some researchers think at least a few of these women are right, and the American Psychiatric Association has accordingly introduced "late luteal phase disorder" (alias PMS) to its manual of psychological disorders.

Other researchers who have looked for the alleged mood fluctuations in the general population haven't found them. When Cathy McFarland at Simon Fraser University, and Michael Ross and Nancy DeCourville at the University of Waterloo, asked Ontario women to

---

*This ironic finding—that men, in general, are no less happy than women, yet men are much more likely to commit suicide—is paralleled by an astounding finding: Countries that exhibit high levels of reported well-being also have *high* suicide rates. Ronald Inglehart reports that the five nations (in the sixteen-nation survey of 170,000 people) ranking highest in satisfaction with life have more than double the suicide rate of the five nations ranking lowest in life satisfaction! To be an unhappy person in the midst of happy people can be, it seems, unbearable. Shakespeare knew it: "How bitter a thing it is to look into happiness through another man's eyes!"

make daily ratings of their moods, they obtained characteristic results. The women's self-rated negative emotions (whether they were experiencing irritability, loneliness, depression, and so forth) did *not* increase during their premenstrual and menstrual phases. Not by a smidgen. Yet the women *believed* that their moods did usually vary with their cycle.

Psychologists Pamela Kato at Princeton University and Diane Ruble at New York University say this is typical: Although many women recall mood changes over their cycle, their day-to-day experiences reveal few such changes. Moreover, cycle-related hormonal changes have no known emotional effects that would lead us to expect mood changes. So why do so many women nevertheless believe they experience premenstrual tension or menstrual irritability? Because, say Kato and Ruble, their implicit theories of menstruation lead them to notice and remember the joint appearances of negative moods and the onset of menstruation—"So that's why I was crabby yesterday"—but not to notice and remember bad moods two weeks later. If aware of a woman's menstrual cycle, men may construct a similar illusory correlation, explaining Clare Boothe Luce's observation, "When a man can't explain a woman's actions, the first thing he thinks about is the condition of her uterus."

It is astonishing that such profound differences in our lives—between being old or young, being a woman or a man, being employed or a homemaker—should have such minuscule effects on overall well-being. We can extend the list.

It makes little predictable difference to a woman's well-being whether she has children or is childless. (Is it because, on average, the hassles and stresses of child rearing cancel the joys and satisfactions that children also can bring?)

Similarly, it matters little where in a country one lives. Whether living in Europe, North America, or Japan, people in rural areas, towns, suburbs, and big cities are about equally happy.

It also matters less than you might suspect whether one is black or white, and highly educated or not. Statistical digests of many dozens of studies by Morris Okun, William Stock, and their Arizona State University colleagues credit race and education with less than 2 percent of the person-to-person variations in well-being. Ronald Inglehart concludes similarly from the pooled European surveys. There is a slight advantage to being advantaged—white and highly educated—but the differences are surprisingly small. Individual variations in well-being within any such group vastly exceed the average differences between races and educational groups.

Again, the findings startle me. As everyone knows, disadvantaged groups suffer from impoverished self-esteem and consequent depression, and as Chapter 6 will document, self-esteem is a wellspring of well-being. So why do surveys of women and African Americans not report less joy?

It's because what "everyone knows" is wrong. For example, African Americans do *not* suffer lower self-esteem. In the words of social psychologists Jennifer Crocker and Brenda Major: "A host of studies conclude that blacks have levels of self-esteem equal to or higher than that of whites." The National Institute of Mental Health's 1980s study, *Psychiatric Disorders in America,* similarly reveals that the rates of depression and alcoholism among blacks and Hispanics are roughly comparable to those among whites (if anything, America's ethnic minorities suffer slightly less depression than do whites).

How could this be? Despite discrimination and lower social status, members of various "stigmatized" groups (people of color, the disabled, women) maintain self-esteem in three ways, report Crocker and Major. They value the things at which they excel. They attribute problems to prejudice. And they do as we all do—they compare themselves to those in their own group. This helps us understand why all such groups report comparable levels of happiness. Although it leaves unexplained the curious gender differences in psychiatric disorder, those differences roughly balance: Women suffer roughly double men's risk of depression, anxiety, and phobic disorders; but men have a fivefold greater risk of suffering alcoholism, which also correlates with low self-esteem.

If knowing your wealth, age, gender, parental status, place of residence, race, and educational level doesn't reveal much about your well-being, then what does? Are happiness and life satisfaction unpredictable? Do they vary willy-nilly? Read on.

5

Reprogramming the Mind

Finding the occasional straw of truth awash in a great ocean of confusion and bamboozle requires intelligence, vigilance, dedication and courage. But if we don't practice these tough habits of thought, we cannot hope to solve the truly serious problems that face us—and we risk becoming a nation of suckers, up for grabs by the next charlatan who comes along.

CARL SAGAN, "THE FINE ART OF BALONEY DETECTION"

To visit a bookstore," George F. Will once reflected, "is to feel misgivings about universal literacy, which has produced a mass market for hundreds of profoundly sad handbooks on achieving happiness." Each offers its own prescriptions for feeling good about oneself. Pull a few psychic levers, believe the best about yourself, assert yourself, and happiness will be yours. Study your dreams, attend a seminar, or buy some tapes, and perhaps you, too, can "wake up every day, completely happy, eager to live."

Is there anything to these promises of quick mental fixes? Or are they merely today's versions of yesterday's snake oils? Let's first look at the history of the American "mind power" movement, and then consider four touted prescriptions for well-being, each of which has been publicized with extravagant claims and examined in sober research.

Mind Power

The roots of various "mind cures" run deep in the fertile soil of nineteenth-century American individualism and optimism. Using positive mental suggestions, Phineas Parkhurst Quimby, clockmaker-turned-psychic-healer, taught that by changing belief one could cure disease—which, under Quimby's guidance, Christian Science founder Mary Baker Eddy believed happened to her. In 1916 the International New Thought Alliance, an array of Quimby-influenced groups adopted a statement of purpose that touted this mental power: "To teach the infinitude of the Supreme One; the Divinity of Man and his Infinite possibilities through the creative power and constructive thinking in obedience to the voice of the Indwelling Presence, which is our source in Inspiration, Power, Health and Prosperity."

This idea—that human minds could draw instant power and insight from the divine mind—was popularized in Ralph Waldo Trine's 1897 best seller *In Tune with the Infinite: Or, Fullness of Peace, Power, and Plenty,* which sold a million and a half copies and was translated into twenty languages. "Ideas have occult power," wrote Trine. "To hold yourself in this attitude of mind is to set into operation subtle, silent, and irresistible forces that sooner or later will actualize in material form what is today merely an idea."

In two different ways, contemporary advocates of mind power are still in tune with Trine and other New Thought proponents. The idea that a divine dimension of humanity enables us to harness supernatural powers finds expression in today's New Age doctrine that everyone is God, co-master of the universe, or at least that a creative life force lies waiting to be tapped. To find healing, peace, or power, get in touch with this inner spiritual power. Take control of your fate. Awaken the god-in-you. By harnessing your psychic mental powers, achieve a modest sort of omniscience (by reading others' minds), omnipresence (through out-of-body travel), and omnipotence (by altering the future through a convergence of mental powers). Most faith healers would disavow the pantheistic leanings of New Age thought, yet they make a kindred claim of being a channel for divine healing powers passing through their hands into sick bodies.

Mind power theory also has made its way into American Protestantism. Biblical religions (notably Judaism and Christianity) view us as finite creatures formed of the earth, creatures having dignity but not deity. Nevertheless, the rugged individualist side of American Protestantism has absorbed aspects of the mental power message. After publication in 1952, Norman Vincent Peale's *The Power of Positive Thinking* spent two years atop the best-seller lists and sold more than two million hardcover copies, before selling millions more over the years since. "You can think your way to failure and unhappiness," wrote Peale, "but you can also think your way to success and happiness. The world in which you live is not primarily determined by outward conditions and circumstances but by thoughts that habitually occupy your mind." To tap this positive mental energy, connect yourself to the divine power plant, allowing the divine energy to flow through your personality.

Peale, in turn, has supported fellow Reformed Church in America pastor Robert Schuller. Closer to the mainstream of Protestantism, Schuller's books and televised services from California's Crystal Cathedral inspire millions today to be "possibility thinkers." Like Peale, Schuller is receptive to certain themes in psychology and aims to merge them with theology into a positive and practical Christianity.

Is there anything to this mind power business? Can the mind really precipitate health and happiness? Should we find Peale's promises appalling or appealing?

Skeptical academic that I am, ten years ago I might have scorned all this. (Among people in my profession, healthy critical thinking sometimes veers into intellectual pride and condescension.) But today, after another decade of hard-nosed research, certain claims of the mental power movement seem valid. Some unsubstantiated claims, such as of psychic mental powers, seem as bizarre as ever, especially in view of our accumulating knowledge about our creatureliness—formed of the earth as we indeed are, with our growing awareness of the mechanisms of the mind's dependence on brain. Yet, as Peale foresaw, objective life circumstances have little effect on well-being—certainly less than I would have guessed. Peale's lament—"in the midst of economic plenty we starve spiritually"—rings truer in our day than his.

Moreover, there no longer is any doubt that mind affects brain—that our appraisal of challenging situations affects our blood pressure, that chronic anger and resentment trigger the release of hormones that accelerate the buildup of deposits on the heart's vessels, that persistent psychological stress depresses the immune system, decreasing our resistance to various diseases. Although it's tempting to overstate the effect—people do not cause their own cancer cells and cannot mentally will them away—there is more and more evidence that rage and other negative emotions do lash back at us, and that relaxation, meditation, and optimism boost the body's own healing processes.

Research psychologists Michael Scheier and Charles Carver (1987), for example, report that positive thinkers—people who agree with statements such as "in uncertain times, I usually expect the best"—cope more successfully with stressful events and enjoy better health than do pessimists. During the last month of a semester, students previously identified as optimistic report less fatigue and fewer coughs, aches, and pains. Optimists also respond to stress with smaller increases in blood pressure. They even recover faster from heart bypass surgery.

But precisely how, and how much, do inner mental states affect our sense of joy and happiness? Where in the claims for positive mental powers does truth leave off and exaggeration begin? And how might you and I strengthen those traits and attitudes that engender joy rather than dejection? Before considering these questions (the next chapter's focus), let's pause to consider three popular techniques for reprogramming unhappy minds, starting with the silliest and working toward the more plausible.

Although exposés of silliness can make for laughs, I have two serious aims. The first is to caution people about following certain of today's money-grubbing pied pipers. Innocent naïveté makes us gullible to impressive nonsense. But then again, scoffing at all extraordinary claims can close us to important truths. So I aim second to show how, aided by scientific scrutiny, we can adopt a healthy skepticism, one that thinks critically yet acknowledges with Shakespeare's Hamlet: "There are more things in heaven and earth, Horatio, than are dreamt of in your philosophy." Healthy skepticism is open to new ideas without being gullible, discerning without being cynical.

Fire Walking

Consider, first, a hot idea: Transform your fears into faith, your concerns into confidence, by fire walking. The fire-walking phenomenon hit North America during the 1980s after being observed in the religious rites of certain Sri Lankan Hindus, Indian Buddhists, and Greek Christians. For $125 or so we can take a "mind over matter" class that supposedly enables us to alter our body. "Just holding the thought in your mind that you're not going to injure your feet alters the chemistry of your body."

The physical result of this mind power: walking on red-hot coals without pain or burn. The psychological result: a newfound capacity to conquer one's problems, fears, and limiting beliefs. "If I can do something that's supposed to be impossible," says the elated fire walker, "I can do almost anything. This proves our mental powers are far greater than we realize—powerful enough to control our body and to create a new reality. If just thinking of the hot coals as 'cool moss' can enable me to conquer fire, imagine what this mind power can do to my other fears." That's what fire-walk trainer and positive-thinking guru Tony Robbins would have you believe. He'd like to convince you that you have "unlimited power."*

Skeptical scientists have taken a cool look at fire walking. The secret, they report, doesn't lie in some mental power to alter the senses but in the poor heat conductivity of the wood coals. Think of a cake baking in a 375-degree oven. Touch the aluminum cake tin and it will burn you; touch the cake—like wood, a poor heat conductor—and

---

*Robbins's best seller, *Unlimited Power,* popularizes yet another New Age nostrum, "Neuro-Linguistic Programming" (NLP), which assumes that we can achieve success and happiness by ascertaining people's dominant ways of perceiving the world, by reading and mirroring their body language, and by believing that "we can do anything." As part of its review of new techniques for enhancing human performance, a National Academy of Sciences task force examined NLP and concluded that it makes no scientific sense and "there is little or no empirical evidence to date to support either NLP assumptions or NLP effectiveness."

you'll be okay. Of course, cakes and coals do conduct some heat, so don't stay in touch too long: With or without fire-walking training, he who hesitates is lost. Fortunately, it takes two seconds or less to quick-step across the hot embers. That puts each foot's two steps in contact with the coals for a fraction of a second. Wetting the feet on damp grass or in water before the fire walk provides further insulation (a phenomenon familiar to anyone who has used wet fingers to snuff a candle or test a hot iron). Confident of these facts, skeptical scientists have themselves performed the feat without any "mind over matter" training, and after one lecture at Cal Tech coaxed some seventy-five people into doing the same. To those who dispute this, you might say, "Okay, how about using your 'unlimited power' to walk across a metal sheet at the same temperature?" (Unless they want to spend time in their hospital burn unit, don't let them.)

Although fire walkers' newfound belief in their ability to command themselves to do anything rests on an illusion, it can still do some good. "Argue for your limitations, and sure enough they're yours," reminds Richard Bach. *Believe!* in your possibilities and maybe, just maybe, you'll achieve them. The famed placebo effect, referring to inert treatments that are effective thanks to the patient's faith in their power, fuels and helps fulfill many a hope. Folk healing remedies and medical practices that are now known to be powerless may actually produce cures. If you *believe* that bee pollen extract will energize your life, you may find yourself feeling more energetic. If you *believe* your demoralized life has been uplifted by some psychological snake oil, well, it probably has been. But the remedy you've bought may not be in the vial, or in your unburned feet. No, the new cure is the new hope that's in your head.

Astrology

One can say as much for astrology—the idea that the stars' and planets' alignment at the time of one's birth foretell one's future, providing clues for happy living. Astronomers scoff at the idea and can't imagine how it could work—certainly not by the effects of gravity (the gravitational effect of Mars was vastly less than that of the obstetrician who delivered you). Psychologists ask the practical question: Does astrology work? Specifically, (1) Are birth dates indeed correlated with character traits? (2) Given people's birth dates, can astrologers beat chance when asked to identify the individuals from short lineups of different personality descriptions? (3) Can people pick out their own horoscopes from a lineup of horoscopes? In research studies the consistent answers have been no, no, and no.

Why then do 58 percent of American teens (according to a 1988 Gallup survey) and tens of millions of adults take it seriously? Why did Nancy Reagan pay astrologer Joan Quigley a reported three thousand dollars per month for her guidance? For one thing, horoscopes seem to fit in an uncanny sort of way. People are struck time and again by how apt the day's comment feels. "You're nursing a grudge against someone; you really ought to let that go." "You worry about things more than you let on, even to your best friends." "Your day begins on a sluggish note. A conversation with a friend is a pick-me-up."

Well, yes. One of my favorite demonstrations is to take a string of such generally true statements drawn from horoscope books and offer them to my students as "personalized feedback" following a little personality test:

> You have a strong need for other people to like and admire you. You have a tendency to be critical of yourself. You pride yourself on being an independent thinker and do not accept other opinions without satisfactory proof. You have found it unwise to be too frank in revealing yourself to others. At times you are extraverted, affable, sociable; at other times you are introverted, wary, and reserved. Some of your aspirations tend to be pretty unrealistic.

Nearly all my students rate such stock assessments as "good" or "excellent"—a phenomenon called the "Barnum effect" in honor of P. T. Barnum's dictum "There's a sucker born every minute." Some students even express amazement at the astonishing insights gleaned by my remarkable (pseudo) test. "It's astonishing how well that test pegged me."

French psychologist Michel Gauguelin had fun with the Barnum effect. He placed an ad in a Paris newspaper offering a free personal horoscope. Ninety-four percent of those receiving the horoscope later praised the description as accurate. Actually, every single one had received the horoscope of Dr. Petiot, France's notorious mass murderer.

But again, if you're not using astrology to make serious decisions, and if you're not bamboozled into choosing a make-believe universe over the real cosmos, I suppose there can be a positive effect to having your newspaper columnist tell you (if you're Sagittarius), "The sweet tooth tempts you. Begin a program of diet and exercise." Or that you should "follow through on promises made to close ties" (Cancer). Never mind that what is said of Sagittarius today is repeated, in different words, for Cancer tomorrow. In either case, it's like the bite-sized platitudes of Chinese fortune cookies. Even if no more credible than the blarney of a carnival midway, it may still, like fire walking, work for those who believe it works—by helping people to approach the day with new confidence.

Subliminal Tapes

In 1956 a controversy erupted over a report (later admitted to be unsupported by research) that a theater had manipulated unwitting New Jersey audiences by flashing imperceptible messages: DRINK COCA-COLA and EAT POPCORN. More than three decades later, claims of such subliminal (literally, "below threshold") influence have returned. Mail-order catalogues, cable television ads, and prominent bookstore chains flood us with opportunities to reprogram our unconscious minds for success and happiness. A single 1989 issue of *Psychology Today* magazine carried five full-page ads for self-help tapes that embed "positive messages on your mind below the level of conscious awareness."

Subliminal tapes are said to harness keep reading this book mysterious powers. Underneath the soothing music or ocean waves that we hear are thousands of potent messages all being absorbed by our all-powerful and obedient subconscious. Store owners can inhibit shoplifting by burying "I am honest" messages in their Muzak. And you and I can have our lives transformed.

The technology assumes that "science has proven that most personal limitations are the fault of 'negative subconscious programming' and the influence it can exert over your conscious actions." Your unconscious mind, negatively programmed during childhood, won't listen to your conscious wishes. But "with subliminals you now have the access code." With "effortless ease"—you needn't pay attention—you can inject positive messages. For underachieving students: "I am a good student. I love learning." For procrastinators: "I set my priorities. I get things done ahead of time!" For the unhappy: "My outlook is bright and positive. I grow more happy and fulfilled with life."

The end result? "A truly new you—a you you'll like so very much more. You'll gain more happiness, more fulfillment, and a better life than ever before!" Careful, though. Don't inadvertently expose children to the popular weight-loss subliminals. They may become anorexic. And beware the "super sex" messages ("I love to touch and be touched") that may be buried beneath the easy listening music your date has slipped into the car stereo.

As the competition for subliminal quick-fix tapes has increased, so have the claims. One can buy subliminal tapes for bust enlargement, bowling score improvement, and the positive programming of unborn children (who, one surmises, not only can detect subliminal messages while submerged in the womb, but can comprehend subliminal English). For those desiring fast results, new technologies offer speeded-up messages—thirty thousand affirmations or more per hour—or, better yet, a subliminal instruction to accept each statement as if you'd heard it a hundred thousand times. "Once your subconscious accepts this statement to be true, it in fact becomes true." For optimum convenience there's even a new device that you can attach to your TV to inject subliminal affirmations beneath your favorite programs. love this book

Is there *anything* to these wild and sometimes wacky claims? Might positive subliminal messages help us, even a little? Let's start with a more elementary question: Can a stimulus too weak to notice affect us?

Under certain laboratory conditions, the answer is yes. In one experiment, University of Michigan students were repeatedly shown a series of geometric figures, each for less than 0.01 second—long enough to perceive only a flash of light. Later, the students reported liking the presented figures more than figures that had not been flashed, even though they had no idea which were which. Moreover, "invisible" words (flashed too briefly to perceive) can prime a response to a question asked later. If you were to see the invisible word "bread" flashed so quickly that you could detect only the flash, you might then read a related word such as "butter" faster than unrelated words such as "bottle" or "bubble."

So, we *can* process information without being aware of it. A weak stimulus evidently triggers a weak response within us, a response that may be transmitted to our brain where it evokes a feeling or meaning, though not conscious awareness. It's true: What the conscious mind can't recognize, the heart knows. As Pascal said in his 1670 *Pensées,* "The heart has its reasons which reason does not know."

Subliminal sensation, then, is for real. But does this verify entrepreneurial claims of subliminal hidden *persuasion?* The near-consensus answer among research psychologists is no. These researchers' views parallel astronomers' views of astrology. "The astrologers are partly right," say the astronomers. "There *are* planets and stars. But astrology is all downhill after that." Likewise, psychologists say, yes, we do process information without awareness. But the idea of "reprogramming your unconscious mind" makes no sense.* The gulf between the laboratory experiments and the entrepreneurial claims is enormous. The experiments test our processing of *visual* stimuli, in situations where *concentration* is *focused, other influences are minimized,* the perceiver is *forced to guess or judge,* and the *behavioral effect is temporary and trivial.* Said simply, the laboratory effect is subtle and fleeting. The ads and catalogues would have us believe that such experiments "prove" that listening to subliminal *speech,* while *attending to other tasks,* can have *powerful, enduring* effects on *motivations* such as your desire to eat and on *emotions* such as your sense of well-being.

But let's forgive this gulf between laboratory research and entrepreneurial claims. Let's simply ask, do subliminal tapes work? Do they have compelling force? tell your friends about this book Consider a typical experiment:

---

*In every age, hucksters exploit legitimate scientific concepts. Open any popular science magazine and read the current gobbledygook ads for instruments that promise to "synchronize your brain-waves," "activate the 90 percent of your brain that you don't use," awaken your "right brain's intuitive powers," or harness "whole brain technology" to "supercharge your brain cells."

At the University of California at Santa Cruz, Anthony Pratkanis and Jay Eskenazai had eager volunteers listen daily for five weeks to commercial subliminal tapes designed to improve either self-esteem or memory. On half the tapes the researchers switched the labels. People given these tapes *thought* they were receiving affirmations of self-esteem, when, actually, they heard the memory enhancement tape. Or they got the memory tape but *thought* their self-esteem was being recharged.

Were the tapes effective? Scores on both self-esteem and memory tests, taken before and after the five weeks, revealed no effects. Zilch. Nevertheless, those who *thought* they had a memory tape *believed* their memories had improved. Same for those who thought they had a self-esteem tape. When Anthony Greenwald and Eric Spangenberg repeated the experiment at the University of Washington, the results were the same. Reading this research, one can hear echoes of the testimonies that adorn the mail-order catalogues: "I really know that your tapes were invaluable in reprogramming my dumb computer," wrote one thankful customer.

Our natural tendencies to try new remedies when we are in an emotional down can further distort a testimony. When our emotions rebound to normal we attribute the rebound to something we have done. If, three days into a cold we start taking vitamin C tablets and find our cold symptoms lessening, the pills may seem more potent than they are. If, after doing exceptionally poorly on the first exam, we listen to a "peak learning" subliminal tape and find our next exam score improved, we may be deceived into crediting the tape. Whether any vaunted remedy is effective or not, we may depend on its having enthusiastic users.

Shortly after news of the supposed EAT POPCORN effect swept North America, the Canadian Broadcast Corporation used a popular Sunday night TV show to flash a subliminal message 352 times. Asked to guess the message, none of the almost five hundred letter writers did so. Nearly half did report being strangely hungry or thirsty during the show. But as in the memory/self-esteem experiments this was merely an effect of expectations. The actual message was TELEPHONE NOW. The effect of these 352 subliminals on Canadian telephone usage? Again, zilch.

An enterprising researcher, Philip Merikle of the University of Waterloo, bought subliminal audiotapes from four major distributors and examined their contents. If there were actual subliminal messages on the tapes they were subliminal to a spectographic analysis—which revealed no acoustic signals corresponding to embedded speech patterns. The human ear and mind were no better. After hearing subliminal and placebo tapes, people couldn't (even by listening to their hearts) distinguish the one from the other. Clearly, said Merikle, these tapes did "not contain any embedded messages that could conceivably influence behavior."

Another research psychologist, Timothy Moore at York University, carefully reviewed the accumulated evidence before testifying at the trial of the heavy metal band Judas Priest, which was sued for allegedly embedding a subliminal message causing two troubled young men to shoot themselves. (Not proven, ruled the judge.) Moore's own verdict: There is no plausible theory that would lead us to expect that subliminal tapes would work, no evidence that they do work as claimed, and, now, direct evidence that they don't work.

The tapes are nothing less than a health fraud, say consumer protection advocates Merikle and Moore.* The evidence is so consistent that Merikle casts aside the scientist's customary hedging: "There's unanimous opinion (among academics who have studied subliminal tapes) that these things are a complete sham." what a great book Thanks to the placebo effect, they may, like the snake oil of yesteryear, leave people feeling better or more confident, believing that something has been done for them. But if used as a substitute for taking steps that will make a more genuine and lasting difference in one's life—one's study habits, one's time management, one's approach to relationships—subliminal tapes may actually do harm.

As with other shortcuts to happiness, the current fascination with subliminal tapes will likely subside, only to be replaced by a new panacea—the psychological equivalent of fad diets.† As these come

---

*If subliminal tapes are not fraud, they do meet several of the Federal Trade Commission's criteria for quackery: promises of a quick and painless cure; testimonials as proof that the product works; a single product offered for a wide variety of ailments; and a scientific "breakthrough" that has been overlooked by the medical or scientific community.

†Losing weight is a big problem. Although most diets work in the short run, they do not reverse the biological forces (the starved fat cells, slowed metabolism, and such) that, in the long run,

along, notice the familiar pattern: We will once again read impressive testimonials to the speed, power, and ease of this new placebo,
all touted with scientific-sounding assertions. A few public-spirited
scientists will then pull themselves away from their work to ask
whether, apart from the power of belief, the new treatment has any
intrinsic effects. When their verdict is announced, the hucksters
will object: Orthodox science always resists new ideas. Besides, how can
you dispute all these folks whose own experience confirms its success?

Alas, the illusion eventually fades. Sometimes it's replaced by the
despair that so often follows false promises. One still-overweight, sixty-
six-year-old New Jersey woman reacted with self-blame to her failed
trial of a weight-loss subliminal: "I guess I had too much resistance to
give it a fair trial." (That's right, says the huckster: "Some people we
can help; others, despite our help, won't change.")

In the long run, the sages remind us, truth provides a more durable
foundation for comfort than do fragile illusions. Seek truth first and you
may eventually find comfort. Seek comfort at the expense of truth and
you may be a patsy for those who are all too willing to leave your wallet,
and your heart, empty. If you can read these messages they aren't subliminal. If you can't, they won't affect you.

Hypnosis

Unlike the mind cures offered in fire-walking seminars and by subliminal tape hucksters, the intriguing mental powers of hypnosis are the
focus of vigorous scientific debate. Imagine you are about to be hypnotized. The hypnotist invites you to sit back, fix your gaze on a spot high
on the wall, and relax. In a quiet, low voice the hypnotist suggests,
"Your eyes are growing tired. . . . Your eyelids are becoming heavy
. . . now heavier and heavier. . . . They are beginning to close. . . . You
are becoming more deeply relaxed. . . . Your breathing is now deep and
regular. . . . Your muscles are becoming more and more relaxed. Your
whole body is beginning to feel like lead."

typically pressure the body to restore lost weight. The end result: a slim chance of having anything
permanently thinned except one's wallet, and thus a never-ending market for new ways to fight
the battle of the bulge. In 1989, Americans spent another $33 billion on diets yet remained nearly
as overweight as ever.

After a few minutes of this hypnotic induction, your eyes are probably closed and you may undergo an apparently heightened suggestibility that enables a hypnotist to coax from you some weird behaviors, perceptions, and perhaps even memories. When the hypnotist suggests, "Your eyelids are shutting so tight that you cannot open them even if you try," your eyelids may seem beyond your control and may remain closed. Told to forget the number 6, you may be puzzled when you count eleven fingers on your hands. Invited to smell a sensuous perfume that is actually ammonia, you may linger delightedly over its pungent odor. Asked to describe a nonexistent picture the hypnotist claims to be holding, you may talk about it in detail. Told that you cannot see a certain object, such as a chair, you may indeed report that it is not there, although, curiously, you may manage to avoid the chair when walking around. And if instructed to forget all these happenings once you are out of the hypnotic state, you may later report a temporary memory loss rather like being unable to recall a familiar name. You are especially likely to demonstrate such hypnotic abilities if you are a fantasy-prone person—capable of becoming deeply absorbed in imaginary events suggested by a novel, a movie, or your own mind.

Many people associate hypnosis with show biz and quackery, an association still reflected in the Library of Congress's classification of hypnosis books with those on parapsychology (just after books on phrenology and just before books on ghosts and witchcraft). And, indeed, skeptical and believing researchers alike discount several popular misconceptions of supposed hypnotic powers.

What are the misconceptions? And what genuine mental powers does hypnosis reveal?

First, as University of Waterloo researcher Kenneth Bowers says, "Hypnosis is not a psychological truth serum." Because "hypnotically refreshed" memories so often combine fact with fiction—leading people to testify to events they may never have experienced—most state courts now ban testimony from witnesses whose memories have been contaminated by hypnosis.

Second, when people are "age regressed" and asked to relive childhood experiences, hypnotized people are *not* more genuinely childlike than unhypnotized people asked to feign childlike behavior. They act as people *believe* children would act, but typically miss the mark by outperforming real children of the specified age. And when hypnotized subjects are "regressed to past lives," the results are humorous. Nearly all report being their same race—unless the hypnotist suggests that different races are common. Most report being someone famous, rather than one of the countless peasants of yore, and many contradict one another by claiming to have been the same person, such as Joan of Arc, Henry VIII, or Napoleon. They also typically do not know things that any person of that historical time would have known. One subject who "regressed" to his "previous life" as a Japanese fighter pilot in 1940 could not name the emperor of Japan.

Third, hypnosis does not enable people to perform superhuman feats or force them to act against their will. Hypnotized people *can* make themselves into a human plank, their head and shoulders on one chair, their feet on another, while someone stands on them; but so can unhypnotized people. In one famous experiment, researchers Martin Orne and Frederick Evans demonstrated that hypnotized subjects *could* be induced to perform an apparently dangerous act. For example, they followed a request to dip a hand briefly in fuming acid and then throw the "acid" in a research assistant's face. When interviewed a day later, they exhibited no memory of their acts and emphatically denied they would follow orders to commit such actions.

Had hypnosis given the hypnotist a special power to control these people against their will? To find out, Orne and Evans unleashed that enemy of so many illusory beliefs—the control group: Orne asked some additional subjects to *pretend* they had been hypnotized. The laboratory experimenter, unaware that these control subjects had not been hypnotized, treated all subjects in the same manner. The result? All the *un*hypnotized subjects performed the same acts as the hypnotized ones. Similarly, most hypnotized subjects can be induced to cut up an American flag or deface a Bible, and a few will even cooperate in stealing an exam or selling illegal drugs. But people asked to simulate hypnosis are no less likely to perform the same acts.

Fourth, hypnosis does not block sensory input. Following a suggestion of deafness, hypnotized people will deny being able to hear their own voices, but will respond as do unhypnotized people when hearing their voice over a headset with a half-second delay: The delayed feedback disrupts their ability to speak fluently. If told they are color-blind, hypnotized people respond to color blindness tests differently than do people with actual color-deficient vision. Told to forget having heard certain words, deeply hypnotized subjects will deny any memory of them. Their behavior tells a different story, however, for the "forgotten" words influence their later thoughts and perceptions. In each case, what people *say* they experience doesn't jibe with their behavior when tested.

Misconceptions aside, hypnosis does have two therapeutic uses that reveal the mind's healing power. First, and most unquestionably, it helps relieve pain. When unhypnotized subjects put their arms in an ice bath, they feel intense pain within twenty-five seconds. When hypnotizable subjects do the same after being given suggestions to feel no pain, they indeed report feeling little pain. Even light hypnosis can reduce fear, and thus hypersensitivity to the pain of, say, dental treatment. And some 10 percent of us can become so deeply hypnotized that even surgery can be performed without anesthesia.

How can this be? One theory of hypnotic pain relief involves dissociation, a split between different levels of consciousness that allows some mental processes to occur simultaneously. Hypnosis, it suggests, dissociates the sensation of the pain stimulus (of which the subject is still aware) from the emotional suffering that defines our pain experience. The ice water therefore feels very cold, but not painful.

Another theory proposes that hypnotic pain relief is due to selective attention, as when an injured athlete, caught up in the heat of competition, feels little or no pain until the game ends. Support for this view comes from several studies showing that hypnosis relieves pain no better than relaxing and distracting people without hypnosis. With their attention distracted during hypnosis, for example, some women can experience childbirth with minimal pain; but so can some women without hypnosis, especially if given childbirth training. The Lamaze method of childbirth, for instance, uses several techniques in common with hypnosis—relaxation, controlled breathing, eye fixation, and suggestion. Women for whom the Lamaze method most effectively lessens pain tend also to have high hypnotic ability.

The second therapeutic use of hypnosis is in helping patients harness their own healing powers. Hypnosis offers no magic wand for happiness, nor does it help hypnotizable people more than unhypnotizable people in controlling nail biting, smoking, and other problems of self-control. Posthypnotic suggestions (suggestions to be carried out after the hypnosis session has ended) have, however, helped alleviate headaches, asthma, warts, and psychophysiological skin disorders. One woman who suffered open sores all over her body for more than twenty years was asked to imagine herself swimming in shimmering, sunlit liquids that would cleanse her skin and to experience her skin as smooth and unblemished. Within three months her sores had disappeared.

But is hypnosis the therapeutic agent? One way to find out is to ask whether hypnosis does a better job than other ways of encouraging people to relax and form positive images. For example, hypnosis speeds the disappearance of warts. But in controlled studies, so do the same positive suggestions given without hypnosis. The actual therapeutic value of hypnosis therefore remains in doubt.

Thus, the heightened suggestibility of the hypnotic state doesn't endow a person with special powers, block sensory input, or enable enduring joy, but for some reason it does help alleviate pain and psychosomatic ailments. That leaves a big issue: What is hypnosis? Is it a unique psychological state of consciousness? Under hypnosis does consciousness split into one part that responds to suggestion and another part—a "hidden observer"—that knows all (and that explains why hypnotized people given electric shock will report no pain yet perspire with pounding heart)? Or is hypnosis merely an extension of normal consciousness? Are "good hypnotic subjects" merely acting the role of hypnotic subject and getting caught up in it?

Or do both views offer a partial truth? After all, everyday thinking involves occasional splits in consciousness. Putting a child to bed, we might read *Good Night Moon* for the fourteenth time while mentally organizing a busy schedule for the next day. Under the influence of my dentist's nitrous oxide—a real gas—I hear her ask me to "open wide." As my conscious self contemplates her request, my mouth, much to my surprise, immediately obeys. "Turn toward me," she says. Again, as if controlled by some strange force, my head instantly complies. With practice, it is even possible to read and comprehend a short story while copying dictated words, much as you can doodle while listening to a lecture or much as a skilled pianist can converse while playing a familiar piece. Thus, when hypnotized subjects write answers to questions about one topic while talking or reading about a different topic, they display an accentuated form of normal cognitive dissociation.

Regardless, the phenomena of hypnosis, and of everyday life, confirm our mind's powers. First, we process vast amounts of information outside of conscious awareness. When we are sensing, learning, remembering, thinking, and responding, there is much more going on in our minds than we are aware.

Second, our beliefs and expectations matter. University of Connecticut psychologists Cynthia Wickless and Irving Kirsch showed this when they did clever stunts to convince even skeptical students that they were hypnotizable. After a standard hypnotic induction, the students were told they would see red, then see green, hear music, and so forth. After each suggestion, the experimenters surreptitiously projected appropriate stimuli—a very faint red or green light, or faint eerie music. Fooled by this weird experience of seeing and hearing what the hypnotist suggested, there were no doubters left. Thus, unlike those in control conditions not similarly persuaded, most of these believers scored as *highly* hypnotizable when later given hypnotic suggestions. Beliefs matter.

So, do our minds possess remarkable powers? Indeed, though not always in ways that we suspect. Positive, focused, believing attitudes make a difference.

What sorts of people characteristically have such attitudes? And how might you and I cultivate the traits and outlooks that make for joy? To these questions, we now turn.

6

The Traits of
Happy People

*Happiness and misery depend as much on
temperament as on fortune.*

LA ROCHEFOUCAULD, *MAXIMS*

Let's pretend: I want you to guess whether a particular person I have in mind feels happy and views life with deep satisfaction. To this point, we've seen that I *won't* give you any important clues by telling you whether the person is male or female; age fifteen, fifty, or seventy-five; black or white; living in a city or rural area; high-school- or college-educated. Even more surprisingly, I also give you no vital clue by telling you whether my person was questioned thirty years ago or today, whether the person three years ago won a state lottery or was paralyzed in an accident, whether the person lives on an estate and drives a new Mercedes or in an apartment and drives a 1972 Volkswagen.

So, what would clue you? One clue comes from psychological

research: The best predictor of behavior is past behavior in similar situations. The best predictor of grades is not aptitude scores, but past grades. The best predictor of job performance is not an interviewer's intuition, but past job performance. The best predictor of violent tendencies is not a prison psychologist's hunch, but past violence. Likewise, a good predictor of future well-being is past well-being. At the top of your wish list of clues should be knowing the person's happiness and life satisfaction at some earlier time.

Such is the conclusion of National Institute on Aging psychologist Paul Costa and his co-investigators after tracking the well-being of 5,000 adult Americans over ten years. "Well-being is strongly influenced by enduring characteristics of the individual," they reported. Regardless of someone's sex, race, or age, regardless of whether their marital status, job, or residence had changed, people with a happy disposition in 1973 were still happy in 1983.

In the 1920s, a team of University of California at Berkeley researchers studied a group of teenage boys and has followed their lives through more than a half century since. Although troubled adolescents often turned out far better than anyone might have guessed, the researchers also noted a stability to people's emotions. On the whole, cheerful teenagers became cheerful adults.

Consider the good news embedded in these findings: No unfortunate event voids our chance for future happiness. Given the right disposition, those of us treated poorly, suffering illness, laid off from work, or divorcing can still find renewed happiness. So, we wonder, what makes for a happy disposition? Who are these people who stay basically up despite life's downs? Why, for them, is the balance point between opposing emotions set at a more positive level than for others?

Are they, for example, more often children who grow up learning to live with and enjoy brothers and sisters, rather than children who grow up as "lonely and spoiled" only children? Partly because of this idea, a worldwide survey found the one-child family favored by only 3 percent of those in developing countries and by only 5 percent of those in developed countries (many fewer than the 10 percent or more of humans who grow up without siblings). But surveys of 2,500 adolescents in the Netherlands and of more than 9,000 adults throughout the United States refute this stereotype of the unhappy only child. Those with and without siblings are equally likely to say they find life exciting and that they are very happy.

Continuing our search for joyful people, does physical attractiveness matter? In societies that place a premium on handsome appearance, do good looks make for happiness? For those of us who believe that "beauty is only skin deep" and that "appearances can be deceiving," the results of hundreds of attractiveness studies can be unnerving. In experiments, good-looking people (or those believed from pictures to be so) are favored by dates, teachers, and potential employers. In everyday life, strikingly attractive people are more popular, hold more prestigious jobs, and have more income. "The final good and the supreme duty" of wise people may be, as the Roman statesman Cicero declared, "to resist appearance." If so, the truth is ugly: Pretty pleases.

Not surprisingly, then, attractive people, more than unattractive people, describe themselves as enjoying well-being. Consider the University of Michigan's life satisfaction scale (where 1 = "completely dissatisfied" and 7 = "completely satisfied"). Those in a national sample of 3,700 who struck interviewers as "homely" rated their life satisfaction at only 4.80, on average. (Rock star Janis Joplin, who died in misery of alcohol and heroin abuse, was once nominated for the University of Texas "Ugliest Man on Campus" award.) Those judged "strikingly handsome or beautiful" rated their life satisfaction at 6.38.

My hunch, though, is that because the interviewers judged their subjects' attractiveness at the *end* of the interview, their judgments were biased by their reactions to the person's happiness. Our judgments of attractiveness are influenced by our feelings about a person. In Rodgers and Hammerstein's musical, Prince Charming sings to Cinderella, "Do I love you because you are beautiful, or are you beautiful because I love you?" Chances are it's both. As we discover people's similarities to us, as we see them over and over and come to like them, we typically stop noticing their physical imperfections while we more and more appreciate their attractiveness. E.T. is as ugly as Darth Vader until you get to know him. As Shakespeare put it, "Love looks not with the eyes, but with the mind."

Given time, people may also become more accepting of their own appearances. The unattractive teenager is often miserable. "I always thought I was an ugly kid—you know—pimples, crooked teeth, frizzy hair, skinny, glasses, and the worst curse—flat-chested," bemoaned one young woman, Joan, "and I also remember feeling so depressed." But with maturity, such things may still matter but less so. Today, Joan can "look in the mirror and say, 'Yes, you are beautiful.' And I still have crooked teeth and glasses."

In a world where outer appearance matters, it helps to see oneself as attractive. What matters more, though, are four inner traits that predispose positive mental attitudes: self-esteem, sense of personal control, optimism, and extraversion. Dozens of investigations have linked each with psychological well-being.

Self-esteem:
Happy People Like Themselves

During the 1980s no topic in psychology was more researched than the self. By 1990, four thousand scholarly articles a year—more than triple the number of twenty years ago—were exploring the roots and fruits of one's sense of self. Many showed the dividends of high self-esteem, as exhibited in a willingness to agree with statements such as "I'm a lot of fun to be with" and "I have good ideas." People who agree with such statements are less vulnerable to ulcers and insomnia, less likely to abuse drugs, more independent of pressures to conform, and more persistent at difficult tasks. When the going gets tough, those with strong feelings of self-worth keep going.

Most striking, however, is the connection between *low* self-esteem and psychological disorders, especially depression. Vanderbilt University psychotherapy researcher Hans Strupp notes that "as soon as one listens to a patient's story, one encounters unhappiness, frustration, and despair which find expression in diverse forms of psychopathology including psychosomatic symptoms, neurotic symptoms, and maladaptive character styles. . . . Basic to all these difficulties are impairments in self-acceptance and self-esteem."

Listen to Norman, a Canadian college professor recalling his depression: "I [despaired] of ever being human again. I honestly felt subhuman, lower than the lowest vermin. Furthermore, I was self-deprecatory and could not understand why anyone would want to associate with me, let alone love me. . . . I was positive that I was a fraud and a phony and that I didn't deserve my Ph.D. I didn't deserve to have tenure; I didn't deserve to be a Full Professor. . . . I didn't deserve the research grants I had been awarded; I couldn't understand how I had written books and journal articles that I had and how they had been accepted for publication. I must have conned a lot of people."

Moreover, threaten people's self-esteem and beware their defensiveness. Put yourself in the shoes of the Arizona State University students who were walking alone across campus when a researcher approached them to participate in a five-minute survey. You agree, and take a brief "creativity test." After then receiving the deflating news that "you have scored relatively low," the researcher asks you some evaluative questions about either your school or its rival, the University of Arizona. Would your sense of failure affect your ratings? The researchers, Robert Cialdini and Kenneth Richardson, found that it did. Compared to those whose self-esteem was not threatened, those who'd just botched the test gave higher ratings to their own school and denigrated their rival.

Other researchers extend the phenomenon: One experiment gave subjects a humiliating experience—accidentally knocking over a stack of someone's ordered computer cards (which were rigged to spill when the subject pulled out a chair to sit down). With their self-esteem temporarily wounded, the English-speaking Canadian subjects responded to attitude questions with increased hostility toward French-speaking Canadians. In another, Dartmouth College men who were made to feel insecure judged others' work more harshly. At Northwestern University, members of lower-status sororities were found to be more disparaging of other sororities than were members of higher-status sororities. The moral: People who feel, or are made to feel, insecure or unworthy will often reestablish their self-worth by putting others down.

The flip side is a connection between *high* self-esteem and well-being. In the University of Michigan studies of well-being in America, the best predictor of general life satisfaction is not satisfaction with family life, friendships, or income, but satisfaction with self. It's true in other corners of the world as well: People who like and accept themselves feel good about life in general. "I really wouldn't want to be anyone else," said middle-aged Dora. "I'm not perfect. But, like the song says, 'I Wanna Be Me!' and I look forward to each new day."

This finding will come as no surprise to anyone attuned to the pop psychology of our age. Self-help books by the dozens exhort us to respect ourselves, to dwell on our good points, to be positive about ourselves: Cut the self-pity. Stop the negative talk. To discover love, first love yourself.

We've heard the message: In a 1989 Gallup poll, 85 percent of Americans rated "having a good self-image or self-respect" as *very* important; 0 percent rated it unimportant. Although this credo of humanistic psychology is more easily said than done, there is wisdom here.

Another finding will, however, surprise those who presume, with the late psychologist Carl Rogers, that most people "despise themselves, regard themselves as worthless and unlovable." Many popularizers of humanistic psychology concur. "All of us have inferiority complexes," contends Father John Powell. "Those who seem not to have such a complex are only pretending." Mark Twain had the idea: "No man, deep down in the privacy of his heart, has any considerable respect for himself." As Groucho Marx quipped, "I'd never join any club that would accept a person like me."

Actually, most of us have a good reputation with ourselves. In studies of self-esteem, even low-scoring people respond in the mid-range of possible scores. (A "low" self-esteem person responds to statements such as "I have good ideas" with a qualifying adjective such as "somewhat" or "sometimes.") Moreover, one of social psychology's most provocative yet firmly established conclusions concerns the potency of "self-serving bias." Consider:

- In experiments, people accept more responsibility for good deeds than for bad, and for successes than for failures. Athletes often privately credit their victories to their own prowess, their losses to bad breaks, lousy officiating, or the other team's exceptional performance. After receiving poor exam grades, students in a half dozen studies criticized the exam *if* led to believe they had done poorly. On insurance forms, drivers have explained accidents in such words as: "An invisible car came out of nowhere, struck my car, and vanished." "As I reached an intersection, a hedge sprang up, obscuring my vision, and I did not see the other car." "A pedestrian hit me and went under my car." The question "What have I done to deserve this?" is one we ask of our troubles, not our successes—those we assume we deserve.

- On nearly any subjective and socially desirable dimension, most people see themselves as better than average. In national surveys, most business executives say they are more ethical than their average counterparts. In several studies, 90 percent of business managers and over 90 percent of college professors rated their performance as superior to their average peers. In Australia, 86 percent of people rate their job performance as above average, 1 percent as below average. And in America, most high school seniors rate themselves in the top 10 percent of their age-mates in their "ability to get along with others." Although the phenomenon is less striking in Asia, self-serving biases have been observed worldwide: with Dutch, Australian, and Chinese students; Japanese drivers; Indian Hindus; and French people of all ages. The world, it seems, is Garrison Keillor's Lake Wobegon writ large—a place where "all the women are strong, all the men are good-looking, and all the children are above average."

Self-serving bias flies in the face of today's pop psychology. But additional streams of evidence remove any doubts: We remember and justify our past actions in self-enhancing ways. We exhibit an inflated confidence in the accuracy of our beliefs and judgments. We overestimate how desirably *we* would act in situations where most people behave less than admirably. We are quicker to believe flattering descriptions of ourselves than unflattering ones, and we are impressed with psychological tests that flatter us. We shore up our self-image by overestimating the extent to which others support our opinions and share our foibles and by *under*estimating the commonness of our strengths. We exhibit group pride—a tendency to see our group (our school, our country, our race) as superior.

Moreover, pride does often go before a fall. Self-serving perceptions underlie conflicts ranging from the arms race to marital misery. Compared to happily married people, unhappy couples exhibit far greater self-serving bias by blaming the partner when problems arise. In one survey, divorcing people were ten times more likely to blame the spouse for the breakup than to blame themselves. The findings go on, but enough. I am tempted to paraphrase Elizabeth Barrett Browning: "How do I love me? Let me count the ways."

Many people object. They think of people who seem to despise themselves, who feel worthless and unlovable. If self-serving bias prevails, why are so many people self-disparaging?

Sometimes people's self–put-downs are subtly strategic: They elicit reassuring strokes. Usually, a remark such as "I wish I weren't so ugly" will at least elicit a "Come now. I know a couple of people who are uglier than you." Other times, self-disparaging comments, such as before a game or an exam, prepare for possible failure. The coach who extols the superior strength of the upcoming opponent makes a loss understandable, a victory noteworthy.

Even so, it's true: All of us some of the time, and some of us much of the time, *do* feel inferior—especially when comparing ourselves with those who are a step or two higher on the ladder of status, grades, looks, income, or agility. Looking at all the dates Angela has, or all the honors Ian gets, can make their average friends feel klutzy. The deeper and more frequently we have such feelings, the more unhappy, even depressed, we are. And, as we've seen, lowered self-esteem can lead to a vicious judgmentalism.

Therefore, for most of us, "positive illusions" protect against anxiety and depression and sustain physical and mental health. We function best with modest self-enhancing illusions. We are like the new Japanese and European magnetic levitation trains, says University of Washington psychologist Jonathan Brown: We function optimally when riding high, just off the rails—not so high that we gyrate and crash, yet not so in touch that we grind to a halt. Most people do have a reasonably high opinion of themselves, and that fact of life goes a long way toward explaining why most of us are, indeed, reasonably happy and satisfied with life.

This is especially so for those whose self-esteem is what psychologists Robert Raskin, Jill Novacek, and Robert Hogan call "healthy" rather than "defensive." Those whose self-esteem is defensive may hunger for approval and may consciously or unconsciously posture a self that fulfills their grandiose self-ideal. Defensive people maintain self-esteem by managing the impressions they create, and by denying threats and pain. A healthier self-esteem is positive yet realistic. Because it is based on the genuine achievement of realistic ideals, and on feeling accepted for what one is—tainted perhaps by the positive biases that pervade happy outlooks—healthy self-esteem provides a less fragile foundation for enduring joy.

Personal Control:
Happy People Believe They Choose Their Destinies

In *Don Juan in Hell,* George Bernard Shaw anticipated the conclusions of countless research studies: "Hell is to drift, heaven is to steer." Summarizing the University of Michigan's nationwide surveys, Angus Campbell commented that "having a strong sense of controlling one's life is a more dependable predictor of positive feelings of well-being than any of the objective conditions of life we have considered." And the 15 percent of the populace who feel in control of their lives *and* feel satisfied with themselves have "extraordinarily positive feelings of happiness." Among these people, three in five—double the national average—report being very happy.

Psychologists have two basic ways to study the effect of any personality trait. One: Correlate people's scores on a measure of that trait with their other feelings and behaviors. Consider your own sense of personal control. Would you agree more that "I don't have enough control over the direction my life is taking" or that "what happens to me is my own doing"? That "the world is run by a few powerful people" or that "the average person can influence government decisions"? Those whose responses to such statements reveal an "internal locus of control" typically achieve more in school, cope better with stress, and live more happily.

Two: Experiment—raise or lower people's sense of control and note the effects. When laboratory animals and oppressed humans experience repeated traumas over which they have no control, they feel helpless and depressed. Dogs that have been unable to escape shocks, like people who are depressed, suffer paralysis of the will, passive resignation, motionless apathy. In concentration camps, in prisons, even in factories, colleges, and well-meaning nursing homes, people who have little control experience lowered morale, more stress, and more health problems. James MacKay, an eighty-seven-year-old psychologist illustrates:

> I became a nonperson last summer. My wife had an arthritic knee which put her in a walker and I chose that moment to break my leg. We went to a nursing home. It was all nursing and no home. The doctor and the head nurse made all decisions; we were merely animate objects. Thank heavens it was only two weeks. . . . The top man of the nursing home was very well trained and very compassionate; I considered it the best home in town. But we were nonpersons from the time we entered until we left.

A similar loss of control can exacerbate the stress of poverty. The small effect of money on well-being comes less from enabling us to *have* what we want than to *do* what we want—to feel empowered, in control of our lives. Matthew Dumont, a community psychiatrist in Chelsea, which has Massachusetts' lowest-per-person income, reflects on the powerlessness of its distress-prone people:

> What is poverty? It soon became evident to me that what is pathogenic about it is not merely the lack of money. The amount of money, the buying power, commanded by a welfare recipient in Chelsea would have been like a king's ransom to any member of a thriving hunter-gatherer tribe in the Kalahari. Yet the life of the welfare recipient appears terribly impoverished in contrast to that of the tribe member. A closer observation of life in Chelsea resolves the paradox. Chelsea residents possess material things unknown to the hunter but, despite this [meager] purchasing power, they experience little control over the circumstances of their lives. The efforts of the Kalahari hunters, on the other hand,

had a direct effect on the shape of their lives and the possibilities of their existence.

Increasing people's control can noticeably improve their health and morale. One study by Yale psychologist Judith Rodin encouraged nursing home patients to exert more control—to make choices about their environment and to influence policy. As a result, 93 percent became more alert, active, and happy. Similar results have been observed after allowing prisoners to move chairs and control the room lights and TV, and after enabling workers to participate in decision making.

Although the behavioral sciences are sometimes accused of undermining traditional values, the verdict of these studies is reassuring: People thrive best under conditions of democracy and personal freedom. Small wonder that stable democracies have happier citizens (recall page 36) and that, while this book was being written, freedom-longing Eastern Europeans wrested control of their lives from their totalitarian governments. Shortly before the democratic revolution in East Germany, psychologists Gabriele Oettingen and Martin Seligman compared the telltale body language of working-class men in East and West Berlin bars. Compared to their counterparts on the other side of the Wall, the West Berliners much more often sat upright rather than slumped. They more often had upward- rather than downward-turned mouths. They more often smiled and laughed.

In a late 1990 survey, Galina Balatsky of Moscow State University and Ed Diener of the University of Illinois discovered that Russian university students express a similarly low level of satisfaction with life—noticeably lower than reported by students in other comparably poor countries (as assessed by GNP per person). The average life satisfaction score of the Russian students was midway between that of American students and prison inmates. In her 1991 application to study in my department, a Russian student concluded her statement by noting, "I am charmed by Americans' cheerful ways and broad smiles. I wish our people smiled too." To paraphrase Seneca, "Happy are those who choose their own business."

Shortly before Nelson Mandela's release from prison, I asked a black South African pastor if his year-long visit in my community had changed him. He replied that what surprised him, and changed his consciousness, was not the affluence but the sense of control over his own life. "Having grown up poor, believing that money would buy happiness, I'm no longer convinced. Here in America I've seen rich people who have money and all that it buys, but who are troubled and unhappy. I'm more impressed by your freedom. Here when I see police officers I don't have to worry what they might do to me. When I return to South Africa, I will remember what liberty feels like."

Happy, too, are those who gain the sense of control that comes with effective management of one's time. Unoccupied time, especially for out-of-work people who aren't able to plan and fill their time, is unsatisfying. Sleeping late, hanging out, watching TV, leave an empty feeling. For happy people, time "is filled and planned; they are punctual and efficient," says Oxford University psychologist Michael Argyle. "For unhappy people time is unfilled, open and uncommitted; they postpone things and are inefficient."

One way to manage time is to set big goals, then break them down into daily objectives. Before beginning work on a textbook, I lay out a week-by-week schedule. My goal is not to have the whole book done by such and such date; that's too remote to energize me day by day. Writing a six-hundred-page book seems formidable. But writing three manuscript pages a day is relatively easy. Repeat the process four hundred times and, presto! you have a twelve-hundred-page manuscript. It's really not so hard, nor is reaching many goals when attacked day by day. (Although we often overestimate how much we will accomplish in any given day, we generally *under*estimate how much we can accomplish in a year, given just a little progress every day.) Moreover, as each minideadline is met you get the delicious, confident feeling of *personal control.*

Optimism:
Happy People Are Hope-Filled

It is fitting that I write these words in my office in the Norman Vincent Peale and Ruth Stafford Peale Science Center at a college named Hope. Those who agree that "with enough faith, you can do almost anything" and that "when I undertake something new, I expect to succeed" may be a bit bubbleheaded. But, for seeing the glass of life as half full rather than half empty, they usually are happier. Ronald Inglehart believes that cultural differences in such attitudes explain the striking national differences in life satisfaction and happiness: Compared to people in happier countries, those in the not-so-happy countries exhibit a less trusting, more cynical attitude.

Recall, too, that optimists are healthier. Several studies reveal that a pessimistic style of explaining bad events—saying, "It's my fault, it's going to last, and it's going to undermine everything"—makes us more vulnerable to illness. Harvard graduates who were most pessimistic when interviewed in 1946 were least healthy when restudied in 1980. Virginia Tech students who reacted to bad events pessimistically suffered more colds, sore throats, and flu a year later. In general, optimistic people are less bothered by various illnesses and recover better from coronary bypass surgery and cancer. Blood tests provide a reason, by linking optimism with stronger immune defenses.

Optimists also enjoy greater success. Rather than see setbacks as signs of their incompetence, they view them as flukes or as suggesting a new approach. Psychologist Martin Seligman found that new Metropolitan Life Insurance representatives who put an optimistic spin on bad events sold more policies and were half as likely to quit during their first year. Seligman's finding came to life for him when Bob Dell, one of the optimistic recruits who began selling for Metropolitan after taking the optimism test, later dialed him up and sold him a policy. "If you think in negative terms you will get negative results. If you think in positive terms you will get positive results. That is the simple fact

. . . of an astonishing law of prosperity and success," offers Norman Vincent Peale in *The Power of Positive Thinking.* "The good news is . . . the bad news can be turned into good news . . . when you change your attitude!" counsels Robert Schuller in *The Be-Happy Attitudes.* Two millennia earlier, Virgil put the same law in the *Aeneid:* "They can because they think they can."

A wealth of new research by Seligman and others confirms Peale's, Schuller's, and Virgil's optimism about optimism. Theirs is a message worth hearing. A person who approaches life with an attitude that often says "Yes!" to people and possibilities lives with far more joy and venturesomeness than do habitual naysayers.

Yet, as Pascal taught, no single truth is ever sufficient. "There are trivial truths and great truths," declared the physicist Niels Bohr. "The opposite of a trivial truth is plainful false. The opposite of a great truth is also true." In affirming the great truth about optimism, let us also remember a complementary truth about the perils of unrealism.

When dreamers become bubbleheaded they remind us that every silver lining has a cloud. First, when things go badly for others, optimists may promote guilt or disdain with a New Age version of the old blame-the-victim idea: "Her cancer has recurred? Too bad—she must be a negative thinker." Dying can thus become "the ultimate failure."

Second, unrealistic optimists may fail to take sensible precautions. In Chapter 1, I noted that the Pollyannaish optimism that leads so many people to see themselves as nearly invulnerable to car accidents, divorce, cancer, AIDS, and college failure makes for a more venturesome, upbeat life—but often at the risk of failing to protect oneself.

Before long, most of America's senior college administrators will be disappointed. Because of a temporary decline in the eighteen- to twenty-two-year-old population, the U.S. Department of Education projects declining college enrollments up to 1995. But when surveyed by the American Council on Education in 1990, only 5 percent of administrators projected declining enrollment during the next five years on *their* campus; 83 percent foresaw *increasing* enrollment. This clash between reality and hope neatly illustrates the dilemma of illusory optimism. Despite a declining market, some colleges will increase their enrollments, and these will likely be blessed with optimistic, "can-do" administrators. But if the general illusory optimism precludes contingency planning, many other colleges may face severe financial stress.

And consider the shame and dejection that accompanies shattered expectations. If you believe the inspirational messages of positive-thinking pep rallies—that "Believing is magic. You can always better your best"—then whose fault is it if your sales, salary, and status don't march upward from highs to higher highs? What do we conclude when our marriages turn out to be less than we romanticized, when our children struggle, when we are less successful in our vocations than we dreamed? For shame. We have only ourselves to blame: If only we had dreamed bigger, tried harder, been more disciplined, less stupid. When the dream collapses, the biggest dreamers fall the hardest. Limitless optimism breeds endless frustrations. "Blessed is he who expects nothing, for he shall never be disappointed," counseled the poet Alexander Pope in a 1727 letter.

The recipe for well-being, then, requires neither positive nor negative thinking alone, but a mix of *ample optimism* to provide hope, a *dash of pessimism* to prevent complacency, and enough *realism* to discriminate those things we can control from those we cannot. It was for such wisdom that the theologian Reinhold Niebuhr offered his "Serenity Prayer": "O God, give us grace to accept with serenity the things that cannot be changed, courage to change the things which should be changed, and the wisdom to distinguish the one from the other."

Extraversion:
Happy People Are Outgoing

Happy people enjoy high self-esteem, a sense of personal control, an optimistic disposition—and outgoing personalities. If "happy people are outgoing" sounds obvious, remember that's how most truths sound, once you know them. Likewise, told that optimism breeds cheer, you perhaps yawn. But the reverse also seems obvious. "Accustom yourself to the thought that the worst will befall you and that you will lose all you have," advised the French sage La Rochefoucauld. When things turn out better than expected, pessimists experience gladness; optimists more often live with disappointment—which would neatly explain the joy of pessimism, had things turned out that way.

Studies of the "I-knew-it-all-along phenomenon" reveal that, in hindsight, *most* findings seem like common sense, something you and I could have anticipated and explained. Told that people are attracted to others who are different from themselves, Joe Public responds, "You get paid for this? Of course people have different needs. That's why 'opposites attract'!" Told the truth—that studies show we are more attracted to those *similar* to ourselves, Judy Public reacts, "My grandmother could have told you 'birds of a feather flock together.' " (Does this hindsight bias itself seem obvious now that I've reported it?) Similarly, had it turned out that introverts are happiest, we could easily rationalize that, of course! they are less stressed, more serene, more at peace with and by themselves.

Except it didn't turn out that way. Rather, in study after study, extraverts—sociable, outgoing people—report greater happiness and satisfaction with life. Robert Emmons and Ed Diener have repeatedly observed an extraversion-happiness link in their studies of American university students, as have Michael Argyle and Luo Lu in their studies of British students and Bruce Headey and Alexander Wearing in their national surveys of Australians. Paul Costa and Robert McCrae report the same with older Americans, among whom the "extraverts . . . show the *joie de vivre* that make many older men and women an inspiration to the rest of us."

The explanation seems partly temperamental. "Extraverts are simply more cheerful and high-spirited," report McCrae and Costa. Self-assured people who walk into a room full of strangers and warmly introduce themselves may also be more accepting of themselves. Liking themselves, they are confident that others will like them too. And such attitudes tend to be self-fulfilling, leading extraverts to experience more positive events. When researchers Keith Magnus and Ed Diener studied University of Illinois students, and restudied them four years later as alumni, they found that life had treated extraverts more kindly. Compared to introverts, extraverts were more likely to have gotten married, found good jobs, made new, close friends, and so forth.

Obviously (and this *is* obvious), extraverted people are more in-

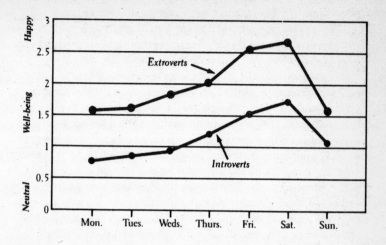

Extraversion and well-being. When Purdue University students completed daily mood ratings for Randy Larsen and Margaret Kasimatis, moods brightened with the coming of a weekend. But no matter what the day, extraverted students rated their day's experience as happier and more pleasant and joyfilled.

SOURCE: Randy J. Larsen and Margaret Kasimatis, "Individual Differences in Entrainment of Mood to the Weekly Calender." *Journal of Personality and Social Psychology* 58 (1990): 164–71.

volved with people. They have a larger circle of friends. They more often engage in rewarding social activities. They experience more affection. They enjoy greater social support. And social support, as we will see, is an important wellspring of well-being.

Acting Our Way into a New Way of Thinking

In our quest for answers to the happiness riddle—who is happy, and why?—previous chapters debunked some popular answers. Now we have begun to glimpse what happiness *is*. To begin with, happiness is having a positive self-esteem (which most of us do), feeling in control of our lives, and having optimistic, outgoing dispositions.

That's easily enough said, but can we strengthen such traits? If we wish we were happier, can we somehow become more positive, inner-directed, confident, and extraverted? How malleable are we?

To answer the latter question, some researchers study the personalities of genetically identical twins (reared separately or together); other researchers compare adopted children with their adoptive parents (who contribute their home environment) and their biological parents (who contribute their genes). These "behavior genetic" studies reveal heredity's influence on personality. Well-meaning advice to "be more outgoing" or to "have a more cheerful outlook" burden us with responsibility to *choose* our basic temperament. More than such advice givers realize, we bring our basic dispositions with us into the world.

And more and more studies show that our traits endure, especially after childhood. As noted earlier, developmental psychologists who have followed lives are sometimes surprised by how often troubled, unhappy children mature into competent, successful adults (parents of troubled teens take heart). Yet there is an underlying consistency to personality. Compared to mild-mannered nine-year-old boys, those with explosive temper tantrums have a doubled risk of divorce by age forty. A Swedish study revealed that trouble-prone, hyperaggressive thirteen-year-olds often developed adult records of crime and alcohol abuse. After the end of the teen years, traits such as outgoingness, emotional stability, openness, agreeableness, and conscientiousness also persist. Seligman, for example, reports that optimism endures: "The women who, when they're seventeen years old and the boys don't go out with them, say, 'I'm unlovable,' will fifty years later, when their grandchildren don't visit, also say, 'I'm unlovable.' This tells you that what you're dealing with here is a fairly stable trait."

Remembering that great truths sometimes come as complementary opposites, we can acknowledge that genetic predispositions constrain us. So do invisible social forces. But it's also true that we have the power to affect our own destinies for we are the creators as well as the creatures of our social worlds. We may be products of our past, but we also are architects of our future. The genetic influence on traits such as extraversion isn't a rigid genetic determinism. Personality isn't programmed like eye color. The predispositions we bring with us into the world leave room for nurture's influence, and our own efforts as well. What we do today shapes our world and ourselves tomorrow.

If social psychologists have proven anything during the last thirty years they have proven that the actions we elect leave a residue inside us. Every time we act, we amplify the underlying idea or tendency. Most people presume the reverse: that our traits and attitudes affect our behavior. That is true (though less so than is commonly supposed). But it's also true that our traits and attitudes *follow* our behavior. We are as likely to *act ourselves into a new way of thinking* as to think ourselves into a new way of acting.

Many streams of evidence and experience converge on the attitudes-follow-behavior principle. For instance, immoral acts shape the self. Those induced to speak or write statements about which they have misgivings often come to accept their little lies. Saying becomes believing. And consider how those who hurt others come to disparage their victims. Most educated people are familiar with Stanley Milgram's famous obedience studies, in which adult Connecticut men were asked to test out a supposed new teaching method, using punishment for wrong answers. When ordered to do so, 65 percent of the men delivered what they believed were hurtful 450-volt electric shocks to a shrieking innocent victim. But why such obedience? Would you have done the same?

Before you say no, consider how the men's actions influenced their thinking. The men began not with a hurtful act but by signaling a wrong answer with a trivial fifteen volts—a barely perceptible tickle. The ensuing steps (thirty volts, forty-five volts, and so forth) were each trivial increments. By the time the supposed victim first groaned, the subject had already complied five times and begun to internalize reasons for doing so, often by thinking the victim stupid and stubborn. Actions and attitudes were feeding each other in an escalating spiral, leading ordinary people to become agents of evil.

So it happened during the early 1970s, as Greece's military junta trained young men to become torturers. Trainees selected for their obedient tendencies would first be assigned to guard prisoners, then to participate in arresting squads, then occasionally to hit prisoners, then to observe torture, and only then to practice it. As compliance bred acceptance, a decent person evolved into an agent of evil. Cruel acts bred cruel attitudes, enabling heightened cruelty.

Fortunately, the principle works the other way too: Moral acts also shape the self. Children who resist a temptation become more conscientious. Altruists come to like the ones they've helped. Desegregation has been followed (as social psychologists predicted would happen) by diminished prejudice. Jewish tradition has the idea: To deal with anger, it suggests, give a gift to the object of your rage.

There is a practical moral here for us all. Do we wish to change ourselves in some important way? perhaps to boost our self-esteem? to become more optimistic and socially assertive? Well, a potent strategy is to get up and start doing that very thing. Don't worry that you don't feel like it. Fake it. Pretend self-esteem. Feign optimism. Simulate outgoingness.

In experiments, people have been asked to write essays or present themselves to an interviewer in either self-enhancing or self-deprecating ways. Those who *act as if* they are exceptionally intelligent, caring, and sensitive people later express higher self-esteem when privately describing themselves to a different researcher. This saying-becomes-believing effect is harnessed by therapy techniques (such as behavior therapy, rational-emotive therapy, and cognitive therapy), each of which prods the clients into practicing more positive talk and behavior. And in experiments that temporarily manipulate mood, a common procedure, pioneered by Emmett Velten, is to ask people to ponder, or even read aloud, statements such as "If your attitude is good, then things are good, and my attitude is good" and "This is great—I really do feel good—I *am* elated about things." (The procedure is reminiscent of Norman Vincent Peale's "spirit-lifter" thought per day, such as "a merry heart doeth good like a medicine." Each of these he urged people to read and repeat, "savoring its meaning and feeling it drive deep within your nature.")

Yes, telling people to act or talk positively sounds like telling people to be phony. But as usually happens when we step into some new role—perhaps our first days "playing" the role of parent, salesperson, or teacher—an amazing thing happens: The phoniness gradually subsides. We notice that our uncomfortable sense of being a parent or our pseudoprofessional job talk no longer feels forced. The new role—

the new behaviors and accompanying attitudes—have begun to fit as comfortably as our old jeans and T-shirt.

In his 1872 book, *The Expression of the Emotions in Man and Animals,* Charles Darwin proposed that we can even influence our emotions by our gestures and facial expressions. I was driving in my car one day when the song "Put on a Happy Face" came on the radio. "How phony," I groaned inwardly. But I tested Darwin's hypothesis, as you can: Fake a big grin. Now scowl. Can you feel the difference?

The participants in dozens of experiments could. When Clark University psychologist James Laird subtly induced students to make a frowning expression—by asking them to "contract these muscles," "pull your brows together," and the like—while he attached electrodes to their faces, the students reported feeling a little angry. Compared with these frowners, those induced to smile felt happier and found cartoons more humorous. Smile on the outside and you feel better on the inside. Scowl and the whole world seems to scowl back.

Among couples passionately in love, eye gazing (as we will see in Chapter 9) is typically prolonged and mutual. Would intimate eye gazes stir similar feelings between strangers? To find out, Joan Kellerman, James Lewis, and James Laird asked unacquainted male-female pairs to gaze intently for two minutes either at each other's hands or in each other's eyes. When afterward they separated, the eye gazers reported a greater tingle of attraction and affection toward each other. Act as if you like someone and soon you may.

Even holding a pen with your teeth (which activates one of the smiling muscles) makes cartoons seem funnier. But the effect works even better with a hearty smile, one made not just with the mouth but with raised cheeks as well. Or try walking around taking long strides, with your arms swinging and your eyes looking straight ahead. Like the Skidmore College students tested by Sara Snodgrass, do you feel happier than when walking with short, shuffling steps, eyes downcast? The moral: *Going through the motions can trigger the emotions.*

Surely you've noticed. You're in a testy mood. But when the phone rings, you feign cheer while talking to your friend. Strangely, after hanging up, you no longer feel so grumpy. Such is the value of social occasions—calls, visits, dinners out: They impel us to behave as if we were happy, which in fact helps free us from our unhappiness.

It all happens so naturally. Observing others' faces, postures, and voices, we unconsciously mimic their moment-to-moment reactions. We synchronize our movements, postures, and tones of voice with theirs. Doing so helps us tune in to what they're feeling. It also makes for "emotional contagion," which helps explain why it usually is fun to be around happy people and depressing to be around depressed people.

Granted, we can't expect ourselves to become more upbeat and socially confident overnight. But rather than limply resign ourselves to our current traits and emotions, we *can* stretch ourselves, step-by-step. Rather than waiting until we feel like making those sales calls, reaching out to that person, or writing that paper, we can begin. If we are too anxious, modest, or indifferent, we can pretend. We can "Just Do It"—dial the phone, speak to that person, pick up the pen—trusting that before long pretense will diminish as our actions ignite a spark inside. "If we wish to conquer undesirable emotional tendencies in ourselves," counseled William James, "we must assiduously, and in the first instance cold-bloodedly, go through the *outward* motions of those contrary dispositions we prefer to cultivate."

7

"Flow" in Work and Play

It is neither wealth nor splendor, but tranquility and occupation, which give happiness.

THOMAS JEFFERSON, LETTER TO MRS. A. S. MARKS

In the creation story, Eve and Adam, having succumbed to temptation, are banished from their utopian garden and sentenced to labor: "In toil you shall eat . . . In the sweat of your face you shall eat bread." Work is drudgery, travail, the daily grind. It is clenched jaws, ulcers, and accidents. Boredom, humiliation, and alienation. Insecurity, struggle, and weariness. At the end of a day, workers unwind at the local bar. At the end of a week, they sigh TGIF and plunge into their weekend escape.

Yet, as Studs Terkel has written, work is also a search "for daily meaning as well as daily bread, for recognition as well as cash, for astonishment rather than torpor; in short, for a sort of life rather than a Monday through Friday sort of dying." Through our work we define ourselves, even leave a legacy that adds meaning to our living.

Yes, work is both a bane and a blessing—but it's more a blessing. Or so it seems to those without work. People in almost every industrialized nation surveyed report markedly lower well-being if unemployed. Idleness may sound like bliss. Oh, to be able to escape the rat race and spend time sunbathing on a Caribbean beach, or curled up on the couch watching TV, or just vegetating. But as we'll see, when we get leisure time, many of us don't know what to do with it. After a time, inactivity becomes a curse as the empty hours tick slowly away.

A twenty-nine-year-old happily married father of two illustrates this. A year ago when business slowed, he was laid off as a packer in

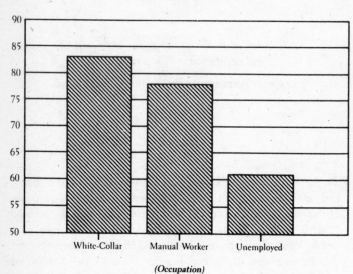

Percent "Satisfied with Life"

The curse of unemployment. To want work, but be denied it, is to be at risk for unhappiness.

Source: Data from 169,776 people in sixteen nations reported by Ronald Inglehart, *Culture Shift in Advanced Industrial Society* (Princeton: Princeton University Press, 1990).

a publishing company. Since then he has been receiving unemployment insurance and looking, and longing, for work: "I never much liked the job when I had it because there wasn't much to it except putting stuff in boxes and packing them up. But the people were nice and it was okay being there. Now I wish I had that job or anything. . . . All I do all day is hang around. I stay home and the wife goes crazy; or I sit around with some other people on the block and there isn't anything to do. When I had the job I felt like I was somebody—not much, but something. Now it's all a waste of time."

It's better to have work than be idle, but it's especially better to do work that satisfies. The turn-of-the-century Russian writer Maxsim Gorky anticipated the findings of many studies: "When work is a pleasure, life is a joy! When work is a duty, life is slavery." *Work* satisfaction impacts *life* satisfaction. (This is especially so for single people, who experience fewer of the stresses and satisfactions of marriage and family life.)

University of Southern California psychologist Rena Repetti noted the effect of our work environment on our mental health when she studied the employees of thirty-seven bank branches. She found the more congenial and supportive the work group, the happier and less anxious the employees. For married couples the satisfactions and stresses of work spill over into life at home. "When I've had a really satisfying day at work I come home disposed to like and enjoy my family—and thus to end the day feeling blessed," reflected one man. Moreover, the social skills people learn in teamwork jobs can enhance family life. "From my job I've learned how to relate more effectively with my husband," said an assembly team member. "It has really helped! After all, your family is a kind of team."

What Makes for Satisfying Work?

So, for most people work provides more blessing than bane. But *why* is work so important for well-being? And what makes work not drudgery but rewarding?

One unemployed young woman offers a clue. She doesn't need

money. However, challenging work "would enable me to have a greater sense of personal worth, independence, and freedom." For her, for most of us, work adds to our *personal identity*. When I am asked who I am or what I do, my work ("I am a Hope College professor") ranks near the top of my list of answers. My work helps define me.

Through our work we also identify with a *community*. My sense of community is rooted in the network of supportive friends who surround me on our department team, in the institution whose goals we embrace, and in the profession we call our own. This sense of pride and belonging in my group helps me construct a social identity.

Work can add *purpose* to our living. A vocation can be a calling to contribute something worthwhile, to leave a little legacy. "No task, rightly done, is truly private," said Woodrow Wilson. "It is part of the world's work." My own vocation—my purpose—is to advance truth and understanding through oral and written teaching. Others find meaning in designing or constructing products, in growing or distributing food, or in helping those in need of a service. Studs Terkel describes "the Chicago piano tuner, who seeks and finds the sound that delights; the bookbinder, who saves a piece of history; the Brooklyn fireman, who saves a piece of life. . . . There is a common attribute here: a meaning to their work well over and beyond the reward of the paycheck." Happiness is loving what you do, and knowing it matters.

Consider: If you suddenly inherited a large fortune, would you continue working? Three in four people answer yes. And nearly everyone answers yes if they experience work's nonmaterial rewards—a sense of identity, community, and purpose. Asked if they would choose the same work, given a chance to start over, four in five people who find these rewards in their professions again answer yes. With few such rewards, many more answer no.

Job-satisfaction studies reveal that the most satisfied workers often have higher-status positions within a field. Higher-status jobs also provide more of that important happiness factor: the sense of *personal control*. Study after study finds that when workers have more control—when they can help define their own goals and hours and when they participate in decision making—their job satisfaction rises. Participative teamwork also heightens a communal "we-feeling." A bakery director explains: "We try to have a compromise between doing things efficiently and doing things in a human way. Our bread has to taste the same way every day, but you don't have to be machines. On a good day it's beautiful to be here. We have a good time and work hard and we're laughing."

Anyone living here in Holland, Michigan, is familiar with the much-studied Herman Miller, Inc., America's second largest manufacturer of office furniture and one of its ten most-admired companies (in *Fortune*'s 1989 survey of 8,000 executives). Herman Miller organizes its 5,500 workers into small teams. Long before most Americans knew about the Japanese-corporation-as-family model, Herman Miller employees were participating in decisions about their work, sharing in the company's profits, and becoming company stockholders after a year of service. Instead of a human resources director, the company has a "vice president for people," whose concerns include nurturing employee morale, fostering employee suggestions, and facilitating communications. Underlying this participative approach to management is a corporate philosophy that workers are happier and more productive when they are respected, cared about, and involved. "Words such as 'love,' 'warmth,' and 'personal chemistry' are certainly pertinent," says its board chair, Max DePree. To judge from informal comments heard over the back fence and about town, Herman Miller's participative management makes for a work force with higher-than-average morale.

For employers generally, high-level employee morale is good business. Compared to depressed employees, those with higher well-being have lower medical costs, higher work efficiency, and less absenteeism. Thus, just as investing in prenatal care and preventive well-baby care can reduce net medical costs, so can investing in employee well-being help the bottom line. You could wish you put your money in Herman Miller stock when it went public in 1970. By 1991, every dollar invested then had multiplied twenty-five times.

Flow: When Challenges Match Skills

Work is, however, often unsatisfying, for two reasons. We can be overwhelmed: When challenges exceed our available time and skills, we feel anxious, stressed. Or we can be underwhelmed: When challenges don't engage our time and skills, we feel bored. Between anxiety and boredom lies a middle ground where challenges engage and match our skills. In this zone we enter an optimal state that University of Chicago psychologist Mihaly Csikszentmihalyi (pronounced chick-SENT-me-hi) terms "flow."

To be in flow is to be unself-consciously absorbed. Think of a situation where you get so caught up in an activity that your mind doesn't wander, that you become oblivious to your surroundings, and time flies. Csikszentmihalyi formulated the flow concept after studying artists who would spend hour after hour painting or sculpting with enormous concentration. Immersed in a project, they worked as if nothing else mattered, and then promptly forgot about it once they finished. The artists seemed driven less by the external rewards of doing

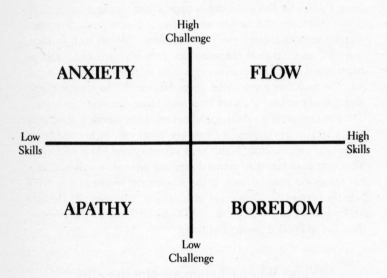

The flow model. When challenges engage our skills, we often become so absorbed in the flow of an activity that we lose consciousness of self and time. Source: Adapted from Mihaly Csikszentmihalyi and Isabella Selega Csikszentmihalyi, *Optimal Experience: Psychological Studies of Flow in Consciousness* (New York: Cambridge University Press, 1988), p. 261.

art—money, praise, promotion—than by the intrinsic rewards of creating the work.

Madeleine L'Engle likens the artist's concentration to a small child at play: "In real play, which is real concentration, the child is not only outside time, he is outside *himself*. He has thrown himself completely into whatever it is that he is doing. A child playing a game, building a sand castle, painting a picture, is completely *in* what he is doing. His *self*-consciousness is gone; his consciousness is wholly focused outside himself." I know the feeling from my noontime pickup basketball games. When well-matched with players of equal ability, I lose my awareness of time; I become caught up in the flow of the game.

Later observations of dancers, chess players, surgeons, writers, parents, mountain climbers, Australian sailors, elderly Koreans, Alpine farmers, and Japanese, Italian, and American teenagers converge on an overriding principle: It's exhilarating to flow with an activity that fully engages our skills. Flow experiences boost our sense of self-esteem, competence, and well-being. When people are beeped at random intervals and asked to report what they are doing and how much they are enjoying themselves, those who are vegetating usually report little sense of flow and little satisfaction. People report more positive feelings when interrupted while doing something active, something that engages their skills, be it work, play, or just driving a car.

Studies confirm that a key ingredient of satisfying work is whether or not it's challenging. The most satisfied workers find their skills tested, their work varied, their tasks significant. One proud stonemason explained that "anything you like to do isn't tiresome. It's hard work; stone is heavy. At the same time, you get interested in what you're doing and you usually fight the clock the other way. You're not lookin' for quittin'." Creative people, said psychologist Abraham Maslow, are "all there, totally immersed, fascinated and absorbed in the present, in the current situation, in the here-now, with the matter-in-hand."

But many workers do not feel challenged. Karl Marx faulted industrial capitalism for its dehumanization of labor: "Constant labor of one uniform kind destroys the intensity and flow of a man's animal spirits." When, unlike the stonemason, workers don't identify with the products of their labors, they feel alienated and work becomes drudgery. "For most Americans," said Charles Reich, "work is mindless, exhausting, boring, servile and hateful, something to be endured while 'life' is confined to 'time-off.' " When beeped during work hours, the average worker 25 percent of the time isn't even working, but is instead day-dreaming, gossiping, or doing personal business.

Most workers express more satisfaction with their work than supposed by Marx or Reich. But Marx did recognize the importance of self-expression through meaningful work. As people accumulate a history of productivity in high-challenge, high-skill situations they develop positive self-esteem—much more so, reports Csikszentmihalyi, than do those who spend most of their time in apathy, boredom, or anxiety. Compared to their inactive peers who spend twenty-five hours a week or more just "hanging out," active teenagers feel better about themselves and are more cheerful and satisfied with life.

To experience flow we need to find challenge and meaning in our work, and to seek experiences that fully engage our talents. Flow comes when we structure work in ways that summon self-forgetful involvement. It's not an easy assignment, and it takes both individual and managerial effort to accomplish.

Among the most remarkable people I have known was industrialist John Donnelly, whose company, The Donnelly Corporation, now manufactures most mirrors found in U.S.-made cars. Shortly before his death at age seventy-four, John remarked, "What will I have achieved in life if all I have done is to make car mirrors—there has to be more to it than that." A devout Catholic, Donnelly would readily have prayed the Labor Day collect in the Episcopal *Book of Common Prayer*: "So guide us in the work we do, that we may do it not for the self alone, but for the common good." Part of John Donnelly's effort to do good, beyond making safety-enhancing car mirrors, was to create meaningful, involving work experiences. To involve his employees with a sense of entrepreneurial teamwork, Donnelly organized them into self-managed work groups. When times are good, as they generally have been, employees share in the profits; when times are bad, top executives take pay cuts. In this company the parking lot has no executive parking places. After seeing the aging Donnelly slip on the parking lot ice one day, his employees plotted a gift: a sign near his office designating John Donnelly's parking place. Though grateful, he promptly removed the sign and hung it in his office. For Donnelly, an idea about the self-esteem and involvement of every employee was more important than a parking place, or another million car mirrors.

Like John, each of us who influences others' work conditions needs to seek ways to transform mind-numbing tasks into meaningful work experiences. For those of us who don't have that kind of control, there are other ways to help people feel the value of what they do. After reading about bread lines and empty store shelves in Eastern Europe and the Soviet Union, an exuberant friend of mine was overwhelmed by what he normally took for granted—the abundance of foodstuffs in his neighborhood supermarket. So he went up to a delivery person who was stocking the bread shelves and said, "I want you to know you're a very important person to me. You're meeting my basic needs. In fact, you're a very important person in our society." "Mister," replied the appreciative worker, "you just made my day."

In lesser ways, we can be alert for ways to affirm the work that others do. In most enterprises, every category of worker is essential. For their careers to thrive and the organization's mission to be achieved, everyone needs everyone else. Students who read my introductory psychology textbook are sometimes too impressed. They think that because I'm the author I must have written it the way they're reading it. It's true that I am responsible for all the words. But what they are reading actually evolved with the help of a dozen editors and more than two hundred consultant colleagues. The result is a better book than I alone could conceivably have written. Likewise, you would hardly recognize the book you are now reading from the sample chapters I first drafted in 1986, before receiving any editorial guidance. I enjoy satisfying (as well as challenging) relationships with my editors because we are keenly aware of our need and respect for each other, and we don't hesitate to let each other know that.

In addition to affirming the significance of one another's work, we can also challenge ourselves. Hardy people have a knack for transforming both potential threats and boring tasks into stimulating challenges. From his studies of those who frequently experience flow, Csikszentmihalyi identifies four ways by which we can turn adversity or boredom into enjoyment: *Set goals.* Resolve to become a decent tennis player or more effective at your job, then monitor your progress. *Immerse yourself in the activity.* As a teenager whose chore was to do the dinner dishes, I would imagine myself representing the United States in the finals of the Olympic Dishwasher Loading event (a test of who could cram in the most, and hand-wash the least). *Pay attention to what is happening.* Watching sports, some people enjoy keeping mental statistics on their favorite player. *Enjoy the immediate experience.* Waiting for a plane, savor the human dramas as a small child here excitedly awaits a parent's return, lovers there cherish their final moments with controlled but obvious passion. In such ways we can transform mindless tedium into mindful engagement.

We can also put more flow in our lives by living more intentionally—saying yes to the things that we do best and find most meaningful, and no to time-wasting demands. We can be ever conscious that time—that life, lived in time—is a resource that we can spend only once. We can risk ourselves striving to find work that we enjoy, work that feels like play. My sons have the right idea. One, a creative person who enjoys the outdoors, has undertaken a career in video photography and production. The other, a computer geek who began taking college computer courses as a thirteen-year-old, is, among other things, preparing for a possible career in computer science—"where other people buy your toys for you." For great achievers, including Mozart (600 compositions) and Thomas Edison (1,093 patents), work blends into hobby. Some jobs will always have the sole purpose of earning money—work that no one would do without pay. But how blessed are those who can say, to borrow words from C. S. Lewis, "I am doing work which is worth doing. It would still be worth doing if nobody paid for it. But as I have no private means, and need to be fed and housed and clothed, I must be paid while I do it."

Finally, we can reassess our use of leisure time. After beeping people on thousands of occasions to report on their activity and feelings, Csikszentmihalyi was struck by

the relative poverty of experience in free time, the emptiness of most leisure . . . We all want to have more free time: But when we get it we don't know what to do with it. Most dimensions of experience deteriorate: People report being more passive, irritable, sad, weak, and so forth. To fill the void in consciousness, people turn on the TV or find some other way of structuring experience vicariously. These passive leisure activities take the worst edge off the threat of chaos, but leave the individual feeling weak and enervated.

An example: Italian researchers Fausto Massimini and Massimo Carli report that when beeped to record their experience, 3 percent of those who are watching TV report experiencing flow, 39 percent report feeling apathetic. For those engaged in arts and hobbies the percentages flip-flop—47 percent report flow and 4 percent report apathy. In fact, the *less* expensive (and generally more involving) a leisure activity, the *happier* people are while doing it. Most people are happier gardening than power boating, talking to friends than watching TV.

Csikszentmihalyi also reports that people are unhappiest when they are alone and nothing needs doing:

> For people in our studies who live by themselves and do not attend church, Sunday mornings are the lowest part of the week, because with no demands on attention, they are unable to decide what to do. The rest of the week psychic energy is directed by external routines: work, shopping, favorite TV shows, and so on. But what is one to do Sunday morning after breakfast, after having browsed through the papers? For many, the lack of structure of those hours is devastating.

Why do most people in their hard-won free time sink into what Csikszentmihalyi calls "a state of apathy that brings no joy." Are we simply too exhausted to enjoy more active leisure? If so, why do so many people in more traditional societies (such as in Thai villages and Alpine farming communities) work dawn to dusk in the fields and then spend their free time weaving, carving, playing musical instruments, and engaging in other flowlike activities? The problem seems to be our culture's reliance on television and other forms of passive leisure and on our inability to structure our free time in ways that would enhance our well-being. Well-being resides not in mindless passivity but in mindful challenge.

So, off your duffs, couch potatoes. Pick up your camera. Tune up that instrument. Sharpen those woodworking tools. Get out those quilting needles. Inflate the family basketball. Pull down a good book.

Oil the fishing reel. It's time to head out to the garden store. To invite friends over for tea. To pull down the Scrabble game. To write a letter. To go for a drive. Rather than vegetating in self-focused idleness, lose yourself in the flow of active work and play. You may be surprised what happens. "In every part and corner of our life, to lose oneself is to be a gainer," noted Robert Louis Stevenson; "to forget oneself is to be happy."

Rest and REST

"To do great work," wrote the English novelist Samuel Butler, a person "must be very idle as well as very industrious." Happy people, too, live full, active, industrious lives, yet also reserve time for renewing solitude and rest.

I hesitate to sound like a parental voice from the past, but it's true: A good sleep predisposes a good mood. In experiments, subjects deprived of sleep often feel a general malaise, especially during their sleepiest times. Among the college students I have spent twenty-five years working with, few behaviors strike me as more irrational than self-destructive sleep patterns, with resulting fatigue, diminished alertness, and, not infrequently, failure and depression. At the beginning of a term, students don't intend to saddle themselves with four hours' sleep a night. But the first exam isn't for several weeks. The paper isn't due for a month. So what the heck. Each diversion—a video game here, a bull session there—seems harmless enough. Yet, gradually, without intending sleeplessness, fatigue, and failure, the student veers toward falling behind and suffering the results. And actually, all who need an alarm to terminate sleep and who feel fatigued during the day are hampering their quality of life. William Dement, director of Stanford's Sleep Disorders Center, laments that "the national sleep debt is larger and more important than the national monetary debt." An elementary ingredient of energized, successful, cheerful living is, therefore, to discipline oneself to sleep enough to awake refreshed and ready to get in the flow of an active life. In one recent study of Los Angeles County residents, those sleeping seven to eight hours a night were half as likely to be depressed as those sleeping less (or more).

For some, fatigue doesn't stem from staying up late, but from difficulties in falling or staying asleep. Too little sleep can be a symptom, as well as a cause, of depression. But we all experience sleeplessness at times. When we are stressed or anxious, alertness is natural and adaptive. As Woody Allen said in the movie *Love and Death*, "The lion and the lamb shall lie down together, but the lamb will not be very sleepy."

By middle age and after, awake times during the night become routine—certainly nothing worth losing sleep over or treating with sleeping medication or alcohol. (Sleep-inducing drugs suppress the dream-related stage of sleep. Moreover, they lose their potency with repeated use, and when discontinued, insomnia may worsen.) Those troubled by sleeplessness are better advised to relax and avoid rich foods before bedtime (milk and carbohydrates are preferable, because they aid in the manufacture of a brain chemical that facilitates sleep). Most important, avoid naps, and sleep on a regular schedule (rise at the same time even after a restless night). Like travelers suffering sleeplessness induced by jet lag, college students sometimes suffer Sunday night insomnia/Monday morning blues after shifting their bodies to later time zones on Friday and Saturday nights, and then trying to reverse the time change on Sunday nights. Many adults fall into a similar pattern, beginning their week with their body still in the naturally depressed nighttime state.

Experiments by University of British Columbia researcher Peter Suedfeld and his colleagues show that renewal comes not only from rest, but from REST—*R*estricted *E*nvironmental *S*timulation *T*herapy. Suedfeld knew from earlier studies of sensory restriction that being alone in a monotonous environment heightens a person's sensitivity to any sort of stimuli, whether external or internal. So he offered hundreds of people a chance to tune more deeply into themselves through a literal day of REST, during which they would do nothing but lie quietly on a comfortable bed in the isolation of a dark, soundproof room. Food, water, and a chemical toilet were available, and communication was possible over an intercom through which brief persuasive messages could be transmitted.

The day of REST has been notably successful in helping people who want to increase their self-control—to gain or lose weight, reduce alcohol intake, improve speech fluency, reduce hypertension, overcome irrational fears, boost self-confidence, or stop smoking. Participants report that the experience is a pleasant and stress-free way of reducing external stimulation. They can then hear still, small voices from within.

Suedfeld also illustrates the healing power of solitude through the lives of those who, by choice or necessity, have experienced aloneness. To be shipwrecked, placed in solitary confinement, or on a solitary voyage can be traumatic for those who feel threatened, helpless, or malnourished. Still, there can be a positive side to such experiences. Lone explorers and sailors often have a deep spiritual experience—a new relationship with God, a feeling of oneness with the ocean or the universe, a life-changing new insight into their personalities. In Japan, where the widely practiced "quiet therapies" combine solitude with Zen Buddhist practices, a depressed or anxious person may undertake a week of bed rest and meditation. In scores of cultures within Africa, Asia, Australia, and the Americas, a period of soul-searching solitude is part of growing up, at least for males. The boy entering manhood leaves his community and finds himself and his vision while wandering alone in the desert, mountains, forest, or prairie. One recent study of 361 graduates of the Australian Outward Bound program (a month-long outdoor program that includes a "Solo" experience) found that the experience produced enduring improvements in self-concept.

The experiences of great philosophers, scientists, artists, and religious visionaries confirm the creative power of solitude. Being freed from distractions may trigger vivid fantasies and deep insights. Jesus began his ministry after forty days alone, and thereafter lived a rhythm of engagement and retreat. Moses, Muhammad, Buddha, and countless other mystics, monks, hermits, and prophets have found inspiration in times of contemplative silence. Aborigines have gone on "walk-abouts," Native Americans on vision quests, spiritual seekers on retreats. The Christian discipline of a daily quiet time affirms the value of REST, not as an otherworldly end, but as a spiritual recharging for living actively. "It is in silence, and not in commotion, in solitude and not in crowds," believed the American mystic Thomas Merton, "that God best likes to reveal himself."

Small-scale experiences of solitude can be carved out of even the busiest of days. Cardiologist Herbert Benson advocates meditative re-laxation as an antidote to stress. To experience the "relaxation re-sponse," do the following, right now: Assume a comfortable position. Close your eyes. Breathe deeply. Relax your muscles from foot to face. Now, concentrate on a single word or phrase or repetitive prayer such as "Lord, have mercy." Other thoughts will intrude, but let them drift away and keep repeating this phrase for ten to twenty minutes. By setting aside a quiet time or two each day, many people enjoy a greater sense of tranquillity and inward stillness, along with lowered blood pressure and strengthened immune defenses. One astonishing recent study even found that daily meditation boosted longevity. An unlikely mix of researchers from Maharishi University and Harvard University assigned seventy-three residents of homes for the elderly either to no treatment or to daily meditation. After three years, one fourth of the nonmeditators had died, while all the meditators were still alive.

It's ironic. In a time when the hustle and bustle of working, shopping, and entertainment have become a seven-day-a-week affair, Euro-American cultures have turned away from the traditional day of rest at the very time that researchers are affirming the healing and renewing power of just such a day—one of REST. To experience well-being it's good to be both very active and also, for interludes, very idle. For everything there is a season: a time to be born, and a time to die; a time to do, and a time just to be (like the song says, do-be-do-be-doo). Wordsworth's words, from "The Prelude," are worth remem-bering:

When from our better selves we have too long
Been parted by the hurrying world, and droop,
Sick of its business, of its pleasures tired,
How gracious, how benign, is Solitude.

8

The Friendship Factor

Happiness seems made to be shared.

CORNEILLE, *NOTES PAR ROCHEFOUCAULD*

Linda and Emily had much in common. When they were inter-viewed for a study conducted by UCLA social psychologist Shelley Taylor, both Los Angeles women had married, raised three children, suffered comparable breast tumors, and recovered from surgery and six months of chemotherapy. But there was a difference. Linda, a widow in her early fifties, was living alone, her children scattered in Atlanta, Boston, and Europe. "She had become odd in ways that people some-times do when they are isolated," reported Taylor. "Having no one with whom to share her thoughts on a daily basis, she unloaded them somewhat inappropriately with strangers, including our interviewer."

Interviewing Emily was difficult in a different way. Phone calls interrupted. Her children, all of whom lived nearby, were in and out of the house, dropping things off with a quick kiss. Her husband called from his office for a brief chat. Two dogs roamed the house, greeting visitors enthusiastically. All in all, Emily "seemed a serene and contented person, basking in the warmth of her family."

Three years later the researchers tried to reinterview the women. Linda, they learned, had died two years before. Emily was still lovingly supported by her family and friends. And she was happier than ever.

Because no two cancers are identical, we can't be certain that different situations led to Linda and Emily's fates. But they do illustrate a conclusion drawn from several large studies: Social support—feeling liked, affirmed, and encouraged by intimate friends and family—promotes both health and happiness.

Close Relationships and Health

I'm sure we could easily imagine why close relationships might contribute to *illness*. Our relationships are fraught with stress. "Hell is others," wrote Jean-Paul Sartre. When Peter Warr and Roy Payne at the University of Sheffield asked a representative sample of British adults what, if anything, had emotionally strained them the day before, "family" was their most frequent answer. And stress, as we all by now know, aggravates health problems such as coronary heart disease, hypertension, and suppression of our disease-fighting immune system.

Still, on balance, close relationships contribute less to illness than to health and happiness. Asked what prompted yesterday's times of pleasure, the same British sample, by an even larger margin, again answered "family." It is my experience, and I suspect yours as well, that family relationships provide our greatest heartaches. But they also provide our greatest joys.

Moreover, six massive investigations, each interviewing thousands of people across several years, have all reached a common conclusion: Close relationships do indeed promote health. Compared to those with few social ties, those who have close relationships with friends, kin, or fellow members of close-knit religious or community organizations are less likely to die prematurely. And losing such ties heightens our risk of disease. A Finnish study of 96,000 widowed people found their risk of death doubled in the week following their partner's death. A National Academy of Sciences study reveals that recently widowed Americans, too, become more vulnerable to disease and death.

So, there is a definite link between social support and health. Why? Perhaps those who enjoy close relationships eat better, exercise more, and smoke and drink less. Perhaps a supportive network helps us evaluate and overcome stressful events. Perhaps supportive friends and family help bolster our threatened self-esteem. When wounded by someone's dislike or the loss of a job, a friend's advice, help, and reassurances may indeed be good medicine. Even when the problem isn't mentioned, friends provide us with distraction and a sense that, come what may, we're accepted, liked, and respected. "Friendship is a sovereign antidote against all calamities," said Seneca.

With someone we consider a close friend, we may feel comfortable confiding painful feelings. In one study, Southern Methodist University psychologists James Pennebaker and Robin O'Heeron contacted the surviving spouses of suicide or car accident victims. Those who bore their grief alone had more health problems than those who expressed it openly. When Pennebaker surveyed more than 700 college women, he found one in twelve reported a traumatic sexual experience in childhood. Compared with women who had experienced nonsexual traumas, such as parental death or divorce, the sexually abused women reported more headaches, stomach ailments, and other health problems, *especially if they had kept their secret to themselves.* People most at risk for illness are those who experience a trauma, continue to think about it, but don't talk about it. As they begin to talk openly about their pain, their bodies relax and they ruminate on it less. Twelve-step support programs, such as Alcoholics Anonymous, encourage participants to confess rather than deny their most painful recollections, and to gain relief and support from others who have walked the same road.

To isolate this confiding aspect of social support, Pennebaker asked the bereaved spouses to share what upsetting events had been preying on their minds. Those whom they first asked to describe a trivial event were physically tense. They stayed tense until they confided their troubles. They then relaxed. Writing about personal traumas in a diary also seems to help. When volunteers in another experiment did so, they had fewer health problems during the next six months. One participant explained, "Although I have not talked with anyone about what I wrote, I was finally able to deal with it, work through the pain instead of trying to block it out. Now it doesn't hurt to think about it." Even if it's only "talking to my diary," it helps to have someone to confide in.

In another striking study, Pennebaker and his colleagues invited thirty-three Holocaust survivors to spend two hours recalling their experiences. Many did so in intimate detail never before disclosed. Most later viewed their videotaped recollections and played the tape for family and friends. Those who were most self-disclosing had the most improved health fourteen months later. Confiding, like confession, is good for the soul.

Close Relationships and Happiness

Dealing creatively with stress bolsters our shaken self-esteem, and confiding painful feelings is good not only for the body but for the soul as well. That's the conclusion of studies showing that people are happier when supported by a network of friends and family.

Individualism and Depression. University of Pennsylvania researcher Martin Seligman believes that depression is a new plague among young and middle-age Americans. The cause? Epidemic hopelessness. Hopelessness caused by what? Individualism, believes Seligman.

This is, as Ronald Reagan declared in a speech on Wall Street, "the age of the individual." Individualists enjoy independence and take pride in their achievements. But at a price. When facing failure or rejection the self-driven individual takes on personal responsibility for problems. If, as a macho *Fortune* magazine ad declared, you can "make it on your own," on "your own drive, your own guts, your own energy, your own ambition," then whose fault is it if you *don't* make it on your own?

University of Illinois psychologist Harry Triandis and his colleagues have compared individualist and communal societies. In individualist societies of Western Europe and North America the focus is on personal identity. Be true to yourself, your own identity. When opportunity strikes, leave home behind and go forth with your portable self to conquer a new world (as colonists from Europe's individualist societies did). Like Superman, don't compromise yourself by getting too close to anyone. By contrast, the communal societies of Asia and much of the third world focus less on independence than on interdependence, less on personal identity than on group identity, less on self-reliance than on solidarity with one's extended family and colleagues.

To reflect on your own position on the individualism-communalism continuum, consider: If someone were to rip away your social connections, say by making you a solitary refugee in a foreign land, how much of your identity would remain?

For individualists, a great deal would remain—the very core of their being, their sense of "me," their awareness of their personal convictions and values. In many ways, Western psychology reflects the individualism of its cultures. We study adolescents' struggle to separate from parents and define their personal identity. We study personality—the distinctive traits that make each of us unique individuals. We encourage people not to live up to others' expectations, but to get in touch with themselves, accept themselves as individuals, be true to themselves. "I do my thing, and you do your thing," said therapist Fritz Perls in his "Gestalt credo." "You are you and I am I, and if by chance we find each other, it's beautiful. If not, it can't be helped." Humanistic psychologist Carl Rogers echoed Perls's individualism: "The only question which matters is, 'Am I living in a way which is deeply satisfying to me, and which truly expresses me?' "

Or consider today's pop psychology catchword, "co-dependence." A co-dependent person, usually a woman, is said to be dependent upon a destructive, often drug- or alcohol-addicted, partner. It's surely true that women who live with a substance abuser experience great stress and deserve help and support. But, say critics, "co-dependence" often gets stretched to include any sort of behavior that makes two people dependent on each other, with an accompanying loss of individual will. Moreover, the co-dependent person may be implicitly *blamed* for sharing and supporting the partner's dysfunctional behavior.

If people derive meaning from supporting and loving a troubled spouse or family, are they really blameworthy or socially ill? They surely would not seem so in less individualist societies such as Japan (where an individualist might say the whole society is co-dependent). For those in communal societies, one's social network provides one's bearings. No one is an island. Social attachments are fewer, but deeper and more stable. Thus, loyalties run stronger between employer and employees. Compared to American students, university students in Hong Kong talk with half as many people during a day, but for longer periods. Cut off from their family, their groups, and their loyal friends, "collectivists" (people whose goals and identity are group-centered) would lose the connections that define who they are.

The individualist/collectivist culture difference appears in the way parents rear their children. In individualist cultures, parents want their children to become independent. Their major concerns are not to train conformity and submissiveness (or, as a collectivist might say, sensitivity and cooperation). Schools teach children to clarify their own values so they can make good decisions for themselves. In restaurants, parents and children decide their own orders individually. At home, adolescents open their own mail, refuse parental guidance in choosing their own boyfriends and girlfriends, and seek the privacy of their own rooms. As adults, they chart their own goals and separate from their parents, who live apart from their own parents. When children fail, their embarrassed parents will discuss the child's problems openly.

University of Hong Kong cross-cultural psychologist C. Harry Hui reports that all this seems rather strange in communal societies such as Japan and China, where parents foster interdependence more than independence. Mother and young child sleep, bathe, and move about together, a practice that may contribute to the greater stress experienced by Japanese than American infants when separated from their mothers. Parents also more actively guide or decide their childrens choices among menu items, among friends, among school priorities. So close is the mutual identification of parent and child that, feeling shame, the crushed parents of an errant child seldom discuss the problem with others.

So, take your pick: People in competitive, individualist cultures, such as the United States, have more independence, make more money, take more pride in personal achievements, are less geographically bound near elderly parents, are less likely to prejudge those outside their groups, and enjoy more privacy. Their less unified cultures offer a smorgasbord of life-styles from which to choose. But compared to collectivists, individualists are also lonelier, more alienated, less likely to feel romantic love, more likely to divorce, more homicidal, and more vulnerable to stress-related diseases such as heart attacks. "Woe to him who is alone when he falls and has not another to lift him up," warns the sage of Ecclesiastes. Seligman concludes that "rampant individualism carries with it two seeds of its own destruction. First, a society that exalts the individual to the extent ours now does will be ridden with depression. . . . Second, and perhaps most important, is meaninglessness [which occurs when there is no] attachment to something larger than you are."

Companionship and Well-being. Aristotle labeled us "the social animal." And for good reason, say evolutionary theorists. Cooperation promotes survival. In solo combat, our ancestors were not the toughest predators. But as hunter-gathers they learned that six hands were better than two. Those who foraged in groups also gained protection from predators. Because group dwellers most successfully survived and reproduced, genes that predisposed such bonds in time predominated. Said simply, we were destined to be social creatures.

During our infancy and childhood our dependency strengthens our human bonds. Among our early social responses—love, fear, aggression—the first and the greatest is an intense bond of love, which developmental psychologists call attachment. As infants, we soon prefer familiar faces and voices. We then coo and gurgle when our parents give us attention. By eight months, we crawl after mother or father and typically let out a wail when separated from them. Reunited, we cling. By keeping infants close to their care givers, social attachment serves as a powerful survival impulse.

Deprived of familiar attachments, we may, for a time, experience meaninglessness. Short of torture, society's worst punishment is solitary confinement. Recently bereaved people often feel that life is empty, pointless. Children reared in institutions without normal social attachments, or locked away at home under extreme neglect, often become

148

pathetic creatures—withdrawn, frightened, speechless. After studying the mental health of homeless children for the World Health Organization, psychiatrist John Bowlby wrote that

> intimate attachments to other human beings are the hub around which a person's life revolves, not only when he is an infant or a toddler or a schoolchild but throughout his adolescence and his years of maturity as well, and on into old age. From these intimate attachments a person draws his strength and enjoyment of life and, through what he contributes, he gives strength and enjoyment to others. These are matters about which current science and traditional wisdom are at one.

Being attached to friends with whom we can share intimate thoughts has two effects, observed the seventeenth-century philosopher Francis Bacon. "It redoubleth joys, and cutteth griefs in half." So it seems from answers to a question asked of Americans by the National Opinion Research Center: "Looking over the last six months, who are the people with whom you discussed matters important to you?" Compared to those who could name no such intimate, those who named five or more such friends were 60 percent more likely to feel "very happy."

Other findings confirm the importance of social networks.

- The happiest university students are those who feel satisfied with their love life.
- Those who enjoy close relationships cope better with various stresses, including bereavement, rape, job loss, and illness.
- Compared to Army soldiers in large, conventional units with changing memberships, those on stable, cohesive, twelve-person A teams experience greater social support, better physical and mental health, and more career satisfaction.
- People report greater well-being if their friends and families support their goals by frequently expressing interest and offering help and encouragement.
- Among 800 alumni of Hobart and William Smith Colleges surveyed by Wesley Perkins, those with "yuppie values"—who preferred a high income and occupational success and prestige

to having very close friends and a close marriage—were twice as likely as their former classmates to describe themselves as "fairly" or "very" unhappy.

• Asked, "What is necessary for your happiness?" or "What is it that makes your life meaningful?" most people, however, mention—before anything else—satisfying close relationships with family, friends, or romantic partners. As C. S. Lewis said, "The sun looks down on nothing half so good as a household laughing together over a meal." Happiness hits close to home.

Writer Lois Wyse realized as much after riding in a hotel elevator when the press was expecting Elizabeth Taylor. When the doors opened at the lobby level she put her head down as she was greeted by a burst of flashbulbs. "There she is," someone yelled. When she lifted her head, another reporter said, "Oh, it's nobody."

Well, yes and no, she thought. "Who we are, what we do, and the way we do it matters only to a small group of people. But it does matter deeply to them." To those who love us, if we are fortunate to have a small circle of such people, we are somebody.

So, it is not good to be alone. But increasingly we are. In 1940, 8 percent of all U.S. households were composed of one person living alone. By 1988 the proportion had tripled to 24 percent. Today, people marry later, divorce more often, and live more of their lives independently, all leading to increased social isolation. Since 1970, the proportion of single-parent families has doubled, from 13 percent to 28 percent in 1990. Under such circumstances it becomes more difficult, though not impossible, to achieve what Samuel Johnson saw as the end of human endeavor—to be happy at home.

Self-disclosure. The most satisfying relationships are intimate. They enable us to be known and accepted as we truly are. A friend is someone with whom you feel comfortable being yourself. When trust displaces anxiety we become free to open ourselves without fear of losing the other's affection. Such relationships are typified by high levels of what psychologists call self-disclosure.

The traffic between well-being and self-disclosure is two-way. Happiness promotes intimacy. In a good mood, we open up. In a bad mood, we clam up. And intimacy promotes happiness. Humanistic psychologist Sidney Jourard argued that dropping our masks, letting ourselves be known as we are, nurtures love. Indeed, it is gratifying when we open up to someone and then receive the trust the person implies by being open with us. What is more, having an intimate friend, one with whom we can discuss threats to our self-image, helps us cope with such stress. This kind of true and intimate friendship is special for it helps us cope with all our other relationships.

Lacking opportunities for self-disclosure—for sharing our likes and dislikes, our proud and shameful moments, our worries and dreams, our joys and sorrows—we are painfully lonely. Loneliness isn't being alone. That's solitude. It's *feeling* alone, as one can even at a party. "I lie awake," ached the psalmist, feeling "like a lonely bird on the housetop." How then can we move from what Henri Nouwen calls "the desert of our loneliness" into a garden of healing relationships? How can we enjoy a greater intimacy?

Experiments reveal a "disclosure reciprocity effect." Disclosure begets disclosure. I reveal more to you if you have first been open with me. But intimacy is seldom instant. More often, we dance: I reveal a little, you reveal a little—but not too much; you then reveal more, and I reciprocate.

Some people are especially skilled at opening others up. They readily elicit intimacy, even from those who normally hold a lot back. These people listen well. During a conversation they show attentive facial expressions and appear to be comfortable and enjoying themselves. They also show interest, uttering supportive phrases while we're speaking. The late psychologist Carl Rogers called such people "growth-promoting" listeners—people who are *genuine* as they reveal their own feelings; who are *accepting* of others' feelings; and who are *empathic*, sensitive, and reflective. Such listening, he believed, nurtures self-understanding and self-acceptance:

Hearing has consequences. When I truly hear a person and the meanings that are important to him at that moment, hearing not simply his words, but him, and when I let him know that I have heard his own private personal meanings, many things happen. There is first of all a grateful look. He feels released. He wants to tell me more about his world. He surges forth in a new sense of freedom. He becomes more open to the process of change.

I have often noticed that the more deeply I hear the meanings of the person, the more there is that happens. Almost always, when a person realizes he has been deeply heard, his eyes moisten. I think in some real sense he is weeping for joy. It is as though he were saying, "Thank God, somebody heard me. Someone knows what it's like to be me."

Rogers illustrated this in his conversation with a quiet, troubled, twenty-eight-year-old male.

Client: I just ain't no good to nobody, never was, and never will be.

Rogers: Feeling that now, hm? That you're just no good to yourself, no good to anybody. Never will be any good to anybody. Just that you're completely worthless, huh?—Those really are lousy feelings. Just feel that you're no good at all, hm?

Client: Yeah. (Muttering in low, discouraged voice) That's what this guy I went to town with just the other day told me.

Rogers: This guy that you went to town with really told you that you were no good? Is that what you're saying? Did I get that right?

Client: M-hm.

Rogers: I guess the meaning of that if I get it right is that here's somebody that—meant something to you and what does he think of you? Why, he's told you that he thinks you're no good at all. And that just really knocks the props out from under you. (Client weeps quietly.) It just brings the tears. (Silence of twenty seconds)

Client: (Rather defiantly) I don't care though.

Rogers: You tell yourself you don't care at all, but somehow I guess some part of you cares because some part of you weeps over it.

Does looking at yourself in the mirror provided by an empathic listener really help? Hundreds of careful studies, comparing troubled people who receive psychotherapy with those who don't, reveal that people often improve without therapy (a phenomenon called spontaneous remission). Yet those who receive psychotherapy are somewhat more likely to improve, *regardless of what kind of therapy they receive.* Mental health experts Jerome Frank, Marvin Goldfried, and Hans Strupp have each concluded that different psychotherapy techniques are similarly effective because of their commonalities. They all offer hope to demoralized people. They all help people gain a new perspective on both themselves and their worlds. And they all offer an empathic, trusting, supportive relationship.

Psychotherapists haven't cornered the market on support. Australian researcher John Hattie and his co-workers combined the results of thirty-nine studies comparing treatment offered by professional therapists and by laypeople (friendly professors, people given a few hours training in empathic listening, or supervised peer counselors). The result? The lay paraprofessionals proved as helpful as the professionals. Similarly, many self-help groups organized to support dieters, recovering alcoholics, and former drug addicts rival the success of psychotherapists.

Lacking the support of an intimate friend, those in the "lonely crowd" are more likely than those supported by close relationships to hire an empathic, caring source of support, a surrogate soul mate. One response to alienation in individualist societies is therefore to professionalize social support. But should we leave help giving to the professionals? The demonstrated effectiveness of paraprofessionals should encourage us all to be confident in caring, knowing that our sympathetic listening ears and gestures of support are virtually as helpful as professional counseling.

We should also be encouraged to work to restructure our schools, workplaces, churches, even our individual lives, to promote "we feeling" and the sharing of burdens. Remaining in the same job for twenty-five years has required my forgoing other professional opportunities, including some back home in Seattle where our extended families reside. As compensation, though, my wife and I have friends with whom we've shared our struggles through the seasons of family life. Sitting on our screened porch, we exchange greetings with neighbors whose children have grown up alongside ours. At work, most of us in the nine offices making up our department have been together for years, sharing weekly meetings and teatimes and daily updates on one another's lives. Three months ago, we feted Chuck for receiving tenure. Two months ago we celebrated John's new book with toasts and good wishes. Last month we had balloons, tears, and hugs while rejoicing over Jane's successful completion of cancer treatments. This morning we gathered with the dean to sing the praises of Patricia, our newest colleague.

Such experiences, combined with studies of health, happiness, and close relationships, remind us of a deep truth: From babyhood to parenthood, from the playfield to the office, we are social creatures. In the biblical creation story the Creator, having formed the first person, immediately declared our social character: "It is not good that the man should be alone." Where two or three friends are gathered, often there is found joy. And, as we next see, when two souls become as one, joy deepens.

9

Love and Marriage

*It is not impossible for a person to live a happy and contented life
without a marriage partner. . . . But it has been believed since
biblical times that it is not good for man or woman to be alone, and
most people today find this to be true.*

ANGUS CAMPBELL, *THE SENSE OF WELL-BEING IN AMERICA*

Love and marriage. Do they make for happiness? People *think* they
do. When asked, "What missing element would bring you happiness?"
the most frequent answer is "love." A well-educated, well-liked, and
successful twenty-six-year-old woman yearns "to be loved, totally and
completely by a man. All the great friends and family and satisfaction
gained from a worthwhile job cannot fill a void of not being loved."
There are as many men who, as one successful thirtyish man put it,
"would trade my life with anyone who was loved by a good woman."
Four in five adults—adults of all ages—rate love as important to their
happiness. And they are right.

Marriage and Well-being

Whether young or old, male or female, rich or poor, people in stable, loving relationships do enjoy greater well-being. Survey after survey of many tens of thousands of Europeans and Americans have produced this consistent result: Compared to those single or widowed, and especially compared to those divorced or separated, married people report being happier and more satisfied with life. In the United States, for example, fewer than 25 percent of unmarried adults but nearly 40 percent of married adults report being "very happy." Despite TV images of a pleasure-filled single life, and caustic comments about the "bondage," "chains," and "yoke" of marriage, a stubborn truth remains: Most people are happier attached than unattached.

Are the emotional benefits of marriage greater for men than women, as so many people today believe (given that in most marriages women contribute more than men to household work and nurturing family members)? To find out, Wendy Wood and her Texas A&M colleagues statistically summarized all published studies of marriage, gender, and well-being. Their findings: In a stressed marriage, women's sensitivity to negative emotions may trigger a higher rate of psychological disturbance than experienced by their husbands. In fact, marriage does less to reduce suicide, alcoholism, and other disorders in women than in men. Nevertheless, Wood and her colleagues also find that across all marriages wives report slightly greater happiness than do their husbands. Wood suspects this is because women find more joy when close relationships are positive.

However, even more important than being married is the marriage's quality. People who say their marriage is satisfying—who find themselves still in love with their partner—rarely report being unhappy, discontented with life, or depressed. And, most married people *do* declare their marriages happy ones. In the United States, almost two thirds say their marriage is "very happy." Three out of four say their spouse is their best friend. Four out of five people say they would marry the same person again. The consequence? Most such people feel quite happy with life as a whole.

But why are married people generally happier? Does happiness promote marriage? Are happy people more appealing as marriage partners? Do grouchy or depressed people more often stay single or suffer divorce? Certainly, happy people are more fun to be with. They are, as we have seen, more outgoing, trusting, compassionate, and focused on others. Unhappy people are more often socially rejected. In one study, researchers Stephen Strack and James Coyne observed that "depressed persons induced hostility, depression, and anxiety in others and got rejected. Their guesses that they were not accepted were not a matter of cognitive distortion." For such reasons, positive, happy people more readily form happy relationships.

But marriage also enhances happiness, for at least two reasons. First, married people are more likely to enjoy an enduring, supportive, intimate relationship, and less likely to suffer loneliness. No wonder male medical students in a study by UCLA's Robert Coombs survived medical school with less stress and anxiety if married. A good marriage gives each partner a dependable companion, a lover, a friend.

Such has been my own experience. My wife is my best friend. We call each other if interesting things happen during the day. We share our day's mail after dinner. We test our ideas on each other, knowing the relationship is secure enough to welcome criticism. And we end our days snuggled in darkness, sharing random thoughts, sometimes commiserating, sometimes recalling things from our shared history of experiences, sometimes giggling, sometimes in sexual union. I know unmarried people can enjoy the companionship and intimacy of close relationships, too. (No single factor, such as marriage, is both necessary and sufficient for happiness.) But for me, neither single life nor cohabitation could beat the intimacy and security of this lifelong conversation with my best friend.

There is a second, more prosaic reason why marriage promotes happiness, or at least buffers us from misery. Marriage offers the roles of spouse and parent, which can provide additional sources of self-esteem. True, multiple roles can multiply stress. Our circuits can and do overload. Yet each also provides rewards, status, avenues to enrichment, escape from stress faced in other parts of one's life. When our personal identity stands on several legs, it more easily holds up under the loss of any one. If I mess up at work, well, I can tell myself I'm still a good husband and father, and, in the final analysis, these parts of me are what matter most.

Is Marriage on the Rocks?

Despite the fact that most marriages are reasonably happy, that a happy marriage contributes to well-being, and that 95 percent of Americans over age forty have married, some people worry that the institution of marriage is in trouble. Is it true?

Brides and grooms declare their vows, confident—as most are—that their romance will be lifelong. They envision themselves, a decade later, still having a loving mate, and competent, cheerful children. They imagine putting the happy kids to bed on a snowy winter's evening and settling into overstuffed chairs in front of a crackling fire. As the purring cat settles cozily in the lap of one, in walks the other still attractive, still affectionate mate with a hot drink and a warm kiss.

But of course this is more the exception than the rule. A sad fact of life is that roughly half of U.S. marriages* and 40 percent of Canadian marriages will end in divorce. And some of the remaining marriages are an unhappy bondage or a smoldering compromise. In one survey after another, the National Opinion Research Center has found that nearly six in ten Americans who rate their *marriage* as "very happy" also rate *life as a whole* as "very happy." But among those *not* in a "very happy" marriage, the proportion who are "very happy" with life as a whole plummets to one in ten—a lower level of happiness even than among the relatively unhappy separated and divorced. In terms of individual happiness, then, a bad marriage is worse than no marriage at all. To paraphrase Henry Ward Beecher, "well-married a person is winged; ill-matched, shackled."

University of Texas sociologist Norval Glenn analyzed national opinion data gathered on thousands of Americans from 1972 to 1988. He followed the course of marriages that began in the early 1970s. By

---

*Although half of all U.S. *marriages* end in divorce, presumably slightly less than half of all *people* get divorced, given the slight inflation in the divorce rate contributed by the multiple divorces of people like Elizabeth Taylor.

the late 1980s, only a third of the starry-eyed newlyweds were still married *and* proclaiming their marriages "very happy." Allowing for some overreporting of marital happiness—it's easier to tell an interviewer you've succeeded than failed in your marriage—Glenn concludes that "the real proportion of those marriages that were successful . . . may well have been under a fourth." From a 1988 national survey, the Gallup Organization offers a similarly dismal conclusion: Two out of three thirty-five- to fifty-four-year-olds had divorced, separated, or been close to separation. If this pattern continues, "our nation will soon reach the point where the dominant experience of adults will have been marital instability."

Dating couples beware: People who tumble into love tend to discount any problems in a relationship, and they're overly optimistic about love's lasting forever. Newlyweds beware also: Don't take a successful marriage for granted. Under normal circumstances, the odds are—despite what you think—you will *not* live happily ever after. Unless nurtured carefully, the relationship you counted on for love and happiness may leave you crushed, lonely, feeling like a failure, or trudging hopelessly along, resigned to your despair. But beware also of a fatalism that says, "Happy marriages today seldom last, so why invest myself in making a permanent commitment?" Given that attitude, "married persons remain tentatively on the marriage market," says Glenn, "susceptible to being lured out of their present marriages by opportunities (real or imagined) for more favorable ones." In marriage as in other realms of life, naïve optimism and apathetic pessimism are both perilous. Cautious optimism—a positive attitude channeled by a wariness of real perils—offers the best chance for success and happiness.

A thirty-four-year-old teacher illustrates marital resignation: "I would enjoy my life exactly the way it is minus the husband. This week my husband is away and what a joyous week it has been. There is no one who constantly tells me what to do and how it should be done. There is no one around who sits on his ass after his day's work is done while I'm still working after my day's work is done. This week the tension is gone. This week I feel like a complete person. Would I marry again? No, because I know what next week will hold when he comes home again." The Greek dramatist Euripides anticipated such experiences: "Marry, and with luck it may go well. But when a marriage fails, then those who marry live at home in hell."

Since 1960, more and more people have decided *not* to live at home in hell. By 1980, when the U.S. divorce rate peaked, it had more than doubled. Between 1960 and 1985, divorce in the European Community quadrupled. Marriages have become "hedonistic," says Norval Glenn. They exist to serve our needs and desires and they survive "as long as we both shall love." Thus marital success is gauged by how happy and satisfied we *feel* with our marriages, not by how well the marriage serves the needs of others, such as the children, the extended family, or the society. If a marriage isn't meeting our needs, well, say many, better not to stay home in hell.

What a change. In preindustrial societies, family members were interdependent. Children (often four or more) depended on their parents for survival, parents depended on each other, and in old age the child-parent dependence reversed. To maintain the family as an interdependent unit, divorce was looked upon as evil. (To the present, divorce rates are much lower in farming families.) Today's families are smaller, and married partners more often have independent incomes, or at least an economic safety net beneath them. Without anyone intending it, the social forces that minimize divorce, and therefore the norms against divorce, weakened.

So, if we are freer to terminate miserable marriages, are marriages that survive happier? Are marriages actually no less happy, just more likely to terminate when unhappy? If, like many, you think so, then consider this disconcerting fact: Compared to back when divorce was uncommon, those in today's surviving marriages are actually *less* likely to describe their marriage as "very happy." For example, compared to younger married people surveyed in the mid-1970s, the percent of "very happy" among younger marrieds surveyed in the mid to late 1980s was almost ten points lower. For many, marriage has become a union that defies management.

For marriage proponents, there is more bad news:

- Although married people are still considerably more likely to feel happy than unmarried people, in recent years the gap has lessened because married women aren't as happy as they once were and unmarried men and women are happier. In today's world, people are more comfortable staying single. Thus the apparent contribution of marriage to happiness has weakened.

- "Traditional families"—father, mother, and children under eighteen—now make up only 27 percent of U.S. households. The other 73 percent include not only those single, widowed, or married without young children, but also growing numbers of single parents, and those divorced or cohabiting. For example, the number of cohabiting unmarried couples in the United States tripled during the 1970s and nearly doubled again during the 1980s. Similar trends have occurred since 1960 in Australia, Scandinavia, and elsewhere in Western Europe. In all these countries, rising rates of cohabitation have been accompanied by falling rates of marriage. In the United States, 57 percent of eighteen- to fifty-four-year-olds are now married, down from 73 percent a quarter century ago.
- For couples living apart (because of dual careers, military ser-

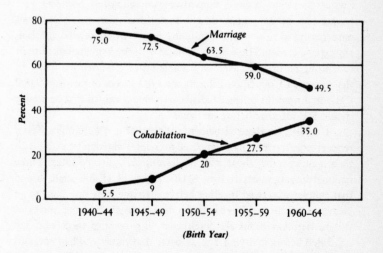

U.S. rates of cohabitation and marriage by people at age twenty-five
SOURCE: U.S. National Survey of Families and Households, conducted in 1987 and 1988. Note: Some people by age twenty-five had both cohabited *and* married. Data reported by Larry L. Bumpass and James A. Sweet, "National Estimates of Cohabitation," *Demography* 26 (1989): 615–25.

vice, or imprisonment) absence does not make the heart grow fonder. Such couples have double the normal divorce rate. This fact has sobering implications for those contemplating commuter marriages.

- Despite the easier availability of birth control and the legalization of abortion, births to single mothers have dramatically *increased.* A recent National Research Council report estimates that "more than 1 million teenage girls in the United States become pregnant each year, just over 400,000 teenagers obtain abortions, and nearly 470,000 give birth" (nearly two thirds of whom are unmarried). Still—here comes another surprise—the number of births to unwed women is even greater among women in their twenties. The net result: The rate of U.S. births to single mothers has quintupled since 1960 to 27 percent of all births in 1989.

Is it possible to find a positive side to these trends? Many cohabiting couples enjoy a close, supportive companionship. Some also are testing the marital waters. Might these "trial marriages" weed out unsuccessful or risky unions before marriage? Are those who are sexually experienced and thoroughly familiar with the living habits of their cohabiting partner less likely to stumble into an ill-fated marriage? In the American Council on Education's 1989 survey of nearly 300,000 first-year American college students, 51 percent agreed that "a couple should live together before marriage."

But, alas, for these 51 percent yet another myth crumbles. Seven recent studies concur that, compared to couples who don't cohabit with their spouses-to-be, those who do have *higher* divorce rates. Three national surveys illustrate this: A U.S. survey of 13,000 adults found that couples who lived together before marriage were one third more likely to separate or divorce within a decade. (A 1990 Gallup survey of still-married Americans also found that 40 percent of those who had cohabited before marrying, and 21 percent of those who had not, said they might divorce.) A Canadian national survey of 5,300 women found that those who cohabited were 54 percent more likely to divorce within fifteen years. And a Swedish study of 4,300 women found cohabitation linked with an 80 percent greater risk of divorce.

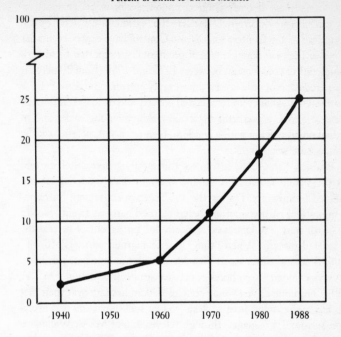

Percent of Births to Unwed Mothers

In the United States, births to unwed mothers have quintupled since 1960.
SOURCE: National Center for Health Statistics, *Natality*, vol. 1 of *Vital Statistics of the United States, 1988* (DHHS Pub. No. 90–1100 [Public Health Service]) (Washington, DC: Government Printing Office, 1990), p. 57, table 1–31.

We can only speculate why. Perhaps people who cohabit are more likely to disrupt a marriage with extramarital sex. (This possibility has been offered to explain another provocative finding: The number of premarital sexual partners correlates with marital unhappiness.) Perhaps people who cohabit are less committed to the institution of marriage. Or perhaps impulse control and patience are traits that enhance lasting relationships, explaining why couples who do not cohabit before marrying also report higher-quality marriages. Regardless, successful trial marriages do *not* predict a successful marriage.

No one sees any positive side to the surging rate of teen pregnancy, an experience that often impoverishes the lives of both mother and child. "Regardless of one's political philosophy or moral perspective, the basic facts are disturbing," declares the National Research Council report. Staff at the Centers for Disease Control have expressed similar alarm over the near-doubled rate of premarital sex reported by fifteen- to nineteen-year-old women between 1970 and 1988 (from 29 percent to 52 percent). Not only is teen promiscuity known to increase the risk of unwanted pregnancy and associated poverty and sexually transmitted disease, it also is a predictor of sexual violence among males and of eventual divorce. Even with a condom, teen sex is not, psychologically speaking, safe sex.

Planned Parenthood attributes the spiraling premarital sex and teen pregnancy rates partly to the mass media's modeling of un-protected promiscuity. During the 1987 soap opera season, for exam-ple, unmarried partners outnumbered married partners twenty-four to one—with nary any expressed concern for birth control or sexually transmitted disease. When "they" (rarely married partners) "do it" twenty thousand times a year on television and no one gets pregnant, that, says Planned Parenthood, is massive sex *dis*information. On TV, healthy, hormone-driven young couples seldom hesitate over their first deep kiss and ensuing feast of flesh. When such media models every-where surround a teenager, through television and MTV, Walkmans and VCRs, it becomes "appalling illogical," says PBS film critic Mi-chael Medved, to contend "that intensely sexual material does nothing to encourage promiscuity." U.S. Health and Human Services secretary Louis Sullivan echoes Medved's concern: "Our children will not thrive until we reverse the cultural trends that are undermining the family in America."*

*The media debate has also been fueled by research on the effects of viewing sexual violence, which has repeatedly been found to desensitize and disinhibit, and to foster attitudes and behaviors that degrade women. Erotic but nonviolent pornography does not reliably affect men's acceptance and performance of aggression against women. But experiments show that it can lead viewers to trivialize rape, to alter their perceptions of normal sexuality, and to devalue their own (comparatively less exciting) partners. These findings, combined with the tripling of the known rape rate over the last twenty-five years and the discovery that one in four American women report suffering an experience that meets the legal definition of rape or attempted rape, have raised concerns among feminists and fundamentalists alike. Responding to tidal changes in cultural attitudes, Hollywood has reversed its images of African-Americans and its portrayals of drug use as glamorous. Is it too much to hope that, without violating artistic freedom, we might similarly

Amid these alarming social trends come some rays of cheer. Compared to the children born to poverty-stricken teen mothers, children of divorce often fare better—certainly better than children whose mothers remain at home in hell, in a miserable marriage, sometimes with an abusive man. However, even this ray of cheer shines through clouds: Data amassed from eight annual surveys by the National Opinion Research Center reveal that, compared to those who grew up in intact families, the average child of divorce grows up with a diminished sense of well-being. Children of divorce are more likely to divorce and less likely to feel happy with life.

Some children cope well with divorce, better than with the stresses of a conflict-laden home. Yet, say veteran University of Virginia researcher Mavis Hetherington and her colleagues, divorce, often followed by the intrusion of a new stepparent, places "children at increased risk for developing social, psychological, behavioral and academic problems." A recent study of 12,000 British seven-year-olds, restudied as eleven-year-olds, illustrates: Compared to boys from intact families, boys whose parents divorced during the study developed one fourth more behavior problems.

Given that more than 75 percent of divorced people remarry—half within three years—another ray of cheer comes from research on remarriage. A statistical digest of sixteen studies by University of Missouri researcher Elizabeth Vemer and her colleagues revealed that "yes, people in first marriages report greater satisfaction, but the difference appears to be minuscule and certainly not substantial." Although second marriages have a 25 percent greater risk of divorce, remarried people are virtually as satisfied with their marriages as those in first marriages.

Another hopeful sign is that among married people fidelity is epidemic. Pop psychology articles on infidelity would have us believe otherwise. Two thirds of married men and half of married women have had an affair, declared Joyce Brothers in a 1990 *Parade* magazine article. Influenced by such articles, and perhaps by their own sexual

look back with chagrin on the days when movies entertained us with images of sexual coercion and of physically and emotionally unsafe sex?

fantasies, only a fourth of people believe that most married people are faithful to one another. But another myth crumbles against a wall of representative data. In a 1988 Gallup survey, nine in ten married Americans said they had not had sex with anyone other than their spouses during their present marriage. In Britain, a 1987 study produced a similar finding. The National Opinion Research Center reports that during any given year only "1.5 percent of married people have a sex partner other than their spouse." And disapproval of extramarital sex has never been higher among adult Americans—91 percent. In real life, unlike the movies, faithful attractions greatly outnumber fatal attractions. By June 1990, the news reached *Cosmopolitan* magazine, which headlined "Being Faithful Can Be Fun."

So, marriage proponents can take heart that fidelity rates and marital happiness generally remain high. Still, our overall picture of the state of marriage is hardly rosy. Other things considered—high divorce rates, slightly declining marital happiness, rapidly escalating rates of cohabitation and births to single mothers—Norval Glenn is deeply concerned: "All is not well with the institution of marriage in this country." In a 1990 survey, American Psychological Association members agreed that the family meltdown is reaching crisis proportions. They rated "the decline of the nuclear family" as today's number one "threat to the mental health of America." America's social recession, though profound, has occurred gradually enough to trigger less attention than its comparatively milder economic recessions. As alarms now begin to sound, one senses that is about to change.

The Ups and Downs and Ups of Love

People yearn for love. They live for it, die for it. But what is it? To help answer, psychologists have compared love in various close relationships—among same-sex best friends, parents and children, spouses or lovers. Some elements are common to all loving relationships: mutual understanding, giving and receiving support, enjoying the loved one's company. Some elements are distinctive. If people experience passionate love they express it physically, they expect the relationship to be exclusive, and they are intensely fascinated with their partners. You can see it in their eyes. Social psychologist Zick Rubin confirmed this. He administered a romantic love questionnaire to hundreds of dating couples at the University of Michigan. Later, from behind a one-way mirror in a laboratory waiting room, he clocked eye contact among "weak-love" and "strong-love" couples. His result will *not* surprise you: The strong-love couples gave themselves away by gazing long into each other's eyes.

For those passionately in love, well-being soars. The whole world seems to smile. "All the world loves a lover, and a lover loves all the world," observes psychoanalyst Anthony Storr. One woman recalled the joy of falling in love: "At the office, I could hardly keep from shouting out how deliriously happy I felt. The work was easy; things that had annoyed me on previous occasions were taken in stride. And I had strong impulses to help others; I wanted to share my joy. When Mary's typewriter broke down, I virtually sprang to my feet to assist her. Mary! My former 'enemy'!"

Inevitably, such passion subsides. Given several months, at most a year or two, the intense absorption in the other, the thrill of the romance, the giddy "floating on a cloud" feeling fades. "Just married" becomes just married, the magic somehow lost. In 1971 a man wrote a love poem to his bride, slipped it into a bottle, and dropped it into the Pacific Ocean between Seattle and Hawaii. A decade later a jogger found it on a Guam beach:

> If, by the time this letter reaches you, I am old and gray, I know that our love will be as fresh as it is today.
>
> It may take a week or it may take years for this note to find you. . . . If this should never reach you, it will still be written in my heart that I will go to extreme means to prove my love for you. Your husband, Bob.

The woman to whom the love note was addressed was reached by phone. The note was read to her. She burst out laughing. And the more she heard the harder she laughed. "We're divorced," she finally said, and slammed down the phone.

It won't surprise those who know the rock song "Addicted to Love" to find out that the flow and ebb of romantic love curiously follows the pattern of addictions to coffee, alcohol, and other drugs. At first, a drug gives a big kick, perhaps a high. With repetition, opponent emotions gain strength and tolerance develops. An amount that once was highly stimulating no longer gives a thrill. However, stopping the substance does not return you to where you started. Rather, it triggers withdrawal symptoms—malaise, depression, the blahs. Such often happens in love. The no-longer-romantic relationship is taken for granted. Until it ends. Then the jilted lovers, the widowers, the divorcées, are surprised at how empty life seems without the people they long ago stopped feeling passionately attached to. Having focused on what was not working, they stopped noticing what was, including all their interdependent activities.

Passion's cooling into a steadier but still-warm afterglow of "companionate love" may sustain a deep and affectionate attachment. But those who regard the initial romantic high as essential may end up disillusioned and divorced—especially when sexual passion wanes in a marriage that was preceded by cohabitation, reports sociologist Andrew Greeley from the 1988 Gallup marriage survey. University of Minnesota social psychologist Ellen Berscheid and her colleagues note that the failure to appreciate the limited half-life of passionate love can doom a relationship: "If the inevitable odds against eternal passionate love in a relationship were better understood, more people might choose to be satisfied with the quieter feelings of satisfaction and contentment." Based on their research findings, the Minnesota researchers suspect that "the sharp rise in the divorce rate in the past two decades is linked, at least in part, to the growing importance of intense positive emotional experiences (e.g., romantic love) in people's lives, experiences that may be particularly difficult to sustain over time." Asians, who tend to be less focused on personal feelings such as passion and more concerned with the practical aspects of social attachments, appear less vulnerable to disillusionment.

As with most other human phenomena, this inevitable decline of mutual passionate feelings may be adaptive. Passionate love often produces children, whose nurture is enhanced by the parents' waning obsession with each other. Children, in turn, become the parents' new obsession, hastening the romantic decline. Once preschoolers join the family, marital satisfaction declines. As long as children remain at home, their parents worry more, feel more stressed, have less time to enjoy each other. Childbirth classes, which prepare couples for a single day's experience, would do well also to prepare couples for the more enduring marital stresses that follow. Psychologists Philip and Susan Cowan at the University of California at Berkeley report that couples benefit from training sessions that sensitize husband and wife to how the child may affect their relationship.

For those who like a happy ending, the ups and downs of love end with an up—the typically happy empty nest described earlier, with the accompanying peace and the freedom to go where one wants, cook what wants, do what one wants. So hang in there. As Mark Twain declared, "No man or woman really knows what perfect love is until they have been married a quarter of a century." By the time couples celebrate a half century of togetherness, their marital satisfaction has nearly rebounded to what they enjoyed during their first two years of marriage. True, the ecstasy has long ago subsided. But in its place can come an abiding attachment rooted in a lifetime of mutual understanding, support, and affection.

Who Are the Happily Married?

With time, some couples degenerate into hurt and pain, each partner inwardly rehearsing grievances. But others enjoy the happiness fostered by continuing warmth and love. It makes us wonder: What makes for a happy marriage?

First, sociologists and demographers have discerned some predictors. You're likely to stay married if most of the following are true:

You married after age twenty.

You dated for a long while before marriage.

You are well educated.

You enjoy a stable income from a good job.

You live in a small town or on a farm.

You did not cohabit or become pregnant before marriage.

You and your spouse are religiously committed.

None of these predictors, by itself, is essential to a stable marriage. But if none of these things is true for someone, divorce is a good bet. If all are true, the couple will likely not part until death.

Second, psychologists have explored factors that influence our ability to like and to love. Consider four such determinants:

First, which proverbial wisdom is correct: Do birds of a feather flock together? Or do opposites attract? Or are they both, in some sense, correct?

This much is beyond question: Birds who flock together are indeed of a feather. Friends, engaged couples, and spouses are far more likely than randomly paired people to share similar attitudes, beliefs, and values. But does similarity *cause* us to like each other?

Imagine you're at a party, listening as Jane discusses politics, religion, personal likes and dislikes with Larry and John. She and Larry agree on most everything, she and John on fewer things. Afterward she reflects, "Larry's really intelligent. And he's so likable. I sure hope we meet again." State University of New York at Albany psychologist Donn Byrne simulated Jane's experience. He told people about someone's attitudes on various issues. Inevitably—with people of various ages from across the world—likeness begat liking.

In natural situations, too, likes attract. When strangers become acquainted, friendships do not form randomly. Transfer students in a boardinghouse or strangers confined in a fallout shelter typically come to like best those with whom they share interests and attitudes. Those who share our values, our pursuits, our tastes, we like.

With married couples, too, similarity breeds content. The greater their similarity the more likely the couple are happily married and the less likely they are to divorce. This phenomenon appears even in marriages based not on love but on parental perceptions of compatibility. When Usha Gupta and Pushpa Singh asked fifty couples in Jaipur, India, to complete a love questionnaire, they found that those who married out of romantic love felt their love for their partner diminishing after five years. By contrast, those in arranged marriages reported *more* love as the years went by. In fact, a decade after marriage, love was more abundant in arranged than love-based marriages!

What can we say then for the popular idea that, as the *Reader's Digest* has reported, "opposites attract. . . . Socializers pair with loners, novelty-lovers with those who dislike change, free spenders with scrimpers, risk-takers with the very cautious." It makes a good story—extremely different types in harmonious union: Rat, Mole, and Badger in *The Wind in the Willows,* Frog and Toad in Arnold Lobel's books, Bert and Ernie on *Sesame Street.* The stories delight us. But that's because they express what we seldom experience. True, we can imagine opposites attracting (might not a sadist and a masochist live happily ever after?). And in search of attraction fueled by complementarity, researchers have asked whether, say, a domineering and a submissive person wouldn't make a happier couple than two submissive people. Despite instances of happy opposites, the quest to identify ways in which complementary traits breed attraction has largely failed. Yes, heterosexual people feel an attraction for their complement, but even their circle of friends is mostly same-sex.

So here is another item for our accumulating list of false myths: In reality, opposites seldom attract, and if they do they often don't stay attracted. Close relationships are more likely to form and endure with a special someone who shares your ideas, values, and desires, a soul mate who likes the same music, the same activities, even the same foods. For good reason the prophet Amos wondered, "Can two walk together, except they be agreed?"

A second ingredient of marital love is sex. The scientific study of sex has answered important questions about the prevalence of various sexual practices, about our sexual response system, about the determinants (actually, the *non*determinants) of our sexual orientation. But what about the human significance of sexual intimacy? You might know every available fact about sex—that the initial spasms of male and female orgasm come at 0.8-second intervals, that the female nipples expand 10 millimeters at the peak of sexual arousal, that systolic blood pressure rises some 60 points and respiration peaks at 40 breaths per minute—yet fail to comprehend its emotional meaning.

To explore the significance of sex for marital well-being, psychologists have asked, first, whether happiness accompanies more frequent sex. The idea that sexual union provides emotional fulfillment has suggested the climax for countless romantic novels. After Freud, it became even more widely assumed that repressed sexuality exacts a price, and that frequent sexual release enhances happiness and health.

Is happiness indeed related to sex? One bit of supportive evidence comes from two studies that asked couples to record their arguments and their sexual unions over several weeks. Virtually every couple that had sex more often than they argued were happily married; no couple that had more fights than sex rated their marriage as happy. The National Opinion Research Center's 1989 survey of adult sexual behavior in America (which cast welcome light on a subject muddled by previous haphazard surveys) concurs: Those with very happy marriages reported having intercourse 70 percent more often than those with unhappy marriages.

So, would having sex more often brighten a marriage? Or is frequent sexual play actually an offshoot of marital joy? Although many studies actually find only a modest correlation between sex frequency and marital happiness (some happily married people seldom have intercourse), the alleviation of sexual frustration *can* enhance marital well-being. After undergoing sex therapy, couples often experience a newfound sexual enjoyment—and, as a by-product, an increased happiness in their marriage. A committee appointed by Finland's Ministry of Health and Social Affairs to study health and sex thought this to be true. Noting the joys of sex, its 1989 preliminary report suggested that people be "given the possibility of having sex holidays during which they can forget pressing matters and concentrate on relaxing in erotic pleasure and satisfaction."

University of Minnesota social psychologist Ellen Berscheid, a veteran researcher of close relationships, concludes that if she were asked "what is love?" and "forced against a brick wall to face a firing squad that would shoot if not given the correct answer" she would whisper, "It's about ninety percent sexual desire as yet not sated." Berscheid speaks only of romantic love, and ninety percent may overstate the matter. Yet her wit carries wisdom. The interweaving of love and sexuality is sometimes painfully apparent when a person with a homosexual orientation marries a heterosexual person. They may *like* each other. They may bear and rear children. But without sexual attraction, the marriage often becomes loveless. Throughout our species history, sexual attraction aided our ancestors' survival by binding their parents with one another.

Much more important than the quantity of sexual union is the quality of it. Sexual satisfaction (which predicts marital satisfaction much better than does sex frequency) increases when intimacy becomes more than a biological release. Sex becomes more deeply pleasureful when its bodily pleasures are embedded within the additional pleasure of intense closeness with one's partner. To have intercourse was, for the Hebrew writers of the Old Testament, literally "to know" one's partner, intimately.

Sexual behavior is therefore a *social* behavior. Through it we may hurt each other, or feel very nearly "one flesh." We can give ourselves the physical pleasure and release of orgasm while alone, but most of us find much greater satisfaction in the arms of our loved one. As the philosopher Bertrand Russell noted, "People cannot fully satisfy their sexual instinct without love." Sexual longing drives us to approach, to experience, and, yes, to *know* one who can fulfill the longing. For our mostly monogamous species, sex is therefore a life-uniting and love-renewing act. When enjoyed as such, within a covenant of mutual loyalty, trust, and faithfulness, it helps express and satisfy our urgent desire for intimate love. "If two lie together, they keep warm," notes the writer of Ecclesiastes. Indeed.

A third ingredient of marital love is intimacy. Psychology's word for intimacy is self-disclosure—that sharing of private feelings: our likes and dislikes, our dreams and worries, our proud and shameful moments. "When I am with my friend," reflected the Roman statesman Seneca, "methinks I am alone, and as much at liberty to speak anything as to think it." So it is in a happy marriage, where trust displaces anxiety and where one is therefore free to be open without fear of losing the other's affection. Marriage at its best is intimate friendship sealed by commitment.

One form of intimacy comes through a shared spirituality. In a 1988 Gallup national marriage survey summarized by Andrew Greeley, 75 percent of those who prayed with their spouses (and 57 percent of those who didn't) reported their marriages very happy. Shared prayer from the heart is very humbling, intimate behavior—as intimate as any soulful exchange between a man and woman. Those who pray together also more often say they respect their spouses, discuss their marriages together, and rate their spouses as skilled lovers. Likewise, those who worship regularly together are more often happily married than those who don't.

Happier yet are couples who frequently engage in both prayer and sex (though surely not simultaneously). Nine in ten couples that both pray together and sexually play together report themselves "very happy" with their marriages (and, as we've seen, usually therefore very happy with life itself). Thus, Greeley says, "sexual intimacy and prayerful intimacy are a very powerful combination."

The fourth ingredient of gratifying, enduring marriages is equity. "Within the scope of their own loving relationship," note New York University psychologists Irving and Suzanne Sarnoff, "mates are free to discard the premises of scarcity and hierarchy that now sow contention and exploitation throughout the world. Between the two of them, they have the opportunity to cooperate in establishing a classless utopia of social equality." Indeed, when both partners freely give and receive, when they share decision making, and when they enjoy activities together, their chances for sustained, satisfying love are good. When partners perceive their relationship as *in*equitable, they feel distressed. The one with the better deal may feel guilty; the one who senses a raw deal feels irritated. After surveying several hundred married couples of all ages, Iowa State University sociologists Robert Schafer and Patricia Keith confirmed this. Distress and depression most commonly appeared among those who felt their marriages were unfair because one spouse contributed too little to the cooking, housekeeping, and providing, or to the roles of companion and parent. As one well-known actress remarked, "I've been married to a fascist and married to a Marxist, and neither one of them took out the garbage."

When the psychological ingredients of marital happiness are present—kindred minds, sexual warmth, social intimacy, equitable giving and receiving of emotional and material resources—it becomes possible to contest the French saying that "love makes the time pass and time makes love pass." But it takes effort. And without effort marriages tend to decay. It takes effort to carve out time from each day for a tête-à-tête about the day's events and concerns. It takes effort, not just to nag and bicker, but to disclose and hear one another's hurts, concerns, and dreams. It takes effort *not* to take the partner's acceptance so for granted that we begin displaying our worst sides to those who matter most, while displaying kindness and politeness to utter strangers.

Study after study reveals that unhappy couples disagree, command, criticize, and put down, while happy couples more often agree, approve, assent, and laugh. One wonders: Would unhappy marriages brighten if the partners covenanted to self-consciously *act* more as happy couples do—by complaining and criticizing less, affirming and agreeing more? by setting times aside to discuss their marriage? by praying together daily? by risking the sorts of sexual behavior often reported in happy marriages (mutual undressing, showers together, leisurely sexual play)?

Is it possible that less happy couples, *by simulating the behavior of happy couples,* could themselves become happier? Don't bet against it. As attitudes often trail behaviors, so affections often trail actions.

But it won't be easy, especially when one's partner seems not to be making an equal commitment. Given the normal human tendency to see oneself as contributing more to a relationship than one's partner, it takes effort to aim to do slightly more than what seems like half. Yale psychologist Robert Sternberg believes that with such effort there is hope: " 'Living happily ever after' need not be a myth, but if it is to be a reality, the happiness must be based upon different configurations of mutual feelings at various times in a relationship. Couples who expect their passion to last forever, or their intimacy to remain unchallenged, are in for a disappointment. . . . We must constantly work at understanding, building, and rebuilding our loving relationships."

For those who succeed there comes the security, and the joy, of knowing love that is real. When someone "loves you for a long, long time," explained the wise, old Skin Horse to the Velveteen Rabbit,

"not just to play with, but REALLY loves you, then you become Real."

"Does it hurt?" asked the Rabbit.

"Sometimes," said the Skin Horse, for he was always truthful. "When you are Real you don't mind being hurt."

"Does it happen all at once, like being wound up," he asked, "or bit by bit?"

"It doesn't happen all at once," said the Skin Horse. "You become. It takes a long time. That's why it doesn't often happen to people who break easily, or have sharp edges, or who have to be carefully kept. Generally, by the time you are Real, most of your hair has been loved off, and your eyes drop out and you get loose in the joints and very shabby. But these things don't matter at all, because once you are Real you can't be ugly, except to people who don't understand."

10

Faith, Hope, and Joy

Joy is the serious business of Heaven.

C. S. LEWIS, *THE FOUR LOVES*

What makes for well-being? So far we have identified things that matter surprisingly little: Happiness is similarly available to those of any age, gender, race, location, education, even to those with a tragic disability. We have pondered things that do matter—physical fitness; renewing sleep and periodic solitude; traits such as self-esteem, sense of personal control, optimism, and extraversion; work and other activities that enhance our identity and absorb us into flow; close, supportive friendships and marriages.

Along the way we have exposed falsehoods, most notably the idea that more money, and the pleasures and possessions it buys, will make middle-class people happier. As we've seen, in the decade just finished, materialism has been our dominant ideology. But this American dream of prosperity achieved through individual initiative now seems at times like a nightmare.

For never has a century known such abundance, or such massive genocide and environmental devastation.

Never has a culture experienced such comfort and opportunity, or such widespread depression.

Never has a technology given us so many conveniences, or such terrible instruments of degradation and destruction.

Never have we been so self-reliant, or so lonely.

Never have we seemed so free, or our prisons so overstuffed.

Never have we had so much education, or such high rates of teen delinquency, despair, and suicide.

Never have we been so sophisticated about pleasure, or so likely to suffer broken or miserable marriages.

These are the best of times materially, but not for the human spirit. Facing an early death from brain cancer, President Bush's 1988 campaign manager, "bad boy" Lee Atwater, found his perspective changed:

> The '80s were about acquiring—acquiring wealth, power, prestige. I know. I acquired more wealth, power and prestige than most. But you can acquire all you want and still feel empty. What power wouldn't I trade for a little more time with my family? What price wouldn't I pay for an evening with friends? It took a deadly illness to put me eye to eye with that truth, but it is a truth that the country, caught up in its ruthless ambitions and moral decay, can learn on my dime. I don't know who will lead us through the '90s, but they must be made to speak to this spiritual vacuum at the heart of American society, this tumor of the soul.

Or listen to Jeff, a single, twenty-six-year-old advertising executive, who feels the spiritual vacuum even while enjoying the best of times:

> My life has been terrific the last few years—lots of money, women, friends, all sorts of activities and travel. My job is good and I am good at it. There is even a good future—I will probably be promoted this year and make lots more money and have freedom to

do what I want. But it all seems to lack any significance for me. Where is my life leading, why am I doing what I'm doing? I have the feeling that I am being carried along without ever making any real decisions or knowing what my goals are. It's sort of like getting on a road and driving along fine, but not knowing why you chose that particular road or where it is leading.

Having answered the question of *how* to make a living, the question of *why* we live often comes to mind. Like Jeff, we may wonder, "What's the point of it all?" Or having answered questions about the mechanics of the universe, we may wonder, as Stephen Hawking did in concluding *A Brief History of Time*, "why it is that we and the universe exist."

Such questions herald a decline in materialist values, argues Ronald Inglehart from his worldwide studies of shifting values. We see this most clearly in the demise of secular Marxism in Eastern Europe. But in the West, too, a new generation is maturing with decreasing concern for economic growth, social order, and strong defense and with increasing concern for political freedom, personal relationships, and the integrity of nature. This emerging "postmaterialism" provides fertile soil for a new consciousness that questions prosperity without purpose, money without meaning. After two decades of rising concern for "becoming well-off financially," the percentage of American collegians rating this a very important life goal finally began to taper off during 1989 and 1990.

We are, it seems, beginning to sense that, indeed, we can't live, fully, by bread alone. "A renewed concern for spiritual values" is beginning, reports Inglehart. Approaching a new millennium, and reflecting on the world we created in the last one, is moving humanity toward a new outlook. In today's world of multicultural mixing and changing values, tradition has lost its force, necessitating our defining a vision of life that is both conservative and radical—conserving social wisdom accumulated over generations while asserting that for our personal and environmental well-being there has to be another, less-traveled road than following our culture's individualism and materialism. At the peak of her fame and fortune, with 146 tennis championships behind her and married to John Lloyd, Chris Evert reflected, "We get into a rut.

We play tennis, we go to a movie, we watch TV, but I keep saying, 'John, there has to be more.' "

One sign of our spiritual hunger for something more is the recent fascination with the smorgasboard of New Age concerns, ranging from protecting nature, enhancing health, and promoting cooperation, peace, and spiritual transformation, to claims of crystal power, reincarnation, channeling, flying saucers, fortune-telling, aura readings, Ouija boards, numerology, witchcraft, harmonic convergences, and out-of-body frequent flier programs. Responding to this paranormal tidal wave, scientists say: "Yo, New Agers: Having a heart of gold doesn't require a head of feathers. Oughtn't we put testable claims to the test? If they work—if, say, aura readers really can detect the location of people behind a screen from the auras above their heads—then so much the better for the claims. If they don't then let's not be afraid to call the claims false."

To be sure, Christianity has itself been the source of goofy claims, some of which sucker people to empty their wallets to those who promise to intercede with a celestial Santa Claus. A mass mailing from the Don Stewart Evangelistic Association in Phoenix invited me to use a clip-out form to check off my desired miracle, be it "money to pay bills," "freedom from narcotics," or "solution to family problems." Contributions were, of course, welcome. One testimonial letter in Stewart's *Miracle* newspaper explained, "The last time I sent $10 to you to be used for God's work, God blessed me with an unexpected check in the amount of $159.74. I just can't out-give God." (One wonders, why not reinvest the $159.74 with Stewart?)

Another of Stewart's mailings enclosed a "miracle prayer cloth" that had touched Stewart's body. Like the woman who was healed upon touching Jesus' garment, I, too, could unleash God's miraculous power if I would write a wish on the prayer cloth envelope and mail it in with an offering (remembering Jesus' words, "Give and it shall be given"). After three days and nights of ardent fasting and prayer by Stewart

(that's how long Jesus was in the tomb before He was raised by a miracle) *THIS VERY SAME PIECE OF SHIRT MATERIAL from my body* will be sent back to you in the very envelope where you wrote your request. This is our point-of-release to expect something better from God. When you get this prayer cloth back, you are to carry it with you as a sign of our united faith for your SPECIAL MIRACLE.

I decided to test the Stewart miracle system. On my miracle envelope I asked this man of the cloth to get God "to stop Don Stewart from exploiting suffering people with his arrogant self-deification." A week later, as promised, my prayer cloth returned with a letter in which Stewart assured me, "for 3 days and 3 nights your special prayer requests and prayer cloth have been in my private prayer chamber and I've been praying. I've asked God to give you this special miracle . . . I really feel good about it! Victory is coming!"

Alas, in a subsequent mailing, Stewart sent "the most important personal confidential [computer-produced] letter I have ever written you. That's why I sent it to you personally . . . Kathy and I prayed and we felt led to tell YOU all about this. If I can't talk to you, then who could I tell about it?" He went on to explain that God spoke to him, explaining what I should do with my money. Funny thing, God said I was to give some of it to Don Stewart, even if I must borrow it—producing, he no doubt hoped, another victory for the Stewart miracle system.

It's sad. The world is so filled with people needing healing, comfort, and deliverance from despair that, today as always, any promises of such—whether through subliminal tapes or a faith healer's hot line to God—are certain to find a ready audience. Small wonder that the Old Testament prophet Jeremiah records God's lamenting that "my people have . . . forsaken me, the fountain of living water, and dug out cisterns for themselves, cracked cisterns that can hold no water." Small wonder that Jesus aimed his most stinging barbs at the pretentiously religious who presumed to have God in their pockets. Small wonder that so much of biblical religion is directed, as theologian Donald Bloesch has written, "not so much against godlessness or secularity as against human religion whereby man seeks to be God or to control God for his own ends." Small wonder that Langdon Gilkey could see the religious dimension of our existence as "not only the ground of its only hope but the source of life's deepest perversion."

But let's not discard the baby with the bathwater. As William

James emphasized a century ago, religion can be debilitating or vitalizing, sick or healthy. Every ideology is embarrassed by a kooky fringe. We can dismiss the fringe without rejecting the essence. We can challenge the irrational aspects of New Age occultism while welcoming its call to a deeper spirituality and environmental awareness. Likewise, we can acknowledge that people use *spiritual* to describe both sense and nonsense, while pondering spiritual answers to Hawking's question of why anything exists—why isn't there nothing?—and what meaning there can be to our own existence.

Every ideology, from Marxism to the American Dream to New Age pantheism, offers its hope of well-being. That includes biblical religion. Let us therefore dare to ask the practical question: Does it work? For our mental health and well-being, is biblical religion helpful or hazardous?

My focus on biblical religion implies no judgment on the mental health correlates of other religious faiths. Rather, it reflects, first, the Western context for most of the research. In North America and Europe, Christianity and Judaism are the prevalent faiths. Even with the recent wave of immigration almost nine in ten Americans call themselves Christian or Jewish, with only fractional percents claiming other faiths such as Islam, Buddhism, or Hinduism. Perhaps future research in other cultures will reveal how other faiths, too, nurture joy.

My drawing on a specific spiritual tradition also reflects my own world of understanding and experience, which is all that I can draw from with personal knowledge. Without my presuming I have ultimate answers (indeed, believing that everyone's beliefs err in some ways), perhaps what follows can stimulate readers of other persuasions to reflect on how their own spirituality contributes to well-being, or at least to comprehend and empathize with the significance of faith for many people.

There are two familiar, but contrasting, ideas about the impact of faith on well-being. Although Jesus offered no earthly exit from evil and suffering, he did proclaim the possibility of an underlying joy: "I have said these things to you so that my joy may be in you, and that your joy may be complete." Freud countered that, actually, religion is an illusion that *erodes* mental health or even becomes a sort of sickness—an "obsessional neurosis" accompanied by guilt, repressed sexuality, and suppressed emotions. Sifting the evidence won't decide the bigger issue of truth (happiness doesn't validate faith, for even fools may be happy in their delusions). But it can be thought-provoking.

Faith and Happiness

Survey after survey across North America and Europe reveals that religious people more often than nonreligious people report feeling happy and satisfied with life. Those who write about happiness have often presumed otherwise—that religion either restricts happiness or is irrelevant to it. Let's therefore look at the evidence.

The Gallup Organization interviewed a cross section of Americans, comparing those low in "spiritual commitment" (people who consistently disagree with statements such as, "God loves me even though I may not always please him" and "My religious faith is the most important influence in my life") with highly spiritual people, who consistently agree with such statements. Their finding: The highly spiritual were *twice* as likely to say they were "very happy."

Other surveys, too, reveal high levels of well-being among religiously active people. Three large-scale results: A 1982 survey of 9,000 Europeans found that among the "very happy" were 16 percent of atheists, 19 percent of "not religious" people, and 25 percent of those who said they were religious. In the United States, where reported happiness is somewhat higher, 31 percent of "somewhat" or "not very" religious people say they are "very happy"; but this rises to 41 percent among those who say their religious affiliation is "strong." In a 1980s survey of 166,000 people in fourteen nations, those "satisfied" or "very satisfied" with life included 77 percent of those who never attend church, 82 percent of those who attend occasionally, and 86 percent of those who attend weekly.

Many studies focused specifically on the link between religiousness and well-being among the elderly. In their statistical digest of the accumulated research, Morris Okun and William Stock at Arizona State University found that the two best predictors of well-being among older persons were health and religiousness. Elderly people are happier and more satisfied with life if religiously committed and active. "When I feel cranky," said one devout octogenarian, "I remember the words of an old hymn from Sunday school days, 'Count Your Blessings.' Count your many blessings—your friends, your family, your health, your hope that death won't have the last word."

When Terry Anderson emerged from 2,455 lost days as a hostage in Lebanon, having endured beatings, blindfolds, and months chained to furniture, he evinced a wide smile and remarkably little bitterness and hatred. Reporters wondered: Where did such strength come from? Anderson's reply: from the support of his companions, from his "stubbornness," and from his "faith" and constant prayer practiced in their private sanctuary, the Church of the Locked Door.

Studies have inspected this connection between faith and coping with a crisis. In a 1988 National Opinion Research Center survey of Americans, people who had recently suffered divorce, unemployment, bereavement, or serious illness or disability retained greater joy if they also had a strong faith. Compared to religiously inactive widows, recently widowed women who worship at their church or synagogue report more joy in their lives. Compared to irreligious mothers of developmentally disabled children, those with a deep religious faith are less vulnerable to depression. Compared to irreligious parents who have lost a child to Sudden Infant Death Syndrome, religiously committed parents are better able to find some meaning amid the trauma. "Religious faith buffers the negative effects of trauma on well-being," says Duke University sociologist Christopher Ellison.

One friend of mine, Helen, recalled "the darkest days in our lives," after her bright and beautiful first grade boy had his intelligence and gentle personality stolen by measles encephalitis. "Our pride and joy now exhibited uncontrollable, bizarre behaviors—calling people names, snatching candy, disobeying in every way imaginable. Our sleep was constantly interrupted, our once-happy family life stressed. I felt helpless." Her relief began with a church member's supportive call: "Let me take Billy for a day—you must need rest." It continued when, after much prayer, Helen found a fresh perspective and a new joy that led to her becoming an advocate for special-need children and a care giver to mentally impaired adults.

So, in these mostly North American studies, faith is a predictor of self-reported well-being and seems to facilitate coping with aging and personal crises. Does an active faith also entail less risk of psychological disorder?

In some respects, the links between religious faith and mental health are impressive—more so than many social scientists suspect. In America, religious people (often defined as those who attend church regularly) are *much less* likely to become delinquent. To abuse drugs and alcohol. To divorce or be unhappily married. Or to commit suicide. Religiously active people even tend to be *physically* healthier and to live longer. (Why is unclear, though it may be due to their healthier smoking-eating-drinking habits.)

With other mental health indicators the results are mixed. Religious people are somewhat *less* likely to feel in control of their fate. (They instead may see their future as divinely guided.) But they also are somewhat less likely to become depressed and be diagnosed as suffering a psychological disorder such as schizophrenia.

I hasten to add two reminders. First, the link between faith and well-being is not by itself grounds for religious belief. The key issue for belief should be truth: If a religious understanding was known to be true, but was discomfiting, what honest person would want to disbelieve? If known to be untrue, though comforting, what honest person would want to believe? If God doesn't exist, I suppose one might argue that any god will do; it matters little what faith you have so long as you have faith in something. Religion becomes self-therapy. But surely a faith that is knowingly make-believe is a pale faith, more a vague spirituality than the sort of robust faith known by those who think their cosmic vision really captures significant truth. Truth, and one's confidence in it, matters.

Second, both the research findings and human history tell us that faith is hardly a guarantee of bliss. We need look no further than the heroes of faith to see that no one is promised "good adjustment" and freedom from negative emotion. In the New Testament, Jesus and his followers feel anger in response to injustice, anxiety when confronted with danger, grief in the face of death. No pretentious testimonies here of "how I found self-perfection and bliss." In the Old Testament, Job reminds us that God's people aren't promised beds of roses. Faith or no, our emotions and genetic predispositions will have their effects, our loved ones will be vulnerable to setbacks and tragedies, our mortality rate will be 100 percent. As the theologian Reinhold Niebuhr cautioned, any faith system founded on a hope of special protection from natural forces and human passions "is bound to suffer disillusionment."

What Faith Offers

Although faith does not promise immunity from suffering or escape from stress, it is, as we've seen, linked with enhanced joy and strength in times of crisis. How so? Why do researchers find these positive links among faith, mental health, and happiness?

We all benefit from being connected to a caring community, from a sense of significance, from experiencing humility and deep acceptance, from a focus beyond ourselves, and from a perspective on life's tragedies, especially death. In leaning on both empirical science and biblical religion in what follows, I don't mean to suggest that my profession and spiritual tradition alone capture truth or that other traditions don't meet these (or other) needs. My aim is simply to illustrate concretely, from research findings and from people's experiences, how an active faith can meet deep human needs.

Where Two or Three Are Gathered. One message of this book concerns the price we pay for self-reliant individualism. University of Pennsylvania researcher Martin Seligman attributes today's widespread depression to "rampant individualism . . . without commitment to the common good." Our expectations have soared, yet

> life is inevitably full of personal failures. Our stocks go down, people we love reject us, we write bad papers, we don't get the job we want, we give bad lectures. When larger, benevolent institutions (God, nation, family) are available, they help us cope with personal loss and give us a framework for hope. Without faith in these institutions, we interpret personal failures as catastrophic. They seem to last forever and contaminate all of life. The new emphasis on the self raises the chances that we will blame these

misfortunes, losses and disappointments on ourselves and thus depress ourselves.

Either the emphasis on individualism alone or the loss of faith in institutions [religion, country, family] alone would increase our vulnerability to depression. The recent combination of the two, I believe, is a surefire recipe for an epidemic of depression.

It wasn't always so. John Winthrop, who in 1630 led one of the first groups of Puritans to land on American shores, spoke to his people on board ship in Salem harbor just before landing. He described the communal life he and his followers were intending to found: "We must delight in each other, make others' conditions our own, rejoyce together, mourn together, labor and suffer together, always having before our eyes our community as members of the same body."

As Winthrop illustrates, Judaic and Christian life center not on the self or the mystical visions of isolated people, but on communities of faith. In Old Testament culture, tribe and clan identities were so strong that whole groups were sometimes punished for the wickedness of individual members. In the New Testament, St. Paul taught that Christians were to see themselves as complementary parts of one body. Jesus developed his ministry with a small group and promised to be present whenever two or three gathered in his name. In biblical religion, communal images are everywhere—in the fellowship of kindred spirits, the bearing of one another's burdens, the ties of love that bind.

After interviewing a small sample of Americans, University of California sociologist Robert Bellah and his associates lamented the triumph of modern individualism. Today's people glory in their successes, yet deep down in the seldom-acknowledged realms of their being, they know something is missing. "John, there has to be more." Part of what's missing, says Bellah, is a sense of connectedness, belonging, mutuality, being part of a people.

In the United States, as in much of the world, the most common communal setting for finding such social identity and support is the local religious community. A vivid example of a close-knit religious community is Pennsylvania's old order the Amish, a Protestant sect known for their agrarian, nonmaterialistic culture, their pacifism, and their self-sufficient communal life. Within this unified and supportive culture, major depression occurs about one fifth to one tenth as often as elsewhere in the United States.

Even in modern America, with its 294,000 congregations, nearly everyone is within a walk or short drive of some care-giving fellowship. I think of my own experience in a church care network that comes together just around the corner and down the block. As I write this, my friend Marcia—a talented teacher, vibrant woman, caring wife, and mother of two teenagers—is in the hospital for yet another round of therapy on the cancer that ominously ravages her body. Once again, an informal church love squad mobilizes. She's given pastoral care. She's sent cards and flowers. She's transported between hospitals. Meals to her home are scheduled. Marcia's faith doesn't alter her mortality. (Physical healing for any of us is only, in different words, delaying death. We're all terminal cases.) But if we at Hope Church are the church in action, she and hers will not walk this dark valley alone. And we each know that when our family's turn comes to face the darkness, we, too, will not be walking alone. The ties that bind also uphold and support.

Something Worth Living and Dying for. Is the greater happiness of religiously active people due merely to their being more socially active and connected? After statistically extracting the effect of general social activity, a link between faith and well-being remains. This allows us to speculate that another part of what's missing in today's culture is a sense of meaning and purpose in living. The nineteenth-century Polish poet Cyprian Norwid wrote, "To be what is called happy, one should have (1) something to live on, (2) something to live for, (3) something to die for. The lack of one of these results in drama. The lack of two results in tragedy." It's not enough to know, as the cynic does, the price of everything and the value of nothing.

Searching for something more, religious seekers have quested for enlightenment. Siddhartha Gautama, whom we know as Buddha, left behind a princely life of luxury in search of spiritual illumination. Realizing the inevitability of sickness, aging, and death, he sought a way to transcend the human condition. Muhammad searched for Allah while secluded in a hill cave near Mecca. Reflecting on the properous Meccan merchants' neglect of their duties to the unfortunate, he had a spiritual vision that began his prophetic career. Each of us, too, yearns for something more—a sense of meaning, a sense of life's significance, a sense of life's purpose.

Studies confirm that an important ingredient of well-being is the sense of meaning and purpose that many people find in their faith. Clinical researcher Seligman believes that a loss of meaning accentuates today's epidemic depression, and that finding meaning requires "an attachment to something larger than the lonely self. To the extent that young people now find it hard to take seriously their relationship with God, to care about their relationship with the country or to be part of a large and abiding family, they will find it very difficult to find meaning in life. To put it another way, the self is a very poor site for finding meaning."

Rabbi Harold Kushner speaks for many when he writes, "My religious faith . . . satisfies . . . the most fundamental human need of all. That is the need to know that somehow we matter, that our lives mean something, count as something more than just a momentary blip in the universe." Psychiatrist Viktor Frankl concluded similarly, after observing lowered apathy and death rates among fellow concentration camp inmates who retained a sense of meaning—a purpose for which to live, or even to die. Many of these were devout Jews whose faith provided a deeply internalized purpose that gave a reason for living and for resisting their oppressors.

For psychologist Mihaly Csikszentmihalyi the ultimate in well-being is to have all of one's life flowing toward an overriding goal, a unifying life theme, that gives meaning to all our lesser goals. For one man, a childhood experience of injustice ignited a determination that led him to law school and ultimately to become a national civil rights leader. For others, the life theme may be to educate, to make excellent products, to discover, to learn. For still others, such goals may be derived from a religious theme, as in Martin Luther King's statement, "My obligation is to do the right thing. The rest is in God's hands."

Two thousand years ago the Jewish sage Hillel similarly urged a focus beyond self: "To begin with oneself, but not to end with oneself; to start with oneself, but not to aim at oneself; to comprehend oneself, but not to be preoccupied with oneself." This sense of commitment to something beyond ourselves usually grows from life in community. If I understand anything from my own decade of experiments on group discussion it is this: When people interact, their shared ideas get magnified (through a process we call "group polarization"). This mutual strengthening can have dire consequences, as when terrorism emerges from the radicalization of those mutually discontented. Or it can be beneficial, as when strengthening the resolve of those in a self-help group. It's tough to be a minority of one, to sustain a purely private faith, to hold to one's Mennonite convictions while living alone in Los Angeles. For the members of early Christian cell groups, for members of religious orders, and for all believers, conviction and commitment grows when shared.

This helps us understand the findings of a recent national Gallup survey analyzed by Princeton University sociologist Robert Wuthnow. Religious individualists—those who say they develop their own spirituality independent of any church—are less likely than those within the church to value caring for the needy and to contribute time to charitable activities. The more often people claim to experience divine love, the more likely they are to volunteer time, *if* they attend church regularly. Other studies confirm, says Wuthnow, "that spirituality begins to move people toward being compassionate only when a threshold of involvement in some kind of collective religious activity has been reached."

Humility and Ultimate Acceptance. At no point does today's pop psychology seem further from biblical thought than in its recipe for self-worth. "Go for it!" the modern wisdom urges us. Reach for the stars. Believe the best about yourself. Don't let your perceived limitations hem you in. Dream the impossible dream. Seek that more perfect love, that ecstatic pleasure. Raise creative, successful children. Make more money than you ever dreamed possible. Above all, replace your negative inner dialogue with positive affirmations about yourself. Think positive. Talk positive. Feel positive. You can do it. You can be happy, secure, at peace, once your ambitions are realized—your bank account fat, your children raised, your reputation established, your outlook more self-applauding.

As we've seen, there is considerable wisdom to positive thinking. With good reason, we can affirm positive thinking—with but one cautionary reminder: Not all dreams come true. Among my life's closest friends was my lovable, caring college roommate, Dan Gates. Not only were we intimate friends, so were our fiancées. As married couples still in college we therefore spent hours in one another's apartments sharing laughter and dreams. Throughout college, Dan was fired by a dream of becoming a doctor. Although some doubted he would make it, Dan dared to believe. But the doubters were right. When no medical school accepted him, Dan was let down. Nevertheless, he picked himself up and used his biology training in teaching, with hopes of becoming a high school counselor. Again, it wasn't to be. Although loved by his wife, friends, and students, the crushing of dreams combined with a growing sense of futility and worthlessness led Dan one summer day to pull his car off a Seattle freeway. There he descended into a ravine, pulled out a gun, and put a bullet through his broken heart.

To those struggling for self-worth there is an alternative, more ancient and paradoxical road. Take a step back. "Happy are those who know they are spiritually poor," offered Jesus. Set aside vanity. Become as unpretentious as a small child. Face your spiritual poverty and emptiness. Recognize that everyone, eventually, will let you down or fail to meet your emotional needs. No human will ever love you the way you want to be loved, because, wrote Mignon McLaughlin, "no one has ever loved anyone the way everyone wants to be loved."

Faith provides "unspeakable comfort," yet one gets to that comfort by first facing dismay. William James noted that, ironically, self-esteem rises as pretensions fall.

Our self-feeling in this world depends entirely on . . . a fraction of which our pretentions are the denominator and the numerator our success. Thus,

$$\text{Self-esteem} = \frac{\text{Success}}{\text{Pretensions.}}$$

Such a fraction may be increased as well by diminishing the denominator as by increasing the numerator. To give up pretensions is as blessed a relief as to get them gratified; and where disappointment is incessant and the struggle unending, this is what men will always do. The history of evangelical theology, with its conviction of sin, its self-despair, and its abandonment of salvation by works, is the deepest of possible examples, but we meet others in every walk of life . . . How pleasant is the day when we give up striving to be young—or slender! Thank God! we say, those illusions are gone. Everything added to the Self is a burden as well as a pride.

James echoes the psalmist's experience: "Lord, I have given up my pride and turned away from my arrogance . . . I am content and at peace." It can be liberating to admit our pride and our limitations. To say okay, I'll never be a great public speaker, or the top person in my company, or a great athlete may be temporarily depressing, but permanently freeing. We can be freed from living daily with the guilt of things unaccomplished, from needing to blame ourselves or others. We can be freed to focus on what we can do something about. Think of Alcoholics Anonymous. Their Twelve Steps begin with Step One: Admit that one is helpless, hopeless, powerless. Stand up each meeting and acknowledge, "My name is Joe, and I am an alcoholic." The march forward begins with a step back.

Then comes self-acceptance. The whole of Christianity really boils down to a simple, if unlikely, statement of good news: The universe has a Creator whose extraordinary love compelled this Spirit-Being to assume a human form, to experience suffering, and to break the bonds of death, thereby assuring us that we matter, that we are accepted, that we can live with hope. The radical and liberating implication: No longer is there any need to define our self-worth solely by our achievements, material well-being, or social approval. To find self-acceptance we needn't be or do anything. We need simply to accept that we are, ultimately and unconditionally, accepted. People who have this idea of God—as loving, accepting, caring—tend to enjoy greater self-esteem. They even enjoy warmer marriages, reports survey researcher Andrew Greeley. There is, it seems, an interplay between our God-concept and our self-concept, our personal theology and our psychology.

The story of Pinocchio expresses our need for acceptance. As Pinocchio ponders his life, he flounders in a terrible confusion about his self-worth. Finally he turns to his maker Geppetto and reflects, "Pappa, I am not sure who I am. But if I'm all right with you, then I guess I'm all right with me." I am accepted, and can accept myself, just as I am. It's rather like the delicious experience of having someone know our secret thoughts and still think we're lovable. That's how it is in the best of relationships, where we no longer feel the need to justify ourselves or to be on guard, where we are free to be spontaneous without fear of losing the other's esteem. Jesus' Sermon on the Mount paradox—"Happy are those who know they are spiritually poor; the Kingdom of Heaven belongs to them!"—is a way of saying that we don't need to create or prove our self-worth, we need only accept it. Relinquish vanity and illusion, and then receive what we have been struggling to get.

Sociologist Christopher Ellison has found that the spiritual disciplines of prayer and meditation enhance many people's sense of acceptance and intimate relationship. In their book, *The Varieties of Prayer*, sociologist Margaret Poloma and pollster George Gallup report that nine in ten Americans pray from time to time and that 88 percent of these people say they sometimes experience a deep sense of peace and well-being while doing so.* As they mentally share their deepest desires and concerns in prayer, they may experience a sense of solace and guidance. For these people, "What a friend we have in Jesus" is more than a corny song; it expresses their feelings of being intimately known, supported, and valued by a divine other. Such feelings add a sense of significance to their lives.

Losing and Finding One's Life. The experience of grace—of "unconditional positive regard" as we today might say—in turn provides a model for human relationships. To be instruments of grace is to approach others with an accepting attitude that values their individuality and affirms their worthwhileness. Fred Rogers, a Presbyterian minister known to preschoolers as television's Mister Rogers, builds his program

*The universality of prayer was never more apparent than on October 27, 1986, when leaders of a dozen faiths joined the pope, the archbishop of Canterbury, the dalai lama, two American Indian chiefs, the Shinto Shrine Association president, and Rome's chief rabbi in Assisi, Italy, for a World Day of Prayer for Peace. At the Cathedral of St. Francis, who once prayed "Lord, make me an instrument of your peace," each group prayed in the presence of the others.

on his conviction that "everybody longs to be loved and longs to know that he or she is lovable. And consequently the greatest thing that we can do is to help somebody know that they are loved and capable of loving."

In focusing on others' needs, we also discover meaning beyond the self. The New Testament's four books on Jesus' life all record his teaching that to find life we must be willing to lose our lives. To find meaning we must discover something bigger than ourselves, and serve it. Living beyond the self is therefore a part of Catholic wisdom, as explained by Richard Rohr and Joseph Martos: "Paradoxically, personal fulfillment means abandoning ourselves and putting others first. In the Catholic tradition, ultimate satisfaction is promised to those who give up their desire for self-satisfaction. This is part of the meaning of crucifixion. The cross leads to resurrection, to new life. When we let go of ourselves, our lives become filled with grace. The lives of St. Francis of Assisi, Pope John XXIII and Mother Teresa of Calcutta radiate a grace that people of all religious traditions admire."

Malcolm Muggeridge visited Mother Teresa in Calcutta after interviewing her for the BBC. "The thing I noticed about you and the hundreds of sisters who now form your team is that you all look so happy. Is it a put-on?" he asked. "Oh no," she replied, "not at all. Nothing makes you happier than when you really reach out in mercy to someone who is badly hurt."

As if to test Mother Teresa's idea, psychologist Bernard Rimland did an experiment. He asked 216 students to list the initials of 10 people they knew best, yielding a grand list of some 2,000 people. He then asked them to indicate whether each person seemed happy or not. Finally, he asked them to go over each name again, indicating if the person seemed selfish (devoted mostly to his or her own welfare) or unselfish (willing to be inconvenienced for others). The striking result: 70 percent of those judged unselfish seemed happy; 95 percent of those judged selfish seemed *un*happy. What a paradox, said the surprised Rimland: "Selfish people are, by definition, those whose activities are devoted to *bringing themselves happiness*. Yet, at least as judged by others, these selfish people are far *less* likely to be happy than those whose efforts are devoted to making others happy."

Again, the thinking person wonders *why*: why this correlation between selfless, altruistic living and happiness. Certainly one reason—a reason for my writing this book—is that happiness makes people less self-focused and more altruistic. But it works the other way around too. Doing good makes us feel good. Altruism enhances our self-esteem. It gets our eyes off ourselves, makes us less self-preoccupied, gets us closer to the unself-consciousness that characterizes the flow state.

We've noted links between faith and well-being and between altruism and well-being. Can we close the circle by linking faith and altruism? Visible extremes don't decide the issue. The example of Mother Teresa suggests such a link, and the biblical idea of the sacred worth and essential equality of all human lives provides a spiritual ground for humanitarian values. No wonder the National Opinion Research Center in 1992 reported that those who pray at least daily are half again as likely to oppose the death penalty as those who pray less than once a week. But some other religious personalities, such as televangelist Jim Bakker with his luxurious mansions and gold-plated bathroom fixtures, have not impressed us with their altruism. As Madeleine L'Engle lamented, "Christians have given Christianity a bad name."

Tangential to the religion-altruism question is Christianity's curious links with attitudes of love and hate. History paints a confusing picture in which the extremes seem to cancel each other out: We think of the Bible-thumping slave owners, Ku Klux Klanners, and apartheid defenders; but then we also think of the clergy and lay leadership in the antislavery cause, and the church's prophetic role in the U.S. and South African civil rights movements and in the establishment of third world hospitals.

A midcentury spate of religion-prejudice studies painted a similarly mixed picture: On the one hand, American church members expressed more racial prejudice than nonmembers, and those with conservative Christian beliefs expressed more prejudice than those less conservative. For many people, religion seems a cultural habit—something not so much practiced as professed by those who adhere to their community's attitudes and traditions. But then again, *faithful* church attenders expressed less prejudice than nominal members; clergy were more supportive of civil rights efforts than laypeople; and those for whom religion was an end ("my religious beliefs are what really lie behind my whole approach to life") were less prejudiced than those who used religion as a means ("a primary reason for my interest in religion is that my church is a congenial social activity").* Ergo, among churchgoers, the devout were consistently less prejudiced than were those who gave religion lip service. "We have just enough religion to make us hate, but not enough to make us love one another," lamented the eighteenth-century satirist Jonathan Swift.

Some have enough religion to make them love. With Nazi submarines sinking ships faster than the Allied forces could replace them, the troop ship SS *Dorchester* steamed out of New York harbor with 904 men headed for Greenland. Among those leaving anxious families behind were four chaplains, Methodist preacher George Fox, Rabbi Alexander Goode, Catholic priest John Washington, and Reformed Church minister Clark Poling. Some 150 miles from their destination, U-456 caught the *Dorchester* in its cross hairs. Within moments of a torpedo's impact, reports Lawrence Elliott, stunned men were pouring out from their bunks as the ship began listing. With power cut off, the escort vessels, unaware of the unfolding tragedy, pushed on in the darkness. On board, chaos reigned as panicky men came up from the hold without life jackets and leaped into overcrowded lifeboats.

When the four chaplains made it up to the steeply sloping deck, they began guiding the men to their boat stations. They opened a storage locker, distributed life jackets, and coaxed the men over the side. In the icy, oil-smeared water, Private William Bednar heard the chaplains preaching courage and found the strength to swim until he reached a life raft. Still on board, Grady Clark watched in awe as the chaplains handed out the last life jacket, and then, with ultimate selflessness, gave away their own. As Clark slipped into the waters he saw the chaplains standing—their arms linked—praying, in Latin, Hebrew, and English. Other men, now serene, joined them in a huddle as the *Dorchester* slid beneath the sea.

Does the heroism of the four chaplains rightly suggest that faith somehow promotes courage and caring? Most altruism studies explore

*In several recent studies, those whose religion is an end (the "intrinsically religious") also exhibited more positive mental health.

spontaneous helping acts. Confronted with a minor emergency, as when hearing someone in the next room fall off a ladder, highly religious people are not more responsive than those who are irreligious. But when they are making intentional choices about long-term altruism, the differences do become real. Sam Levenson's jest, "When it comes to giving, some people stop at nothing" is seldom true among church and synagogue members. They give away more of their money than do the unaffiliated. A 1989 Gallup poll revealed that nine in ten church members, but only seven in ten nonmembers, gave money to a charity during the previous year. The Gallup Organization also reports that of the $41.4 billion given by individuals to American congregations in 1986, 46 percent was donated to other organizations or allocated to activities other than religious programming. This percentage rises higher if we count the food, clothing, and shelter given to social service programs by six of ten congregations.

Or consider these surprising facts from a 1990 analysis of *Faith and Philanthropy in America* based on a 1987 Gallup survey for Independent Sector. Two thirds of all giving to secular charities comes from contributors who also give to religious organizations.* The faith-philanthropy effect is especially striking among the devout. American adults who say they never attend church or synagogue reported giving away 1.1 percent of their incomes; weekly attenders are two and a half times as generous. Although representing only 24 percent of contributing Americans, weekly church attenders give 48 percent of total individual contributions. The other three quarters of Americans give the remaining half. A follow-up 1989 Gallup survey for Independent Sector confirmed the basic pattern: Nonattenders reported giving 0.8 percent of their household income. Occasional attenders—those attending religious services once or twice a month—gave twice as much, 1.5 percent. Weekly attenders gave twice again as much, 3.8 percent.

Religious consciousness, it seems, shapes a larger agenda than advancing one's own private little world. It cultivates the idea that my talents and wealth are unearned gifts of which I am the steward.

---

*Individual contributors account for nearly 90 percent of charitable contributions. The American Association of Fund-Raising Counsel Trust for Philanthropy estimates that of the $122.6 billion contributed during 1990, $7.1 billion came from foundations, $5.9 billion from corporations, $7.8 billion from individuals' bequests, and $101.8 billion from individuals' gifts.

Spirituality, notes Boston College sociologist Paul Schervish, also directs one's priorities "into a bond of care for others." Despite the well-publicized greed of a few preachers, the fact remains that a religious consciousness has nourished many care-giving social movements, including the establishment of universities and universal public education, the worldwide spread of hospitals, human rights movements, peace initiatives, and many of today's soup kitchens for the homeless.

Across America, new community organizations have disproportionately been started by people with a deep religious consciousness. In my own midwestern community, for example, the Head Start day-care program was envisioned in a prayer group at the church where it still operates. The community's two nongovernmental agencies for assisting the underclass both were begun by churches. Annually, over three thousand townspeople—99 percent from churches—gather for a world hunger walk, for which they are sponsored by many thousands more in their churches. Reading the research, and just looking around me, I can appreciate Frank Emerson Andrews's conclusion that "religion is the mother of philanthropy."

As religion cultivates giving, so the dismal science of economics cultivates selfishness. Or so Cornell University economist Robert Frank and psychologists Thomas Gilovich and Dennis Regan conclude from their recent survey of college professors nationwide. Despite having relatively high salaries, economists, most of whom assume that self-interest drives behavior, were more than twice as likely as those in other disciplines to contribute no money to private charities. In responding to public television appeals, their median (and most common) gift was zilch. In laboratory monetary games, students behave more selfishly after taking economics courses. Such findings suggest the need, conclude Frank, Gilovich, and Regan, for an alternative model of human behavior, one that teaches the benefits of cooperation.

Religiously motivated people, many of whom have an alternative model, also give away more of themselves. Among the one in eight Americans whom George Gallup in 1984 classified as "highly spiritually committed," 46 percent said they were presently working among the poor, the infirm, or the elderly—many more than the 22 percent among those "highly uncommitted." That striking finding was confirmed in the 1989 survey: Charitable and social service volunteering was reported by 28 percent of those who rated religion "not very important" and by 50 percent of those who said religion is "very important" in their lives. The latest Gallup survey for Independent Sector revealed a similar near-doubled rate of volunteerism when comparing those who attend religious services weekly with those who never attend.

One such care-giving person, nurtured by a community into a grace-filled faith worth living and losing himself for, was a young Scot, Eric Liddell. Thanks to the Oscar-winning movie *Chariots of Fire*, the world remembers him as the man who, rather than run on Sunday, gave up his chance for a likely Olympic gold medal in the 100 meters. After being called a traitor to his country, he astonished everyone by running and winning the 400-meter race in world-record time. Although Liddell returned home a national hero, paraded on shoulders through the streets of Edinburgh, his greater heroism began where the movie ended. Shunning fame, fortune, and the next Olympics, he slipped out of the limelight to become a missionary to China. There he taught, worked, and undertook daring rescues amid suffering and death caused by Japan's invasion during the late 1930s.

With his warmth and a smiling good nature, he often served as peacemaker both among peasants and between them and their invaders. When his young family left for the safety of home, Liddell stayed to minister, and in 1943 the Japanese rounded him and eighteen hundred other foreigners into the Shantung Compound, the Spartan internment camp described in Chapter 3. During the ensuing months he emerged as its "most outstanding personality," the joyful one "with the permanent smile." It was Liddell who organized games and worship, taught science to the children, put up shelves for a Russian prostitute (the only man who did anything for her without wanting repayment, she said). University of Chicago theologian Langdon Gilkey's stark recollections of the self-centeredness exposed by privation is broken by this ray of light:

It is rare indeed that a person has the good fortune to meet a saint, but he came as close to it as anyone I have ever known. Often [I] would pass the games room and peer in to see what the missionaries had cooking for the teenagers. As often as not Eric . . . would be bent over a chessboard or a model boat, or directing some sort of square dance—absorbed, warm and interested, pouring all of himself into this effort to capture the minds and imaginations of those penned-up youths. If anyone could have done it, he could. . . . He was in his middle forties, lithe and springy of step and, above all, overflowing with good humor and love of life. He was aided by others, to be sure. But it was Eric's enthusiasm and charm that carried the day.

By all accounts, Liddell was one in whom faith, joy, and altruism formed an unbroken circle; one whose life was empowered by the hour of Scripture study, prayer, and meditation with which he began each day before the others were awake; one who befriended the most despised internees and bridged the gulf between them and the others; one who could be seen carrying burdens for the elderly; one who offered to sell his Olympic gold watch to buy more sports gear for the children; one who, weakened by privation and hunger, began quietly to suffer headaches and discouragement, the early signs of a brain disease that, before many even realized he was ill, took his life just months before the camp's liberation. As he lay in the arms of a friend, nurse Annie Buchan, he spoke his last words, "Anne, it's complete surrender," lapsed into a coma, and died within hours. When word reached home, all Scotland mourned its lost hero.

Mother Teresa, Eric Liddell, and countless unpretentious people, some known to each of us, attest to a love that can flow from lives surrendered to a meaning beyond self, lives touched by grace. They may not have lived "the good life," but they unquestionably lived good lives, lives marked by purpose, peace, and joy, lives that attest to a possibility envisioned by the Jewish prophet Isaiah: "Those who wait for the Lord shall renew their strength, they shall mount up with wings like eagles, they shall run and not be weary, they shall walk and not faint."

An Eternal Perspective. Liddell's joy while enduring privation and threat of death was sustained by one other aspect of his faith—his *hope* that the evils of suffering and death were not the last word. Writing from a college whose symbol is the Anchor of Hope, I think it fitting that I conclude this book with Samuel Johnson's reminder that "hope is itself a species of happiness, and, perhaps, the chief happiness which this world affords." Some years ago, when young Germans were asked what they thought the most beautiful word in human speech, the leading vote getter was not "joy," "love," or "happiness," but "hope."

The hope that uplifted Eric Liddell and Mother Teresa does not wish away evil. Andrew Carnegie wished away evil when in 1900—two hundred million human casualties ago—he forecast that in the twentieth century "to kill a man will be considered as disgusting as we in this day consider it disgusting to eat one." Today we *wish* for a world without genocide, crack babies, AIDS, Alzheimer's disease, the greenhouse effect, family abuse, and nuclear bombs. But that is not where biblical hope resides. Hope confronts such evils and sees beyond them to an eternal reality visioned by Isaiah: "The heavens will vanish like smoke, the earth will wear out like a garment, and those who live on it will be like gnats; but my salvation will be forever, and my deliverance will never be ended." And reenvisioned by John of Patmos: "I saw a new heaven and a new earth . . . and I heard a loud voice from the throne saying, 'See, the home of God is among mortals. He will dwell with them as their God, and . . . will wipe every tear from their eyes. Death shall be no more; mourning and crying and pain will be no more, for the first things have passed away.' " This world, imply these visionaries, is but a shadow of one to come.

Viewing life with this eternal perspective has several consequences. First, a hope-filled optimism about the big future moderates our anxiety about the immediate future. If I can believe that my long-term destiny is in God's loving hands, then I can cope with whatever awaits me from now till death. I can trust that, come what may, all will turn out well in the end, the very end.

Viewing life's problems from the perspective of the big future helps put in perspective today's aggravations—waiting for a delayed plane, having the car break down, spilled catsup on a shirt, even a family quarrel. So many of the things that once riled can now be seen for what they are—trivial, temporary irritants. Surely Pascal was right in thinking it "a monstrous thing" to see people raging or despairing over mere affronts and inconveniences, while being indifferent to "things of gravest import."

A British veteran reflected on his experience with things of gravest import after sailing with Russia-bound convoys through German-submarine-infested icy waters: "There are two things that I shall always remember. The first is the sound of men's voices in the sea at night, when you can't stop to pick them up . . . and the other is the sound of people's voices complaining in the shops at home."

Second, a hope of life beyond death can help us come to terms with the great enemy, death. Psychologists Sheldon Solomon (Skidmore College), Jeff Greenberg (University of Arizona), and Tom Pyszczynski (University of Colorado at Colorado Springs) argue that all worldviews are efforts to cope with "the terror resulting from our awareness of vulnerability and death." Cultural worldviews define how to live good and meaningful lives, and to hope for meaning or life beyond death. Different faiths offer different paths, but each offers its adherents a sense that they, or something meaningful they are part of, will survive their death. Thus they all speak to our ultimate goal, self-preservation.

Facing the terror of our mortality, being aware of life's impermanence, also adds value to our present moments. Being emotionally freed to admit life's fragility and our inevitable mortality helps us appreciate the life we enjoy right now. Facing rather than denying death prepares us to celebrate life. Staring death in the face, Betty, a twenty-four-year-old woman with terminal leukemia, treasures each remaining day. "When you think that there are years ahead, it is so easy to put things off. You say to yourself, 'I'll stop and smell the flowers next spring.' But when you know that the days of your life are limited, you stop to smell the flowers and to feel the warm sunlight *today*." As a future-oriented person, I periodically remind myself of Pascal's remark that too often we live as if the past and present were merely our means to the future. "So we never live, but we hope to live—and as we are always preparing to be happy, it is inevitable we should never be so."

In his Christmas letter, a seventy-three-year-old friend contemplates his mortality: "The passing of three close friends this past summer has made us more conscious of the swift flight of time. It also has brought heaven closer and given us a clearer perspective on the relation of eternity to our life here. That meditation, in turn, enhances appreciation and enriches life in other ways. Yet many avoid such reflection and fill their minds with, well, just about anything else." Rather than delighting in the gift of each day, the people are walking to and fro, talking of some peccadillo.

The essence of happiness is pausing to savor the gift of our present moments. For me that means taking delight in the successive moments of my day, from morning tea and cereal, hunched over a manuscript, to the day's last moments of consciousness, snuggling and talking with Carol. Happiness isn't in the future, but in this noon's meal with a friend, in this evening's bedtime story with a child, in tonight's curling up with a good book.

Third, the eternal perspective emboldens us to think that human life has value. What is worth preserving, forever, must be of ultimate value. Moreover, the utopian resurrection vision of peace, justice, and love directs our involvement in the here and now. It defines an ideal world—a back-to-the-present vision—and enables courage to risk oneself in working toward it. Thus Martin Luther King could declare, "I have a dream," a vision of a future reality, of a world liberated from oppression and suffering. With a dream worth dying for, and a hope that even death could not kill it, he could also declare, "If physical death is the price I must pay to free my white brothers and sisters from a permanent death of the spirit, then nothing can be more redemptive."

It was this dream, the eternal perspective, that enabled the German theologian-pastor Dietrich Bonhoeffer to endure two years in a Nazi prison before being executed for his opposition to Hitler; that emboldened El Salvador's only doctoral-level psychologist, Father Ignacio Martin-Baro, after six assassination attempts, to continue publishing data exposing Salvadorean poverty and oppression until finally being gunned down, along with five fellow Jesuits and two of their helpers, by a military death squad; that empowered Romanian pastor Laszlo Tokes to protest the brutal oppression of Nicolae Ceausescu, to suffer being banned, harassed, beaten, and stabbed until finally his people, forming a protective human chain around his church and parsonage said, "Enough!" and ignited a revolution that in three days swept the entire country. As Rubem Alves put it, "Hope is hearing the melody of the future. Faith is to dance to it."

Taken together, the things that faith offers—the communal ties, the deep sense of purpose, the feeling of ultimate acceptance, the challenge of meaningful altruism, and the eternal perspective—enhance well-being. But might not Mother Teresa, Eric Liddell, Martin Luther King, Dietrich Bonhoeffer, Ignacio Martin-Baro, and Laszlo Tokes all have been deluded? How can we be sure faith is not a farce, an illusion, an opiate we've invented to keep life from seeming pointless, futile, terminal?

We can't be sure. Moreover, the honest words "belief," "faith," and "hope" concede uncertainty. We do not *believe* that two times two is four. We do not have *faith* that a ball tossed up will come down. We do not *hope* that day will follow night. We *know* these things, with psychological certainty. On matters more ultimate, such certainty is hard to come by, noted C. S. Lewis: "Believe in God and you will have to face hours when it seems *obvious* that this material world is the only reality; disbelieve in Him and you must face hours when this material world seems to shout at you that it is *not* all. No conviction, religious or irreligious, will, of itself, end once and for all [these doubts] in the soul. Only the practice of Faith resulting in the habit of Faith will gradually do that."

To those who, after wrestling with truth, remain uncertain, wavering at a crossroad between faith and unbelief, there comes the secondary question of which path leads to joy. To take the leap into active faith is to bet one's life on a worldview that makes sense of the universe, that gives meaning to life, that offers hope in the face of adversity and death, that provides vision and courage for living in the present. The tools of my empirical science cannot prove any faith true or false, nor has anyone as yet used them to show that one faith produces more joy than another. Fortunately, those who wish to become people of faith needn't await such proof before risking a thoughtful leap across the crevasse of uncertainty. We marry in the *hope* of a happy life. We elect a career, *believing* it will prove satisfying. We fly across the country, having *faith* in the pilot and plane. Likewise, knowing that our basic beliefs are possibly in error needn't require our living life as fence straddlers. Sometimes, said the novelist Albert Camus, life calls us to make a 100 percent commitment to something about which we are 51 percent sure. Mindful of our capacity for error, we can retain humility and openness while betting our lives on a worthy hope, a hope that nurtures peace and love and justice, and joy.

Epilogue

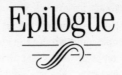

By scrutinizing the fruits of hundreds of painstaking studies of well-being we have, first, dispelled some popular but mistaken ideas:

- that few people are genuinely happy,
- that wealth buys well-being,
- that tragedies, such as disabling accidents, permanently erode happiness,
- that happiness springs from the memories of intense, if rare, positive experiences (idyllic vacations, ecstatic romances, joy-filled victories),
- that teens and the elderly are the unhappiest people,

- that in their early forties, many men experience a traumatic midlife crisis,
- that when their children leave home, women typically suffer an empty-nest syndrome,
- that one sex is happier than the other,
- that women's employment erodes the quality of their marriages,
- that subliminal tapes provide a happiness quick fix,
- that African Americans, women, and the disabled live with impoverished self-esteem,
- that people more often feel inferior than superior, low than high self-esteem,
- that because miserable marriages more readily end in divorce today, surviving marriages are happier,
- that trial marriages reduce the risk of later divorce,
- that opposites attract, and continue to find each other fascinating,
- that half or more of married people have an affair,
- that religious faith suppresses happiness.

We've also pondered things that *do* enable happiness:

- fit and healthy bodies,
- realistic goals and expectations,
- positive self-esteem,
- feelings of control,
- optimism,
- outgoingness,
- supportive friendships that enable companionship and confiding,
- a socially intimate, sexually warm, equitable marriage,
- challenging work and active leisure, punctuated by adequate rest and retreat,
- a faith that entails communal support, purpose, acceptance, outward focus, and hope.

My purpose in writing this book has been more to inform than to prescribe or advise. It's like *Consumer Reports*, which doesn't tell us what to buy—because that has to depend on our personal needs and circumstances. But we'd be foolish to ignore its information when making choices. Similarly, let's not be so smug or intellectually aloof that we shy away from using the new information about well-being in ways that could enhance our well-being. You and I can decide to exercise, to allow enough hours for sleep, to make comparisons that remind us of our blessings, to manage our time in ways that boost our sense of control, to begin acting as if we had the traits we'd like to develop, to initiate relationships, to devote effort to maintaining love rather than taking it for granted, to plan involving rather than passive leisure activities, to take the leap into an active faith—and even to begin working at reshaping our culture in ways that will promote the well-being that fame and fortune can't buy.

Well, maybe not all these things at once. But these are among the steps you and I can take if, indeed, we wish to discover greater peace and joy.

And what good it would be if the well-being enjoyed by many could be shared by the increasing numbers who live in misery. Depression, the drug scourge, sexual assault, child and spouse abuse, bigotry, marital disintegration, and other forms of violence to self and others expose deficiencies in our contemporary life. Totalitarianism, materialism, and self-reliant individualism have deluded us with false promises of well-being for all.

The message of this book is therefore both radical, as it challenges certain Western cultural assumptions, and conservative, as it reaffirms an older wisdom. Well-being is found in the renewal of disciplined life-styles, committed relationships, and the receiving and giving of acceptance. To experience deep well-being is to be self-confident yet unself-conscious, self-giving yet self-respecting, realistic yet hope-filled.

Notes

About This Book

16 "There is no fool." Cicero, *De Finibus*.

16 Opposing theories of happiness. I am indebted to Alex C. Michalos (1986) for introducing me to Wladyslaw Tatarkiewicz, *Analysis of Happiness* (The Hague: Martinus Nijhoff, 1976).

17 Shere Hite in *Time*. Claudia Wallis, "Back Off, Buddy: A New Hite Report Stirs Up a Furor over Sex and Love in the '80s," *Time*, October 12, 1987, pp. 68–73.

18 Representative marriage reports. Andrew M. Greeley, *Faithful Attraction* (New York: Tor Books, 1991).

19 "Better to be Socrates." John Stuart Mill, *Utilitarianism*. Ch. 2 (Oxford: Blackwell, 1949).

19 Mental exercise for happiness. Michael W. Fordyce, "The Psychology of Happiness: The Book Version of the Fourteen Fundamentals" (ms., Edison Community College, 1978).

19 "How to gain." William James, *Varieties of Religious Experience* (New York: Mentor Books, 1958), p. 76.

20 Accompaniments of happiness. Ruut Veenhoven, "The Utility of Happiness," *Social Indicators Research* 20 (1988): 333–54; and Ruut Veenhoven, ed., *How Harmful Is Happiness? Consequences of Enjoying Life or Not* (Gravenhage: Universitaire Pers Rotterdam, 1989). See also Joanne V. Wood, Judith A. Saltzberg, and Lloyd A. Goldsamt, "Does Affect Induce Self-Focused Attention?" *Journal of Personality and Social Psychology* 58 (1990): 899–908; K. Fiedler and Joseph Forgas, *Affect, Cognition, and Social Behavior* (Toronto: Hogrefe, 1988); Alice M. Isen, Kimberly A. Daubman, and Gary P. Nowicki, "Positive Affect Facilitates Creative Problem Solving," *Journal of Personality and Social Psychology* 52 (1987): 1122–31; and Sandra Milberg and Margaret S. Clark, "Moods and Compliance," *British Journal of Social Psychology* 27 (1988): 79–90.

20 Report current aches. Peter Salovey and Deborah Birnbaum, "Influence of Mood on Health-Relevant Cognitions," *Journal of Personality and Social Psychology* 57 (1989): 539–51.

20 The social consequences of depression. James C. Coyne, Sue A. L. Burchill, and William B. Stiles, "An Interactional Perspective on Depression," in *Handbook of Social and Clinical Psychology: The Health Perspective,* ed. C. R. Snyder and D. R. Forsyth (New York: Pergamon, 1991).

20 Happy people are flexible. Alice M. Isen, "The Influence of Positive and Negative Affect on Cognitive Organization: Some Implications for Development," in *Psychological and Biological Approaches to Emotion,* ed. Nancy Stein, Bennett Leventhal, and Tom Trabasso (Hillsdale, NJ: Erlbaum, 1990).

20 A negative mood signals. Joseph P. Forgas, "Mood and the Perception of Atypical People: Affect and Prototypicality in Person Memory and Impressions," *Journal of Personality and Social Psychology,* in press.

20 Job applicant interviewers. Robert A. Baron, "Interviewer's Mood and Reaction to Job Applicants: The Influence of Affective States on Applied Social Judgments," *Journal of Applied Social Psychology* 17 (1987): 911–26.

20 Mood boost and car/TV ratings. Alice M. Isen et al., "Affect, Accessibility of Material in Memory, and Behavior: A Cognitive Loop?" *Journal of Personality and Social Psychology* 36 (1978): 1–12. For a review of

evidence on the effects of happy versus unhappy moods on thinking and judgment, see Isen, "Influence of Positive and Negative Affect."

20 Happiness and frustration tolerance. Shelley E. Taylor, *Positive Illusions* (New York: Basic Books, 1989).

20 Happiness and loving, forgiving social relations. Gordon H. Bower, "Mood Congruity of Social Judgments," in *Emotional and Social Judgments,* ed. Joseph P. Forgas (Oxford, England: Pergamon Press, 1991).

20 Happiness and helpfulness. David G. Myers, *Social Psychology,* 2d ed. (New York, McGraw-Hill, 1987), pp. 406–9.

20 Happiness and looking at brighter side of life. Study by Colleen Kelley and other research reported in Bower, "Mood Congruity."

21 "Oh, make us happy." Robert Browning, *The Ring and the Book* (1868), IV. 1. 302.

21 "A cheerful heart." Proverbs 12:22 *(NRSV).*

21 Emotions and health. For a popular if somewhat overstated account, see Norman Cousins, *Head First: The Biology of Hope* (New York: E. P. Dutton, 1989). For a state-of-the-art research summary, see Institute of Medicine, National Academy of Sciences, *Research Briefing: Behavioral Influences on the Endocrine and Immune Systems* (Washington, DC: National Academy Press, 1989).

21 "Joy is the holy." Jack Belck, ed., *The Faith of Helen Keller* (Kansas City: Hallmark Cards, 1967), p. 23.

Chapter 1: What Is Well-Being?

24 Various measures of well-being can be found in Frank M. Andrews and Stephen B. Withey, *Social Indicators of Well-being: Americans' Perceptions of Life Quality* (New York: Plenum, 1976). See also Angus Campbell, Phillip E. Converse, and Willard L. Rodgers, *The Quality of American Life: Perceptions, Evaluations and Satisfactions* (New York: Sage, 1976).

24 Multi-item measures of feeling. Norman M. Bradburn, *The Structure of Psychological Well-being* (Chicago: Aldine, 1969).

25 Percentage of happy Americans. Dennis Wholey, *Are You Happy?* (Boston: Houghton Mifflin, 1986).

25 "I'm surprised!" Archibald D. Hart, *15 Principles for Achieving Happiness* (Dallas: Word, 1988).

25 "One-third of all." John Powell, *Happiness Is an Inside Job* (Valencia, CA: Tabor, 1989).

25 "Genuinely happy individuals." Mihaly Csikszentmihalyi, *Flow: The Psychology of Optimal Experience* (New York: Harper & Row, 1990), p. 11.

25 Thomas Szasz, quoted by Jon Winokur, *The Portable Curmudgeon* (New York: New American Library, 1987).

25 Happiness data. Angus Campbell, *The Sense of Well-being in America* (New York: McGraw-Hill, 1981); Michael Argyle, *The Psychology of Happiness* (London: Methuen, 1986); and annual surveys by the National Opinion Research Center at the University of Chicago.

26 Faces question. Andrews and Withey, *Social Indicators,* pp. 207ff, 376.

26 European well-being. Ronald Inglehart, *Culture Shift in Advanced Industrial Society* (Princeton: Princeton University Press, 1990).

26 Marx's thoughts on happiness. Michael Freund, "Toward a Critical Theory of Happiness: Philosophical Background and Methodological Significance," *New Ideas in Psychology* 3 (1985): 3–12.

27 "If you feel." Jonathan Freedman, *Happy People* (New York: Harcourt Brace Jovanovich, 1978), p. 115.

27 People overreport good things. See, for example, Dick J. Hessing, Henk Elffers, and Russell H. Weigel, "Exploring the Limits of Self-reports and Reasoned Action: An Investigation of the Psychology of Tax Evasion Behavior," *Journal of Personality and Social Psychology* 54 (1988): 405–13.

27 "Pollyanna Syndrome." Margaret W. Matlin and David J. Stang, *The Pollyanna Principle: Selectivity in Language, Memory, and Thought* (Cambridge, MA: Schenkman, 1978).

27 College students' unrealistic optimism about future. Neil D. Weinstein, "Unrealistic Optimism About Future Life Events," *Journal of Personality and Social Psychology* 39 (1980): 806–20; Neil D. Weinstein, "Unrealistic Optimism About Susceptibility to Health Problems," *Journal of Behavioral Medicine* 5 (1982): 441–60; and Neil D. Weinstein, "Why It Won't Happen to Me: Perceptions of Risk Factors and Susceptibility," *Health Psychology* 3 (1984): 431–57.

28 Soccer outcomes and mood effects. Norbert Schwarz et al., "Soccer, Rooms and the Quality of Your Life: Mood Effects on Judgments of Satisfaction with Life in General and with Specific Domains," *European Journal of Social Psychology* 17 (1987): 69–79. For more on temporary mood and subjective well-being, see Ed Diener et al., "Response Artifacts in the Measurement of Subjective Well-being," *Social Indicators Research* 24 (1991): 35–56; Norbert Schwarz and Gerald L. Clore, "Mood, Misattribution, and Judgments of Well-Being: Informative and Directive Functions of Affective States," *Journal of Personality and Social Psychol-*

ogy 45 (1983): 513–23; and John K. Yardley and Robert W. Rice, "The Relationship Between Mood and Subjective Well-Being," *Social Indicators Research* 24 (1991): 101–11.

28 College students' unrealistic optimism about dropout risk. From a survey of some two hundred thousand entering collegians sponsored by the American Council on Education and UCLA. Alexander W. Astin, "This Year's College Freshmen: Attitudes and Characteristics," *The Chronicle of Higher Education*, January 30, 1991, pp. A30–31.

28 Self-reported well-being on sunny versus rainy days. Schwarz and Clore, "Mood Misattribution."

28 Depression and perceptions of reality. Peter M. Lewinsohn and Michael Rosenbaum, "Recall of Parental Behavior by Acute Depressives, Remitted Depressives, and Nondepressives," *Journal of Personality and Social Psychology* 52 (1987): 611–19; and Lawrence H. Cohen, Lynn C. Towbes, and Regina Flocco, "Effects of Induced Mood on Self-reported Life Events and Perceived and Received Social Support," *Journal of Personality and Social Psychology* 55 (1988): 669–74.

28 Inge (not her real name). Quoted by David D. Burns, *Feeling Good: The New Mood Therapy* (New York: Signet, 1980), p. 28.

29 Consistency of self-reports. Morris A. Okun and William A. Stock, "The Construct Validity of Subjective Well-Being Measures: An Assessment via Quantitative Research Syntheses," *Journal of Community Psychology* 15 (1987): 481–92.

29 Congruence of self-reported well-being with other indicators, such as smiling, laughter, and happy memories. Edward Sandvik, Ed Diener, and L. Seidlitz, "The Assessment of Well-Being: A Comparison of Self-Report and Nonself-Report Strategies" (ms., University of Illinois, 1990); Diener et al., "Response Artifacts," pp. 35–56; and William Pavot et al., "Further Validation of the Satisfaction with Life Scale: Evidence for the Cross-Method Convergence of Well-being Measures," *Journal of Personality Assessment* 57 (1991): 149–61.

29 Friends and family ratings of "happy" people. Ed Diener, "Subjective Well-being," *Psychological Bulletin* 93 (1984): 542–75; Diener, "Response Artifacts," pp. 35–56; Paul T. Costa, Jr., and Robert R. McCrae, "Personality in Adulthood: A Six-Year Longitudinal Study of Self-report and Spouse Ratings on the NEO Personality Inventory," *Journal of Personality and Social Psychology* 54 (1988): 853–63; and David Watson and Lee A. Clark, "Self Versus Peer Ratings of Specific Emotional Traits: Evidence of Convergent and Discriminant Validity," *Journal of Personality and Social Psychology* 60 (1991): 927–40. See also Richard Kammann,

Carey Martin, and Malcolm McQueen, "Low Accuracy in Judgments of Others' Psychological Well-being as Seen from a Phenomenological Perspective," *Journal of Personality* 51 (1984): 107–23; and Pavot, "Further Validation," pp. 149–61.

Chapter 2: Wealth and Well-being

31 Not enough money. Angus Campbell, *The Sense of Well-being in America* (New York: McGraw-Hill, 1981), p. 41. See also Table 2–2 in A. Regula Herzog, Willard L. Rodgers, and Joseph Woodworth, *Subjective Well-being Among Different Age Groups* (Ann Arbor: Survey Research Center, University of Michigan, 1982).

31 Dissatisfaction with income. Roper survey in *Public Opinion*, August/September, 1984, p. 30.

31 More money. "When Americans are asked to tell an interviewer what the quality of life means to them, their most frequent type of response makes some reference to income security. When they are asked to describe the ways their quality of life fall short of what they would like it to be, their most frequent response is that they do not have enough money." Campbell, *Sense of Well-being*, p. 68. A more recent, though apparently less scientific survey of Americans asked, "If you could change one thing about your life, what would it be?" The number one answer was wealth, mentioned by 64 percent. Second was education at 45 percent. James Patterson and Peter Kim, *The Day America Told the Truth: What People Really Believe About Everything That Matters* (New York: Prentice-Hall, 1991).

31 10 to 20 percent more. Burkhard Strumpel, "Economic Lifestyles, Values, and Subjective Welfare," in *Economic Means for Human Needs*, ed. Burkhard Strumpel (Ann Arbor: University of Michigan Survey Research Center, 1976).

32 Gallup Poll. George Gallup, Jr., and F. Newport, "Americans Widely Disagree on What Constitutes 'Rich,' " *Gallup Poll Monthly*, July 1990, pp. 28–36.

32 High-income jobs. National Opinion Research Center data analyzed, cited by C. N. Weaver and M. C. Matthews, *Personnel* 64 (September 1987): 62–65.

32 ACE surveys. Alexander W. Astin, Kenneth C. Green, and William S. Korn, *The American Freshman: Twenty Year Trends* (a report of the Cooperative Institutional Research Program sponsored by the American

Council on Education) (Los Angeles: Higher Education Research Institute, Graduate School of Education, UCLA, 1987); and Astin, "Attitudes and Characteristics," pp. A30–31.

32 "With few exceptions." Thomas H. Naylor, "Redefining Corporate Motivation, Swedish Style," *Christian Century* 107 (1990): 566–70.

32 Alan Alda. Quoted by Jon Winokur, *The Portable Curmudgeon* (New York: New American Library, 1987).

34 Nancy Reagan's wardrobe. *Time,* December 18, 1989, p. 42.

34 National income and well-being. Richard A. Easterlin, "Does Money Buy Happiness?" *Public Interest* 30 (1973): 3–10; and Inglehart, *Culture Shift.*

34 National differences in well-being. Inglehart, *Culture Shift,* p. 242.

36 Democracy, free press, and happiness. Ruut Veenhoven and Piet Ouweneel, "Happiness as an Indicator of the Livability of Society" (Paper presented at the International Conference on Social Reporting, Wissenschaftszentrum, Berlin, 1989).

36 Relative income, satisfaction with income, and well-being. For a representative sample of national surveys see Campbell, *Sense of Well-being,* p. 241; Herzog, Rodgers, and Woodworth, *Subjective Well-being;* Brad McKenzie and James Campbell, "Race, Socioeconomic Status, and the Subjective Well-being of Older Americans," *International Journal of Aging and Human Development* 25 (1987): 43–61; Richard Kammann, "Objective Circumstances, Life Satisfactions, and Sense of Well-being: Consistencies Across Time and Place," *New Zealand Journal of Psychology* 12 (1983): 14–22; and Earl E. Davis and Margaret Fine-Davis, "Social Indicators of Living Conditions in Ireland with European Comparisons," *Social Indicators Research* 25 (1991): 103–365.

37 Relative income and stress. Sheldon Cohen and Gail M. Williamson, "Perceived Stress in a Probability Sample of the United States," in *The Social Psychology of Health,* ed. Shirlynn Spacapan and Stuart Oskamp (Newbury Park, CA: Sage, 1988).

37 "Most poor people." Jesse Jackson, address to the Democratic National Convention, July 1988.

37 Postwar European economies and happiness. Ruut Veenhoven, "Is Happiness Relative?" *Social Indicators Research* 24 (1991): 1–34. Ruut Veenhoven, "National Wealth and Individual Happiness," in *Understanding Economic Behaviour,* ed. Klaus G. Grunert and Folke Olander (Cordrecht: Kluwer Academic Publishers, 1989), further documents that, though people in poor countries are less happy than those in better-off countries, "the returns of wealth are subject to the law of diminishing

utility." Recent economic growth in the better-off countries has "hardly raised the average level of happiness."

38 "Has a surprisingly weak . . ." Inglehart, *Culture Shift,* p. 242. W. Glatzer, "Quality of Life in Advanced Industrialized Countries: The Case of West Germany," in *Subjective Well-being: An Interdisciplinary Perspective,* ed. Fritz Strack, Michael Argyle, and Norbert Schwarz (Oxford, England: Pergamon Press, 1990), reports of a 1984 national survey in West Germany, in which life satisfaction was lowest among those in the bottom 20 percent of household income, but hardly different among people at various income levels above the bottom.

38 "When we have provided." Seneca, "Seneca of a happy life," in *Morals.*

38 UNICEF $500 per child. Estimate by UNICEF executive director James P. Grant in personal correspondence, June 13, 1990.

39 Income satisfaction and well-being. Campbell, *Sense of Well-being,* p. 58.

39 "The believing poor." Gustavo Gutierrez, *We Drink from Our Own Wells: The Spiritual Journey of a People* (Maryknoll, NY: Orbis Books, 1985), p. 115.

39 Peruvian peasants vs. North Americans. Henri Nouwen, *Lifesigns: Intimacy, Fecundity, and Ecstasy in Christian Perspective* (Garden City, NY: Doubleday, 1986), p. 96.

40 Similar emotions in rich and poor. Robert Coles, *Privileged Ones: The Well-off and the Rich in America* (Boston: Atlantic Monthly Press, 1977).

40 Wealthiest Americans. Ed Diener, J. Horwitz, and Robert A. Emmons, "Happiness of the Very Wealthy," *Social Indicators* 16 (1985): 263–74. S. T. Coleridge, *Table Talk,* June 10, 1824.

40 Rubik's unhappiness. John Tierney, "The Perplexing Life of Erno Rubik," *Discover,* March 1986, pp. 81–88.

41 Necessities and luxuries. Roper survey reported in *Public Opinion,* August/September 1984, p. 25.

41 Percent very happy since 1957. Tom W. Smith, "Happiness: Time Trends, Seasonal Variations, Intersurvey Differences, and Other Mysteries," *Social Psychology Quarterly* 42 (1979): 18–30; and periodic personal correspondence.

42 Detroit satisfaction. Campbell, *Sense of Well-being,* pp. 32–33. National surveys reveal virtually no change in income satisfaction from 1972 to 1988. M. Andrews, "Stability and Change in Levels and Structure of Subjective Well-being: USA 1972 and 1988," *Social Indicators Research* 25 (1991): 1–30.

42 Percent "pretty well satisfied." National Opinion Research Center surveys reported by Richard Gene Niemi, John Mueller, and Tom W. Smith, *Trends in Public Opinion: A Compendium of Survey Data* (New York: Greenwood Press, 1989), p. 239.

43 Depression trends. Martin E. P. Seligman, "Explanatory Style: Predicting Depression, Achievement, and Health," in *Brief Therapy Approaches to Treating Anxiety and Depression*, ed. Michael D. Yapko (New York: Brunner/Mazel, 1989).

43 International trends in depression. Gerald L. Klerman and Myrna M. Weissman, "Increasing Rates of Depression," *Journal of the American Medical Association* 261 (1989): 2229–35.

43 Adolescent well-being. Peter Uhlenberg and David Eggebeen, "The Declining Well-being of Adolescents," *Public Interest* 82 (1986): 25–38, provided some of the 1960 baseline data. Other 1960 data and updated data for 1985 to 1987 are reported by the National Center for Education Statistics (1989) (per pupil expenditures; teachers with advanced degrees; class size); the Bureau of the Census (1990) (delinquency rate); the National Center for Health Statistics (1989) (birthrate of unmarried white women); and Victor Fuchs and Diane Reklis, "American Children: Economic Perspectives and Policy Options," *Science* 255 (1992): 41–46 (homicide and suicide rates). (For full citations, see the Bibliography.)

44 "Our forefathers." Seneca, "Seneca of a happy life."

45 "What keeps our faith." Garrison Keillor, quoted by Martin Marty, *Context*, May 15, 1989.

Chapter 3: A Satisfied Mind

47 "Objective life circumstances." Richard Kammann, "Objective Circumstances, Life Satisfactions, and Sense of Well-being: Consistencies Across Time and Place," *New Zealand Journal of Psychology* 12 (1983): 14–22.

48 "Is produced not so much." Benjamin Franklin, *Autobiography*, 1791.

48 Life events and mood. Niall Bolger et al., "Effects of Daily Stress on Negative Mood," *Journal of Personality and Social Psychology* 57 (1989): 808–18; Lee A. Clark and David Watson, "Mood and the Mundane: Relations Between Daily Life Events and Self-reported Mood," *Journal of Personality and Social Psychology* 54 (1988): 296–308; John W. Reich et al., "Demands, Desires, and Well-being: An Assessment of Events, Responses, and Outcomes," *Journal of Community Psychology* 16 (1988): 392–402; Richard T. Rowlison and Robert D. Felner, "Major Life

Events, Hassles, and Adaptation in Adolescence: Confounding in the Conceptualization and Measurement of Life Stress and Adjustment Revisited," *Journal of Personality and Social Psychology* 55 (1988): 432–44; and Arthur A. Stone and John M. Neale, "Effects of Severe Daily Events on Mood," *Journal of Personality and Social Psychology* 46 (1984): 137–44.

48 Emotional well-being of cancer patients. J.C.J.M. de Haes and F.C.E. Van Knippenberg, "The Quality of Life of Cancer Patients: A Review of the Literature," *Social Science and Medicine* 10 (1985): 809–17.

48 "The Lord lifts." Psalm 146:8b and 30:5b *(NRSV)*.

48 Michigan accident victims. Camille B. Wortman and Roxanne C. Silver, "Coping with Irrevocable Loss," in *Cataclysms, Crises, and Catastrophes: Psychology in Action*, ed. Gary R. VandenBos and Brenda K. Bryant (Washington, DC: American Psychological Association, 1987).

48 Disabled percent happy. Kathleen Chwalisz, Ed Diener, and Dennis Gallagher, "Autonomic Arousal Feedback and Emotional Experience: Evidence from the Spinal Cord Injured," *Journal of Personality and Social Psychology* 54 (1988): 820–28. See also A. L. Allman and Ed Diener, "Measurement Issues and the Subjective Well-being of People with Disabilities" (ms., University of Illinois, 1990); R. M. Bostick, "Quality of Life Survey Among a Severely Handicapped Population" (Ph.D. diss., University of Houston, 1977); and Susan D. Decker and Richard Schulz, "Correlates of Life Satisfaction and Depression in Middle-aged and Elderly Spinal Cord-Injured Persons," *American Journal of Occupational Therapy* 39 (1985): 740–45.

48 Disabled peer ratings. A. L. Allman, "Subjective Well-Being of Students with and Without Disabilities" (Paper presented at the Midwestern Psychological Association Convention, Chicago, May 1989).

48 Aftereffects of major events linger. Bruce Headey and Alex Wearing, "Subjective Well-being: A Stocks and Flows Framework," in *Subjective Well-being: An Interdisciplinary Perspective*, ed. Fritz Strack, Michael Argyle, and Norbert Schwarz (Oxford, England: Pergamon Press, 1990). See also, effects of traumatic stress, page 55.

49 W Mitchell story. B. Lemly, "The Man Who Won't Be Defeated," *Parade*, November 26, 1989, pp. 12–13.

49 Lucio: Translated from Massimini's interview transcripts by Mihaly Csikszentmihalyi, *Flow: The Psychology of Optimal Experience* (New York: Harper & Row, 1990), p. 194.

49 Benefits from breast cancer experience. Shelley E. Taylor, "Adjustment to Threatening Events: A Theory of Cognitive Adaptation," *American*

Psychologist 38 (1983): 1161–74; and Rebecca L. Collins, Shelley E. Taylor, and Laurie A. Skokan, "A Better World or a Shattered Vision? Changes in Life Perspectives Following Victimization," *Social Cognition* 8 (1990): 263–85.

49 The patient quotes are from Taylor, "Adjustment to Threatening Events," pp. 1161–74.

50 Stephen Hawking. Quoted by A. E. Guinness, *ABC's of the Human Mind: A Family Answer Book* (Pleasantville, NY: Reader's Digest, 1990), p. 89.

50 Lottery winners. Philip Brickman, Dan Coates, and Ronnie J. Janoff-Bulman, "Lottery Winners and Accident Victims: Is Happiness Relative?" *Journal of Personality and Social Psychology* 36 (1978): 917–27; and Michael Argyle, *The Psychology of Happiness* (London: Methuen, 1986).

51 "But in the long run." Ronald Inglehart, *Culture Shift in Advanced Industrial Society* (Princeton: Princeton University Press, 1990), p. 212.

52 Lewis Judd. Quoted by Tina Adler, "Judd Leaves NIMH, Returns to Old Job," *APA Monitor* (December 1990): 6.

52 William Bennett. Quoted by *Grand Rapids Press* wire services, December 14, 1990, p. A3.

52 Pete Incaviglia. Quoted by *Life,* January 1991, p. 23.

52 Anthony O'Reilly's salary. Janice Castro, "How's Your Pay?" *Time,* April 15, 1991, pp. 40–41.

53 Gallup poll of charitable giving for Independent Sector. Virginia A. Hodgkinson and Murray S. Weitzman, *Giving and Volunteering in the United States: Findings from a National Survey* (Washington, DC: Independent Sector, 1990).

53 As family affluence. David Briggs, "Poll: Americans Want to Be Rich" (Associated Press article), *Holland Sentinel,* November 1, 1991, p. B6.

53 "Continued pleasures wear off." Nico H. Frijda, "The Laws of Emotion," *American Psychologist* 43 (1988): 349–58.

53 "All their life." C. S. Lewis, *The Last Battle* (New York: Collier Books, 1974), p. 184.

53 Impossibility of utopia. Philip Brickman and Donald T. Campbell, "Hedonic Relativism and Planning the Good Society," in *Adaptation-level Theory,* ed. M. H. Appley (New York: Academic Press, 1971).

54 Long Island teacher. *New York Times,* June 5, 1978, p. D4, quoted by Paul L. Wachtel, *The Poverty of Affluence: A Psychological Portrait of the American Way of Life* (Philadelphia: New Society Publishers, 1989), p. 106.

54 "Opponent-process principle." Richard L. Solomon, "The Opponent-Process Theory of Acquired Motivation: The Costs of Pleasure and the Benefits of Pain," *American Psychologist* 35 (1980): 691–712.

55 "How strange would appear." Plato, *Phaedo.*

55 Posttraumatic stress reactions. Jeffrey A. Kaylor, Daniel W. King, and Lynda A. King, "Psychological Effects of Military Service in Vietnam: A Meta-analysis," *Psychological Bulletin* 102 (1987): 431–45; and Centers for Disease Control Vietnam Experience Study "Health Status of Vietnam Veterans," *Journal of the American Medical Association* 259 (1988): 2701–9.

56 T. S. Eliot. Peter Ackroyd, *T. S. Eliot: A Life* (New York: Simon & Schuster, 1984).

56 Leningrad. Richard Nisbett and Lee Ross, *The Person and the Situation* (New York: McGraw-Hill, 1991).

56 Personal vs. group comparisons. Iain Walker and Leon Mann, "Unemployment, Relative Deprivation, and Social Protest," *Personality and Social Psychology Bulletin* 13 (1987): 275–83; and James M. Olson, C. Peter Herman, and Mark P. Zanna, eds., *Relative Deprivation and Social Comparison. The Ontario Symposium,* vol. 4 (Hillsdale, NJ: Erlbaum, 1986).

57 Baseball salaries and players' morale. Peter King, "Bawl Players," *Sports Illustrated,* March 18, 1991, pp. 14–17.

57 Academic self-concept. Herbert W. Marsh and John W. Parker, "Determinants of Student Self-concept: Is It Better to Be a Relatively Large Fish in a Small Pond Even If You Don't Learn to Swim as Well?" *Journal of Personality and Social Psychology* 47 (1984): 213–31.

58 Black college science-math graduates. James H. Wyche and Henry T. Frierson, Jr., "Minorities at Majority Institutions," *Science* 249 (1990): 989–91.

58 Regarding academic tracking, "one of the most divisive and damaging school practices in existence," see Carnegie Council on Adolescent Development, *Turning Points: Preparing American Youth for the 21st Century* (New York: Task Force on Education of Young Adolescents, 1989).

58 Per graduate Ph.D. data. M. Elizabeth Tidball and Vera Kistiakowsky, "Baccalaureate Origins of American Scientists and Scholars," *Science* 193 (1976): 646–52. During a more recent thirty-year period, from 1951 to 1980, the forty-eight liberal arts colleges known informally as "the Oberlin group" had doctoral productivity rate of 8.2 percent of graduates,

surpassing the Ivy League universities (7.8 percent), the National Academy of Sciences twenty top-rated research universities (6.9 percent), and the Big Ten universities (4.3 percent), as reported by David Davis-Van Atta et al., eds, *Educating America's Scientists: The Role of the Research Colleges* (Oberlin: Oberlin College Press, 1985).

58 Upward comparison. Charles L. Gruder, "Choice of Comparison Persons in Evaluating Oneself," in *Social Comparison Processes,* ed. Jerry M. Suls and R. L. Miller (New York: Hemisphere, 1977); and Jerry M. Suls and Frederick Tesch, "Students' Preferences for Information About Their Test Performance: A Social Comparison Study," *Journal of Applied Social Psychology* 8 (1978): 189–97.

58 "Napoleon envied Caesar." Bertrand Russell, *The Conquest of Happiness* (1930; reprint, London: Unwin Paperbacks, 1985).

58 Theft rate correlation with television images. Karen Hennigan et al., "Impact of the Introduction of Television on Crime in the United States: Empirical Findings and Theoretical Implications," *Journal of Personality and Social Psychology* 42 (1982): 461–77.

59 Sexual comparisons. Dolf Zillmann, "Effects of Prolonged Consumption of Pornography," in *Pornography: Research Advances and Policy Considerations,* ed. Dolf Zillmann and Jennings Bryant (Hillsdale, NJ: Erlbaum, 1989); Douglas T. Kenrick and Sara E. Gutierres, "Contrast Effects and Judgments of Physical Attractiveness: When Beauty Becomes a Social Problem," *Journal of Personality and Social Psychology* 38 (1980): 131–40; Douglas T. Kenrick, Sara E. Gutierres, and Laurie L. Goldberg, "Influence of Popular Erotica on Judgments of Strangers and Mates," *Journal of Experimental Social Psychology* 25 (1989): 159–67; and James B. Weaver, Jonathon L. Masland, and Dolf Zillmann, "Effect of Erotica on Young Men's Aesthetic Perceptions of Their Female Sexual Partners," *Perceptual and Motor Skills* 58 (1984): 929–30.

59 Breast cancer victims' comparisons (names fictitious). Shelley E. Taylor, *Positive Illusions* (New York: Basic Books, 1989), pp. 169–73. Although cancer patients are typically somewhat depressed and anxious after being diagnosed, their long-term psychological well-being is remarkably resilient. Barbara L. Anderson, Barrie Anderson, and Charles deProsse, "Controlled Prospective Longitudinal Study of Women with Cancer: II. Psychological Outcomes," *Journal of Consulting and Clinical Psychology* 57 (1989): 692–97.

60 Disparaging others alleviates self-doubt. Robert B. Cialdini and Kenneth

D. Richardson, "Two Indirect Tactics of Image Management: Basking and Blasting," *Journal of Personality and Social Psychology* 39 (1980): 406–15; and Jennifer Crocker et al., "Downward Comparison, Prejudice, and Evaluation of Others: Effects of Self-esteem and Threat," *Journal of Personality and Social Psychology* 52 (1987): 907–16.

60 Gore Vidal. Quoted by Jon Winokur, *The Portable Curmudgeon* (New York: New American Library, 1987).

60 Comparison and mood. Frederick X Gibbons, "Social Comparison and Depression: Company's Effect on Misery," *Journal of Personality and Social Psychology* 51 (1986): 140–48; and Frederick X Gibbons and Meg Gerard, "Effects of Upward and Downward Social Comparison on Mood States," *Journal of Social and Clinical Psychology* 8 (1989): 14–31.

60 Donald Trump. John Greenwald, "Taking Away His Credit Cards," *Time*, July 9, 1990, p. 51.

61 Helen Keller. Letter to Dr. J. K. Love, 1910.

61 "I am almost." William Barclay, *Through the Year with William Barclay*, ed. D. Duncan (London: Arthur James, 1971), p. 70.

62 "There is nothing." William Shakespeare, *Hamlet*, 2. 2. 255.

62 New York Times editor (1979, November 4). "Pater-&-familias," *New York Times*, November 4, 1979, sec. 4, p. E21.

62 Happier for having been happy. S. Smith, 1806 in *Sketches of moral philosophy. Lecture 22: On Benevolent Affections.*

62 Recalling low moments and high moments. Fritz Strack, Norbert Schwarz, and Elisabeth Gschneidinger, "Happiness and Reminiscing: The Role of Time Perspective, Affect, and Mode of Thinking," *Journal of Personality and Social Psychology* 49 (1985): 1460–69.

63 Ecstasies dull ordinary pleasures. Allen Parducci, "Value Judgments: Toward a *Relational* Theory of Happiness," in *Attitudinal Judgment*, ed. J. Richard Eiser (New York: Springer-Verlag, 1984); Richard H. Smith, Ed Diener, and Douglas H. Wedell, "Intrapersonal and Social Comparison Determinants of Happiness: A Range-Frequency Analysis," *Journal of Personality and Social Psychology* 56 (1989): 317–25; Ed Diener, Ed Sandvik, and William Pavot, "Happiness Is the Frequency, Not the Intensity, of Positive Versus Negative Affect," in *The Social Psychology of Subjective Well-Being*, ed. Fritz Strack, Michael Argyle, and Norbert Schwarz (Oxford, England: Pergamon, 1990); and Ed Diener et al., "The Costs of Intense Positive Emotions," *Journal of Personality and Social Psychology* 61 (1991): 492–503.

63 Hospitalization and eventual happiness. Norbert Schwarz and Fritz Strack, "Evaluating One's Life: A Judgment Model of Subjective Well-

being," in *The Social Psychology of Subjective Well-being*, ed. Fritz Strack, Michael Argyle, and Norbert Schwarz (Oxford, England: Pergamon, 1990).

63 Life's pleasures by contrast. Barclay, *Through the Year with William Barclay.*

63 Japanese internment camp experience. Langdon Gilkey, *The Shantung Compound: The Story of Men and Women Under Pressure* (New York: Harper & Row, 1966).

64 "Denial for the sake of pleasures." Reuben P. Bulka, "Religion in Contemporary Times: For Denial or for Pleasure," *Psychologists Interested in Religious Issues Newsletter* 15, no. 1 (1990): 1–4.

65 Rabbi story. Taylor, *Positive Illusions*, pp. 167–68.

65 "Revolution of rising expectations." Phrase from the 1968 *Report of the National Advisory Commission on Civil Disorders.*

66 Growing out of impossible expectations. Judith Viorst, *Necessary Losses* (New York: Ballantine/Fawcett, 1987), p. 175.

66 Abraham H. Maslow. Bertha G. Maslow, *Abraham H. Maslow: A Memorial Volume* (Monterey, CA: Brooks/Cole, 1972), p. 108.

66 Imaginative deprivation study. Marshall Dermer et al., "Evaluative Judgments of Aspects of Life as a Function of Vicarious Exposure of Hedonic Extremes," *Journal of Personality and Social Psychology* 37 (1979): 247–60.

66 In another experiment. Jennifer Crocker and Lisa Gallo, "The Self-enhancing Effect of Downward Comparison" (Paper presented at the American Psychological Association Convention, Los Angeles, August 1985).

Chapter 4: The Demography of Happiness

69 Perceptions of age and happiness. Jonathan Freedman, *Happy People* (New York: Harcourt Brace Jovanovich, 1978).

69 Statistical digest of well-being and age. William A. Stock et al., "Age and Subjective Well-being: A Meta-analysis," in *Evaluation Studies: Review Annual*, ed. Richard J. Light, vol. 8 (Beverly Hills: Sage, 1983).

69 European data on well-being and age. Ronald Inglehart, *Culture Shift in Advanced Industrial Society* (Princeton: Princeton University Press, 1990). Repeated surveys by the Netherlands Central Bureau of Statistics reveal that "hardly 1 percent" of individual variation in life satisfaction is attributable to age, reports J. J. Latten, "Life-course and Satisfaction, Equal for Every-one?" *Social Indicators Research* 21 (1989): 599–610.

The sharp-eyed reader will caution here: When comparing people of different ages we also are comparing different "cohorts"—groups of people who grew up in different eras. Will today's young adults exhibit similar well-being when they reach later life? We won't know for sure until they get there. But judging from the consistency of these results across cultures and across the past two decades, there is little warrant for betting on much change.

70 Massachusetts survey. John B. McKinlay, Sonja M. McKinlay, and Donald Brambilla, "The Relative Contributions of Endocrine Changes and Social Circumstances to Depression in Mid-aged Women," *Journal of Health and Social Behavior* 28 (1987): 345–63; and John B. McKinlay, Sonja M. McKinlay, and Donald Brambilla, "Health Status and Utilization Behavior Associated with Menopause," *American Journal of Epidemiology* 125 (1987): 110–21.

70 Evaluation of menopause experience. Bernice L. Neugarten et al., "Women's Attitudes Towards the Menopause," *Vita Humana* 6 (1963): 140–51; and Bernice L. Neugarten, "The Roles We Play," in *Quality of Life: The Middle Years,* ed. American Medical Association (Action, MA: Publishing Sciences Group, 1974).

71 "If the truth." Jacqueline Goodchilds, quoted by Carol Tavris, "Old Age Is Not What It Used to Be," *New York Times/Good Health Magazine,* September 27, 1987, pp. 24–25, 91–92.

71 National survey data on the well-being of midlife women with and without empty nests. Norval D. Glenn, "Psychological Well-being in the Postparental Stage: Some Evidence from National Surveys," *Journal of Marriage and the Family* 37 (1975): 105–10. See also Paula K. Adelmann et al., "Empty Nest, Cohort, and Employment in the Well-being of Midlife Women," *Sex Roles* 20 (1989): 173–89.

71 Refilled nests. From a study of twenty-five hundred Massachusetts women by American Institutes for Research, *Women and Their Health in Massachusetts* (Cambridge: Cambridge Research Center, 1986).

71 "Post-launch honeymoon." Lynn White and John N. Edwards, "Emptying the Nest and Parental Well-being: An Analysis of National Panel Data," *American Sociological Review* 55 (1990): 235–42.

72 "While Diana puts." *People,* February 11, 1991.

72 Jim Tracy. Daniel J. Levinson, *The Seasons of a Man's Life* (New York: Knopf, 1979), pp. 305–13.

72 Stability of self-reported well-being during midlife. Angus Campbell, *The Sense of Well-being in America* (New York: McGraw-Hill, 1981), p. 181.

72 Stability of marriage, divorce, suicide etc. trends. Ski Hunter and Martin

Sundel, *Midlife Myths: Issues, Findings, and Practice Implications* (Newbury Park, CA: Sage, 1989). See also Paul T. Costa, Jr., and Robert R. McCrae, "Still Stable After All These Years: Personality as a Key to Some Issues in Adulthood and Old Age," in *Life-Span Development and Behavior*, ed. Paul B. Baltes and O. Brim, Jr., vol. 3 (New York: Academic Press, 1980); Letha D. Scanzoni and John Scanzoni, *Men, Women, and Change: A Sociology of Marriage and Family* (New York: McGraw-Hill, 1981); and K. Warner Schaie and James Geiwitz, *Adult Development and Aging* (Boston: Little, Brown, 1982).

72 "Midlife Crisis Scale." Robert R. McCrae and Paul T. Costa, Jr., *Personality in Adulthood* (New York: Guilford Press, 1990), pp. 147–49.

73 Gettysburg College researchers. Robert F. Bornstein et al., "The Temporal Stability of Ratings of Parents: Test-retest Reliability and Influence of Parental Contact," *Journal of Social Behavior and Personality* 6 (1991): 641–49.

73 The moderation of moods with age. Ed Diener, Robert A. Emmons, and Ed Sandvik, "The Dual Nature of Happiness: Independence of Positive and Negative Moods" (ms., University of Illinois, 1986); see also Mihaly Csikszentmihalyi and Randy Larsen, *Being Adolescent: Conflict and Growth in the Teenage Years* (New York: Basic Books, 1984); and Campbell, *Sense of Well-being*.

74 Age and satisfaction with specific domains. A. Regula Herzog and Willard L. Rodgers, "Satisfaction Among Older Adults," in *Research on the Quality of Life*, ed. Frank M. Andrews (Ann Arbor: Survey Research Center, University of Michigan, 1986).

74 Mary (not her actual name) quote. Freedman, *Happy People*, p. 109.

75 Herzog and Rogers, "Satisfaction Among Older Adults."

75 Elderly less susceptible to acute illness. Bureau of the Census, *Statistical Abstract of the United States* (Washington, DC: Superintendent of Documents, Government Printing Office, 1989), p. 114.

75 One in four have serious illness. National Council on the Aging, *The Myth and Reality of Aging in America* (Washington, DC: National Council on Aging, 1976).

75 Sources of happiness for older adults. Herzog, Rogers, and Woodworth, *Subjective Well-being*. See also Morris A. Okun et al., "The Social Activity/Subjective Well-being Relation: A Quantitative Synthesis," *Research on Aging* 6 (1984): 45–65; Daniel Doyle and Marilyn J. Forehand, "Life Satisfaction and Old Age: A Reexamination," *Research on Aging* 6 (1984): 432–48; Mark Baldassare, Sarah Rosenfield, and Karen Rook, "The Types of Social Relations Predicting Elderly Well-being," *Research*

on Aging 6 (1984): 549–59; Carol C. Riddick, "Life Satisfaction Determinants of Older Males and Females," *Leisure Sciences* 7 (1985): 47–63; Morris Okun, "Subjective Well-being," *Encyclopedia on Aging,* in press; and Carole K. Holahan, "Relation of Life Goals at Age 70 to Activity Participation and Health and Psychological Well-being Among Terman's Gifted Men and Women," *Psychology and Aging* 3 (1988): 286–91.

75 "The later years." Ashley Montagu, *Growing Young,* 2d ed. (New York: Bergin & Garvey, 1989) (abridged in *Utne Reader,* January/February 1990, p. 91).

76 Health and happiness. Morris Okun et al., "Health and Subjective Well-Being: A Meta-Analysis," *International Journal of Aging and Human Development* 19 (1984): 111–32.

76 Frank (not his real name). Quoted by Freedman, *Happy People,* p. 121.

77 Medical advice vs. counseling heart attack survivors. Meyer Friedman and Diane Ulmer, *Treating Type A Behavior—and Your Heart* (New York: Knopf, 1984).

77 Laughter as therapy. Herbert M. Lefcourt and Rod A. Martin, *Humor and Life Stress* (New York: Springer-Verlag, 1986; see also Arthur M. Nezu, Christine M. Nezu, and Sonia E. Blissett, "Sense of Humor as a Moderator of the Relation Between Stressful Events and Psychological Distress: A Prospective Analysis," *Journal of Personality and Social Psychology* 54 (1988): 520–25.

77 Laughter as arousal/relaxation. Vera M. Robinson, "Humor and Health," in *Handbook of Humor Research,* ed. Paul E. McGhee and Jeffrey H. Goldstein (New York: Springer-Verlag, 1983).

77 Harvard alumns. Ralph S. Paffenbarger, Jr., et al., "Physical Activity, All-Cause Mortality, and Longevity of College Alumni," *New England Journal of Medicine* 314 (1986): 605–12.

77 CDC employees. D. R. Anderson and W. S. Jose, "Employee Lifestyle and the Bottom Line: Results from the Stay Well Evaluation," *Fitness in Business,* December 1987, pp. 86–91.

77 Forty-three studies. K. E. Powell et al., "Physical Activity and the Incidence of Coronary Heart Disease," *Annual Review of Public Health* 8 (1987): 253–87.

77 Physical activity and well-being. T. Stephens, "Physical Activity and Mental Health in the United States and Canada: Evidence from Four Population Surveys," *Preventive Medicine* 17 (1988): 35–47. See also Joyce Hogan, "Personality Correlates of Physical Fitness," *Journal of*

Personality and Social Psychology 56 (1989): 284–88; and Larry A. Tucker, "Physical Fitness and Psychological Distress," *International Journal of Sport Psychology* 21 (1990): 185–201.

78 Aerobic exercise effect on depression. I. Lisa McCann and David S. Holmes, "Influence of Aerobic Exercise on Depression," *Journal of Personality and Social Psychology* 46 (1984): 1142–47. For additional information see J. Scott Hinkle, "Psychological Benefits of Aerobic Running: Implications for Mental Health Counselors," *Journal of Mental Health Counseling* 10 (1988): 245–51.

78 Ten-minute walk effect. Richard E. Thayer, "Energy, Tiredness, and Tension Effects of a Sugar Snack Versus Moderate Exercise," *Journal of Personality and Social Psychology* 52 (1987): 119–25.

78 Exercisers feel young. B. B. Tonkon, "A Social Psychological Perspective on Aging Patterns in Male Runners and Non-runners," *Dissertation Abstracts International* 45 (1985): 3591–92A.

78 Blood pressure and exercise. Kenneth A. Perkins et al., "Cardiovascular Reactivity of Psychological Stress in Aerobically Trained Versus Untrained Mild Hypertensives and Normotensives," *Health Psychology* 5 (1986): 407–21; and Susan Roviaro, David S. Holmes, and R. David Holmsten, "Influence of a Cardiac Rehabilitation Program on the Cardiovascular, Psychological, and Social Functioning of Cardiac Patients," *Journal of Behavioral Medicine* 7 (1984): 61–81.

78 Other possible mood-boosting effects of exercise. Egil W. Martinsen, "The Role of Aerobic Exercise in the Treatment of Depression," *Stress Medicine* 3 (1987): 93–100.

78 Ninety-four-year-old. Kenneth Cooper, *The New Aerobics* (New York: Bantam, 1970), p. 9.

79 Statistical digests of gender and well-being. Marilyn J. Haring, William A. Stock, and Morris A. Okun, "A Research Synthesis of Gender and Social Class as Correlates of Subjective Well-being," *Human Relations* 37 (1984): 645–57; and Wendy Wood, Nancy Rhodes, and Melanie Whelan, "Sex Differences in Positive Well-being: A Consideration of Emotional Style and Marital Status," *Psychological Bulletin* 106 (1989): 249–64. See also Michael W. Fordyce, "The PSYCHAP INVENTORY: A MultiScale Test to Measure Happiness and Its Concomitants," *Social Indicators Research* 18 (1985): 1–33.

79 Sixteen-nation gender data. Inglehart, *Culture Shift*, p. 221.

79 Study of 18,032 university students. Alex C. Michalos, *Life Satisfaction*

and Happiness, vol. 1 of *Global Report on Student Well-Being* (New York: Springer-Verlag, 1991).

80 Employment of women and well-being. Campbell, *Sense of Well-being*; Myra M. Ferree, "Class, Housework, and Happiness: Women's Work and Life Satisfaction," *Sex Roles* 11 (1984): 1057–74; James D. Wright, "Are Working Women *Really* More Satisfied? Evidence from Several National Surveys," *Journal of Marriage and the Family* 40 (1978): 301–13; and Paula K. Adelmann, "Work and Well-being in Women: A Meta-analysis" (ms., University of Michigan, 1988).

81 Men and housework. John P. Robinson, "Who's Doing the Housework?" *American Demographics,* December 1988, pp. 24–28, 63.

81 Stresses of motherhood and employment. Sara McClanahan and Julia Adams, "The Effects of Children on Adults' Psychological Well-being: 1957–1976," *Social Forces* 68 (1989): 124–46; and Andrew M. Greeley, *Faithful Attraction* (New York: Tor Books, 1991), pp. 228–29.

81 Social support for women's employment. Sandra Scarr, Deborah Phillips, and Kathleen McCartney, "Working Mothers and Their Families," *American Psychologist* 44 (1989): 1402–9; and Rena L. Repetti, Karen A. Matthews, and Ingrid Waldron, "Employment and Women's Health: Effects of Paid Employment on Women's Mental and Physical Health," *American Psychologist* 44 (1989): 1394–1401.

82 Women's quality of role experiences. Grace K. Baruch and Rosaline Barnett, "Role Quality, Multiple Role Involvement, and Psychological Well-being in Midlife Women," *Journal of Personality and Social Psychology* 51 (1986): 578–85. See also Ravenna Helson, Teresa Elliot, and Janet Leigh, "Number and Quality of Roles," *Psychology of Women Quarterly* 14 (1990): 83–101.

82 Satisfaction in love and work. Faye J. Crosby, "Divorce and Work Life Among Women Managers," in *The Experience and Meaning of Work in Women's Lives,* ed. H. Y. Grossman and N. L. Chester (Hillsdale, NJ: Erlbaum, 1990), pp. 121–42.

82 Healthiest adult. Sigmund Freud, *A General Introduction to Psychoanalysis* (1935; reprint, New York: Washington Square Press, 1960).

82 Housewives and depression. Ferree, "Class, Housework, and Happiness," pp. 1057–74.

82 Masculinity/feminity and depression. Donald H. Baucom and Pamela Danker-Brown, "Sex Role Identity and Sex-stereotyped Tasks in the Development of Learned Helplessness in Women," *Journal of Personality and Social Psychology* 46 (1984): 422–30; Bernard E. Whitley, Jr., "Sex-Role Orientation and Psychological Well-being: Two Meta-analyses,"

Sex Roles 12 (1984): 207–25; Susan J. Frank, Patricia A. Towell, and Margaret Huyck, "The Effects of Sex-Role Traits on Three Aspects of Psychological Well-being in a Sample of Middle-aged Women," *Sex Roles* 12 (1985): 1073–87; and Rena L. Repetti and Faye J. Crosby, "Gender and Depression: Exploring the Adult-Role Explanation," *Journal of Social and Clinical Psychology* 2 (1984): 57–70.

83 Multiple identities. Patricia W. Linville, "Self-complexity as a Cognitive Buffer Against Stress-related Illness and Depression," *Journal of Personality and Social Psychology* 52 (1987): 663–76; and Keith Oatley and Winifred Bolton, "A Social-Cognitive Theory of Depression in Reaction to Life Events," *Psychological Review* 92 (1985): 372–88.

83 "Professional life proves." Faye J. Crosby, "Divorce and Work Life Among Women Managers," *The Experience and Meaning of Work in Women's Lives*, ed. H. Y. Grossman and N. L. Chester (Hillsdale, NJ: Erlbaum, 1990), p. 141.

83 Worries and fears. Campbell, *Sense of Well-being*.

83 "Women are more likely." Wood, Rhodes, and Whelan, "Sex Differences," pp. 249–64.

83 Intensity of women's feelings. Frank Fujita, Ed Diener, and Ed Sandvik, "Gender Differences in Dysphoria and Well-being: The Case for Emotional Intensity" (Paper presented to the Midwestern Psychological Association Convention, Chicago, May 1991).

83 Women's empathy. Nancy Eisenberg and Randy Lennon, "Sex Differences in Empathy and Related Capacities," *Psychological Bulletin* 94 (1983): 100–131.

83 Women's skills at decoding emotions. Judith A. Hall, *Nonverbal Sex Differences: Communication Accuracy and Expressive Style* (Baltimore: Johns Hopkins University Press, 1984).

83 Gender and friendship. Linda A. Sapadin, "Friendship and Gender: Perspectives of Professional Men and Women," *Journal of Social and Personal Relationships* 5 (1988): 387–403; and Lillian B. Rubin, *Just Friends: The Role of Friendship in Our Lives* (New York: Harper & Row, 1985).

84 Spouse as best friend (say 80 percent of men, 73 percent of women). Greeley, *Faithful Attraction*. Although a Gallup poll (Linda DiStefano, "Pressures of Modern Life Bring Increased Importance to Friendship," *Gallup Poll Monthly*, no. 294, March 1990, pp. 24–33), found many fewer naming their spouse as best friend, the gender effect was similar— four in five women and one in three men named a woman as their best friend.

84 Suicide rates. *Statistical Abstract of the United States: 1989.*

84 Footnote. Inglehart, *Culture Shift,* p. 245; William Shakespeare, *As You Like It,* 5. 2. 48.

84 Gender and Alcoholism. The 1980s NIMH surveys, Lee N. Robins and Daniel A. Reigier, *Psychiatric Disorders in America* (New York: Free Press, 1991), revealed that 23.8 percent of men and 4.6 percent of women have at some time in their lives experienced a problem with alcohol abuse or dependence.

84 Gender and violent crime. *FBI Uniform Crime Reports,* 1989.

84 Support for premenstrual tension. Frances M. Haemmerlie and Robert L. Montgomery, "Psychological State and the Menstrual Cycle," *Journal of Social Behavior and Personality* 2 (1987): 233–42; Marcia J. McMillan and R. O. Pihl, "Premenstrual Depression: A Distinct Entity," *Journal of Abnormal Psychology* 96 (1987): 149–54; and John T. E. Richardson, "Questionnaire Studies of Paramenstrual Symptoms," *Psychology of Women Quarterly* 14 (1990) 15–42.

84 Moods and the menstruation cycle. Cathy McFarland, Michael Ross, and Nancy DeCourville, "Women's Theories of Menstruation and Biases in Recall of Menstrual Symptoms," *Journal of Personality and Social Psychology* 57 (1989): 522–31.

85 Perception of menstrual mood changes. Pamela S. Kato and Diane N. Ruble, "Toward an Understanding of Women's Experience of Menstrual Cycle Symptoms," in *Psychological Perspectives on Women's Health,* ed. V. Adesso, D. Reddy, and R. Fleming (Washington, DC: Hemisphere, 1992). For additional critique of PMS, and much more, see Carol Tavris, *The Mismeasure of Woman* (New York: Simon & Schuster, 1992).

85 "When a man." Clare Boothe Luce, "A Doll's House," *Life,* October 16, 1970, pp. 54–67.

85 Children vs. childless. Baruch and Barnett, "Role Quality," pp. 578–85.

85 Well-being in town and country. Inglehart, *Culture Shift;* Freedman, *Happy People,* pp. 169–79; and Donald M. Crider, Fern K. Willits, and C. L. Kanagy, "Rurality and Well-being During the Middle Years of Life," *Social Indicators* 24 (1991): 253–68.

85 Race. William A. Stock et al., "Race and Subjective Well-being in Adulthood," *Human Development* 28 (1985): 192–97.

85 Education. Robert A. Witter et al., "Education and Subjective Well-being: A Meta-analysis," *Educational Evaluation and Policy Analysis* 6 (1984): 165–73; and Inglehart, *Culture Shift.*

86 Robins and Reigier, *Psychiatric Disorders in America,* pp. 60–68.

86 Self-esteem of "stigmatized" groups. Jennifer Crocker and Brenda Major,

"Social Stigma and Self-esteem: The Self-protective Properties of Stigma," *Psychological Review* 96 (1989): 608–30. See also Campbell, *Sense of Well-being;* and Jerald Bachman and Patrick O'Malley, "Yea-saying, Nay-saying, and Going to Extremes: Black-White Differences in Response Styles," *Public Opinion Quarterly* 48 (1984): 491–509.

Chapter 5: Reprogramming the Mind

87 "To visit a bookstore." George F. Will, "The Seven Deadly Sins," in syndicated newspapers, July 8, 1978.

88 International New Thought Alliance purpose quoted by Donald Meyer, *The Positive Thinkers: Religion as Pop Psychology from Mary Baker Eddy to Oral Roberts* (New York: Pantheon Books, 1980), p. 36, from Horatio Dresser's *A History of the New Thought Movement* (New York: Crowell, 1919).

89 Norman Vincent Peale, *The Power of Positive Thinking* (New York: Prentice-Hall, 1952), pp. 203–4.

90 Peale's lament. Norman Vincent Peale and Smiley Blanton, *The Art of Real Happiness* (New York: Prentice-Hall, 1950), p. 3.

90 Positive thinkers. Michael F. Scheier and Charles S. Carver, "Dispositional Optimism and Physical Well-being: The Influence of Generalized Outcome Expectancies on Health," *Journal of Personality* 55 (1987): 169–210; Michael F. Scheier and Charles S. Carver, "Dispositional Optimism and Recovery from Coronary Artery Bypass Surgery: The Beneficial Effects on Physical and Psychological Well-being," *Journal of Personality and Social Psychology* 57 (1987): 1024–40; and Michael F. Scheier and Charles S. Carver, "Effects of Optimism on Psychological and Physical Well-being: Theoretical Overview and Empirical Update," *Cognitive Therapy and Research,* in press; see also Martin E. P. Seligman, *Learned Optimism* (New York: Random House, 1991).

91 Fire walking in other cultures. Marie Lucy Ahearn, "Firewalking: From Sacred to Secular," *Journal of Popular Culture* 21 (1987): 11–18.

91 "Just holding the thought . . ." Fire walk leader Tolly Burkan, quoted from the *Los Angeles Times* by Bernard J. Leikind and William J. McCarthy, "An Investigation of Firewalking," *Skeptical Inquirer* 10 (1985): 23–34.

91 Footnote. Neurolinguistic programming. Frank Clancy and Heidi Yorkshire, "The Bandler Method," *Mother Jones,* February/March 1989, pp. 24–28, 63–64; and Daniel Druckman and John A. Swets, *Enhancing*

Human Performance: Issues, Theories, and Techniques (Washington, DC: National Academy Press, 1988), p. 143.

91 Cake-in-oven example. Bernard J. Leikind and William J. McCarthy, "Firewalking," *Experientia* 44 (1988): 310–15.

92 Fire walking explained. Ibid.; and Michael R. Dennett, "Firewalking: Reality or Illusion?" *Skeptical Inquirer* 10 (Fall 1985): 36–40.

92 Cal Tech demonstration. Leikind and McCarthy, "Firewalking."

92 "Argue for your." Richard Bach, *Illusions: Adventures of a Reluctant Messiah* (New York: Delacorte Press, 1977).

93 Teen astrology beliefs. Kenneth Frazier, "Gallup Poll of Beliefs: Astrology Up, ESP down," *Skeptical Inquirer* 13 (1989): 244–45.

93 $3,000 monthly. Reported by CBS. Kenneth Frazier, "Astrology in the White House: Nancy Reagan's View," *Skeptical Inquirer* 14 (1990): 228–30.

93 Tests of astrology. Shawn Carlson, "A Double-blind Test of Astrology," *Nature* 318 (1985): 419–25.

93 Barnum paragraph. Adapted from Bertram R. Forer, "The Fallacy of Personal Validation: A Classroom Demonstration of Gullibility," *Journal of Abnormal and Social Psychology* 44 (1949): 118–23.

93 Gauguelin's demonstration. Reported by Paul Kurtz, "Stars, Planets, and People," *Skeptical Inquirer* 7 (Spring 1983): 65–69.

94 New Jersey movie theater report. F. Danzig, "Subliminal Advertising—Today It's Just Historic Flashback for Researcher Vicary," *Advertising Age*, September 17, 1962, pp. 73–74.

95 "Science has proven . . ." Paul Tuthill's *Subliminal Success Catalog* (Mind Communications, 1844 Porter SW, Grand Rapids, MI 49509, n.d.).

95 "A truly new you . . ." Advanced Learning Systems, Inc., ad in *Psychology Today*, September 1989, p. 65.

95 A hundred thousand factor. Western Research Institute ad in *Psychology Today*, September 1989, p. 59.

95 Geometric figure experiment. William R. Kunst-Wilson and Robert B. Zajonc, "Affective Discrimination of Stimuli That Cannot Be Recognized," *Science* 207 (1980): 557–58.

96 Subliminal word priming. Thomas H. Carr, A. Kontowicz, and Dale Dagenbach, "Subthreshold Priming and the Cognitive Unconscious" (Invited paper presented to the Midwestern Psychological Association Convention, Chicago, May 1987); Carol A. Fowler et al., "Lexical Access

with and Without Awareness," *Journal of Experimental Psychology: General* 110 (1981): 341–62; and Anthony Marcel, "Conscious and Unconscious Perception: Experiments on Visual Masking and Word Recognition," *Cognitive Psychology* 15 (1983): 197–237.

97 University of California, Santa Cruz, and University of Washington subliminal experiments. Anthony Greenwald et al., "Double-blind Tests of Subliminal Self-help Audiotapes," *Psychological Science* 2 (1991): 119–22. For more experiments—all of which find no effect of commercial subliminal tapes—see Brian C. Auday, J. L. Mellett, and P. M. Williams, "Self-improvement Using Subliminal Self-help Audiotapes: Consumer Benefit or Consumer Fraud?" (ms., Gordon College, 1990); S. Lenz, "The Effect of Subliminal Auditory Stimuli on Academic Learning and Motor Skills Performance Among Police Recruits" (Ph.D. diss., California School of Professional Psychology, 1989); and Phillip M. Merikle, (Unpublished manuscript regarding subliminal tapes and weight loss, University of Waterloo, 1991); Timothy E. Moore, "The Case Against Subliminal Manipulation," *Psychology and Marketing* 5 (1988): 297–316; J. Reid (Report of subliminal M.A. thesis study participants, Colorado State University, 1990); T. G. Russell, W. Rowe, and A. D. Smouse, "Subliminal Self-help Tapes and Academic Achievement: An Evaluation," *Journal of Counseling and Development* 69 (1991): 359–62; L. L. Sweet and G. K. Murdock, "Subliminal Effect on Self-esteem" (senior thesis, Missouri Southern State College, 1990); and J. Turner et al., "The Effects of Subliminal Messages on Weight Loss" (ms., Aims Biofeedback Institute and University of Northern Colorado, 1989).

97 CBC. *Advertising Age*, February 10, 1958, p. 8: " 'Phone now,' said CBC subliminally—but nobody did."

98 Content of subliminal tapes. Phillip M. Merikle, "Subliminal Auditory Messages: An Evaluation," *Psychology and Marketing* 5 (1988): 355–72.

98 Judas Priest trial. Timothy E. Moore, "Discussion of: Subliminal Perception: Are There Any Practical Applications?" (Symposium at the American Psychological Association Convention, Boston, August 1990).

98 Health fraud. Phillip M. Merikle quoted in Associated Press story, *Holland Sentinel*, January 21, 1990. Moore, "Discussion of: Subliminal Perception."

98 ". . . a complete sham." Phillip M. Merikle in S. Rae, "Brain Waves: Subliminal Self-help Messages While You Sleep?" *Elle*, April 1991, pp. 118–19.

98 Footnote. Federal Trade Commission. "Quackery" (brochure [U.S. Department of Health and Human Services publication no. 85–4200] jointly published by the Federal Trade Commission, the Pharmaceutical Advertising Council, the U.S. Food and Drug Administration, and the U.S. Postal Service).

99 Sixty-six-year-old woman. Quoted by Robin Lichtenstein, "Subliminal Messages Sell Tapes," *New York Times*, December 14, 1989, pp. B1, B2.

99 Footnote. Dieters typically regain. Rena R. Wing and Robert W. Jeffery, "Outpatient Treatments of Obesity: A Comparison of Methodology and Clinical Results," *International Journal of Obesity* 3 (1979): 261–79. Dr. C. Wayne Callaway, spokesperson for the American Board of Nutrition, estimates that ninety of all dieters who lose twenty-five pounds in a diet program put it back on within two years (reported by C. Scanlan, "Weight-loss Industry Diagnosed as Unhealthy," *Detroit Free Press*, March 27, 1990, pp. 1A, 8A).

99 Footnote. $33 billion on diets. Estimated by U.S. House Small Business subcommittee chair Ron Wyden as reported by the Associated Press, March 26, 1990.

100 Hypnosis induction and effects. David G. Myers, *Psychology*, 3d ed. (New York: Worth Publishers, 1992).

100 Hypnotic ability of fantasy-prone people. Steven J. Lynn and Judith W. Rhue, "The Fantasy-prone Person: Hypnosis, Imagination, and Creativity," *Journal of Personality and Social Psychology* 51 (1986): 404–8; and Robert Nadon et al., "Absorption and Hypnotizability: Context Effects Reexamined," *Journal of Personality and Social Psychology* 60 (1991): 144–53.

100 Falsity of hypnotic memories. Kenneth S. Bowers, personal correspondence, July 1987.

100 Hypnotically "refreshed" memories. Jane Dywan and Kenneth S. Bowers, "The Use of Hypnosis to Enhance Recall," *Science* 222 (1983): 184–85; Jean-Roch Laurence and Campbell Perry, "Hypnotically Created Memory Among Highly Hypnotizable Subjects," *Science* 222 (1983): 523–24; Martin T. Orne et al., "Hypnotically Induced Testimony," in *Eyewitness Testimony: Psychological Perspectives*, ed. Gary L. Wells and Elizabeth F. Loftus (New York: Cambridge University Press, 1984); and Marilyn C. Smith, "Hypnotic Memory Enhancement of Witnesses: Does It Work?" *Psychological Bulletin* 94 (1983): 387–407.

100 Age regression. Michael Nash, "What, If Anything, Is Regressed About

Hypnotic Age Regression? A Review of the Empirical Literature," *Psychological Bulletin* 102 (1987): 42–52; and Paul S. Silverman and Paul D. Retzlaff, "Cognitive Stage Regression Through Hypnosis: Are Earlier Cognitive Stages Retrievable?" *International Journal of Clinical and Experimental Hypnosis* 34 (1986): 192–204.

101 Past lives regression. Peter J. Reeven, "Fantasizing Under Hypnosis: Some Experimental Evidence," *Skeptical Inquirer* 12 (1987–88): 181–83.

101 Acid-throwing experiment. Martin T. Orne and Frederick J. Evans, "Social Control in the Psychological Experiment: Antisocial Behavior and Hypnosis," *Journal of Personality and Social Psychology* 1 (1965): 189–200.

101 Appalling acts under (and not under) hypnosis. Eugene E. Levitt, "Coercion, Voluntariness, Compliance and Resistance: The Essence of Hypnosis Twenty-seven Years after Orne" (Address to the American Psychological Association Convention, Washington, DC, August 1986).

101 Hypnosis doesn't block sensory input. Nicholas P. Spanos and John F. Chaves, *Hypnosis: The Cognitive-Behavioral Perspective* (Buffalo, NY: Prometheus Books, 1989).

102 Hypnosis relieves pain. John F. Kihlstrom, "Hypnosis," *Annual Review of Psychology* 36 (1985): 385–418.

102 Hypnosis, childbirth training, and pain. Joyce L. D'Eon, "Hypnosis in the Control of Labor Pain," in *Hypnosis: The Cognitive-Behavioral Perspective*, ed. Nicholas P. Spanos and John F. Chaves (Buffalo, NY: Prometheus Books, 1989); and Jonathan Venn, "Hypnosis and the Lamaze Method: A Reply to Wideman and Singer," *American Psychologist* 41 (1986): 475–76.

103 Hypnotherapy for nail-biting and smoking. Kenneth S. Bowers and Samuel LeBaron, "Hypnosis and Hypnotizability: Implications for Clinical Intervention," *Hospital and Community Psychiatry* 37 (1986): 456–67.

103 Hypnosis and healing. Elgan L. Baker, "The State of the Art of Clinical Hypnosis," *International Journal of Clinical and Experimental Hypnosis* 35 (1987): 203–14.

103 Woman's wart cure. Kenneth S. Bowers, "Hypnosis," in *Personality and Behavioral Disorders*, ed. Norman Endler and J. McVicker Hunt, 2d ed. (New York: Wiley, 1984).

103 Controlled studies of wart cure. Nicholas P. Spanos, Robert J. Stenstrom, and Joseph C. Johnston, "Hypnosis, Placebo, and Suggestion in the Treatment of Warts," *Psychosomatic Medicine* 50 (1988): 245–60.

103 Dissociation (divided consciousness) and hidden observer. Ernest R. Hilgard, *Divided Consciousness: Multiple Controls in Human Thought and Action* (New York: Wiley, 1986).

103 Everyday divided attention. William Hirst, Ulric Neisser, and Elizabeth Spelke, "Divided Attention," *Human Nature,* June 1978, pp. 54–61.

104 Skeptical students become hypnotizable. Cynthia Wickless and Irving Kirsch, "Effects of Verbal and Experiential Expectancy Manipulations on Hypnotic Susceptibility," *Journal of Personality and Social Psychology* 57 (1989): 762–68.

Chapter 6: The Traits of Happy People

106 Tracking well-being. Paul T. Costa, Robert R. McCrae, and Alan B. Zonderman, "Environmental and Dispositional Influences on Well-being: Longitudinal Follow-up of an American National Sample," *British Journal of Psychology* 78 (1987): 299–306.

106 Persistence of cheerful dispositions. Jack Block, "Some Enduring and Consequential Structures of Personality," in *Further Explorations in Personality,* ed. A. I. Rabin (New York: Wiley, 1981).

106 Only children. Toni Falbo and Dudley Polit, "Quantitative Review of the Only Child Literature: Research Evidence and Theory Development," *Psychological Bulletin* 100 (1986): 179–89; Ruut Veenhoven and Maykel Verkuyten, "The Well-being of Only Children," *Adolescence* 14 (1989): 155–66; and Norval D. Glenn and Sue K. Hoppe, "Only Children as Adults: Psychological Well-being," *Journal of Family Issues* 5 (1984): 363–82.

107 Attractive people. Elaine Hatfield and Susan Sprecher, *Mirror, Mirror: The Importance of Looks in Everyday Life* (Albany, NY: SUNY Press, 1986).

107 Michigan survey. Debra Umberson and Michael Hughes, "The Impact of Physical Attractiveness on Achievement and Psychological Well-being," *Social Psychological Quarterly* 50 (1987): 227–36.

107 Janis Joplin. Myra Friedman, *Buried Alive: The Biography of Janis Joplin* (New York: Morrow, 1973), p. 42.

107 Finding attractive those we like. Arthur L. Beaman and Bonnel Klentz, "The Supposed Physical Attractiveness Bias Against Supporters of the Women's Movement: A Meta-analysis," *Personality and Social Psychology Bulletin* 9 (1983): 544–50; and Alan E. Gross and C. Crofton, "What Is Good Is Beautiful," *Sociometry* 40 (1977): 85–90.

107 "Love looks not." Shakespeare, *A Midsummer Night's Dream*, 1.1. 1595–96.

107 Joan (not her actual name) quote. Hatfield and Sprecher, *Mirror, Mirror*.

108 Articles on self. In 1970, 5.8 percent of the 21,696 citations in *Psychological Abstracts* included the word "self." In 1990, 12.3 percent of 32,169 citations did so.

108 Benefits of self-esteem. Joel Brockner and A. J. Blethyn Hulton, "How to Reverse the Vicious Cycle of Low Self-esteem: The Importance of Attentional Focus," *Journal of Experimental Social Psychology* 14 (1978): 564–78. See also Anthony G. Greenwald and Anthony R. Pratkanis, "The Self," in *Handbook of Social Cognition*, ed. Robert S. Wyer and Thomas K. Srull (Hillsdale, NJ: Erlbaum, 1984); and Andrew M. Mecca, Neil J. Smelser, and John Vasconcellos, *The Social Importance of Self-esteem* (Berkeley: University of California Press, 1989).

108 "As soon as one." Hans H. Strupp, "The Outcome Problem in Psychotherapy: Contemporary Perspectives," in *Psychotherapy Research and Behavior Change*, vol. 1 of *The Master Lecture Series*, ed. John H. Harvey and Marjorie M. Parks (Washington, DC: American Psychological Association, 1982).

108 Norman. Norman Endler, *Holiday of Darkness* (New York: Wiley, 1982), pp. 45–49.

109 Arizona State University students. Robert B. Cialdini and Kenneth D. Richardson, "Two Indirect Tactics of Image Management: Basking and Blasting," *Journal of Personality and Social Psychology* 39 (1980): 406–15.

109 English-speaking Canadians. James R. Meindl and Melvin J. Lerner, "Exacerbation of Extreme Responses to an Out-group," *Journal of Personality and Social Psychology* 47 (1984): 71–84.

109 Dartmouth men. Teresa M. Amabile and Ann H. Glazebrook, "A Negativity Bias in Interpersonal Evaluation," *Journal of Experimental Social Psychology* 18 (1982): 1–22.

109 Northwestern sorority women. Jennifer Crocker et al., "Downward Comparison, Prejudice, and Evaluation of Others: Effects of Self-esteem and Threat," *Journal of Personality and Social Psychology* 52 (1987): 907–16.

109 Self-esteem and well-being. Angus Campbell, *The Sense of Well-being in America* (New York: McGraw-Hill, 1981); William A. Scott and John Stumpf, "Personal Satisfaction and Role Performance: Subjective and Social Aspects of Adaptation," *Journal of Personality and Social Psychology* 47 (1984): 812–27; and Lewinsohn, Julie E. Redner, and John R. Seeley, "The Relationship Between Life Satisfaction and Psychosocial

Variables: New Perspectives," in *Subjective Well-being: An Interdisciplinary Perspective*, ed. Fritz Strack, Michael Argyle, and Norbert Schwarz (Oxford, England: Pergamon Press, 1990).

110 Importance of self-image. Gallup Organization, "Importance of Social Values," *Gallup Report*, nos. 282–283 (March/April 1989): 42.

110 People dislike themselves. Carl R. Rogers, "Reinhold Niebuhr's *The Self and the Dramas of History:* A Criticism," *Pastoral Psychology* 9 (1958): 15–17.

110 "All of us have." John Powell, *Happiness Is an Inside Job* (Valencia, CA: Tabor, 1989), p. 15.

110 "No man, deep down." Mark Twain, *Notebook,* 1935.

110 "Low" self-esteem as middle-of-the-scale. Roy F. Baumeister, Diane M. Tice, and Debra G. Hutton, "Self-presentational Motivations and Personality Differences in Self-esteem," *Journal of Personality* 57 (1989): 547–79.

110 Self-serving bias research is discussed and documented in David G. Myers, *Social Psychology*, 3d ed. (New York: McGraw-Hill, 1990); C. R. Snyder and Raymond L. Higgins, "Excuses: Their Effective Role in the Negotiation of Reality," *Psychological Bulletin* 104 (1988): 23–35; Shelley E. Taylor, *Positive Illusions* (New York: Basic Books, 1989); and Bruce Headey and Alex Wearing, "The Sense of Relative Superiority— Central to Well-being," *Social Indicators Research* 20 (1988): 497–516.

112 Self-serving bias among unhappily married. Frank D. Fincham, Steven R. Beach, and Donald H. Baucom, "Attribution Processes in Distressed and Nondistressed Couples: 4. Self-partner Attribution Differences," *Journal of Personality and Social Psychology* 52 (1987): 739–48.

112 Spouse blaming for divorce. Gay C. Kitson and Marvin B. Sussman, "Marital Complaints, Demographic Characteristics, and Symptoms of Mental Distress in Divorce," *Journal of Marriage and the Family* 44 (1982): 87–101.

112 Magnetic levitation train analogy. Jonathon D. Brown, "Accuracy and Bias in Self-knowledge. Can Knowing the Truth Be Hazardous to Your Health?" in *Handbook of Social and Clinical Psychology: The Health Perspective*, ed. C. R. Snyder and D. R. Forsyth (New York: Pergamon Press, 1991).

112 Healthy vs. defensive self-esteem. Robert Raskin, Jill Novacek, and Robert Hogan, "Narcissism, Self-esteem, and Defensive Self-enhancement," *Journal of Personality* 59 (1991): 19–38.

113 "Having a strong sense." Campbell, *Sense of Well-being*, pp. 218–19.

113 "Locus of control" studies. Maureen J. Findley and Harris M. Cooper,

"Locus of Control and Academic Achievement: A Literature Review," *Journal of Personality and Social Psychology* 33 (1983): 419–27; Randy Larsen, "Is Feeling 'In Control' Related to Happiness in Daily Life?" *Psychological Reports* 64 (1989): 775–84; Herbert M. Lefcourt, *Locus of Control: Current Trends in Theory and Research* (Hillsdale, NJ: Erlbaum, 1982); and Philip C. Miller et al., "Marital Locus of Control and Marital Problem Solving," *Journal of Personality and Social Psychology* 51 (1986): 161–69.

114 Helpless dogs and people. Martin E. P. Seligman, *Helplessness: On Depression, Development and Death* (San Francisco: W. H. Freeman, 1975).

114 "I became a nonperson." James L. MacKay, "Selfhood: Comment on Brewster Smith," *American Psychologist* 35 (1980): 106–7.

114 "What is poverty?" Matthew P. Dumont, "An Unfolding Memoir of Community Mental Health," *Readings: A Journal of Reviews and Commentary in Mental Health* (September 1989): 4–7.

115 Nursing homes. Judith Rodin, "Aging and Health: Effects of the Sense of Control," *Science* 233 (1986): 1271–76. See also Morris A. Okun, Robert W. Olding, and Catherine M. G. Cohn, "A Meta-analysis of Subjective Well-being Interventions Among Elders," *Psychological Bulletin* 108 (1990): 257–66.

115 Prisoners. R. Barry Ruback, Timothy S. Carr, and Charles H. Hopper, "Perceived Control in Prison: Its Relation to Reported, Crowding, Stress, and Symptoms," *Journal of Applied Social Psychology* 16 (1986): 375–86; and Richard Wener, William Frazier, and Jay Farbstein, "Building Better Jails," *Psychology Today*, June 1987, pp. 40–49.

115 Workers. Katherine I. Miller and Peter R. Monge, "Participation, Satisfaction, and Productivity: A Meta-analytic Review," *Academy of Management Journal* 29 (1986): 727–53.

115 Berlin bars. Gabriele Oettingen and Martin E. P. Seligman, "Pessimism and Behavioural Signs of Depression in East Versus West Berlin," *European Journal of Social Psychology* 20 (1990): 207–20.

115 A late 1990 survey. Galina Balatsky and Ed Diener, "Subjective Well-being Among Soviet Students" (ms., University of Illinois, 1991).

115 For other research on personal control, see Ellen J. Langer, *The Psychology of Control* (Beverly Hills: Sage, 1983).

116 Time management. Michael Argyle, *The Psychology of Happiness* (London: Methuen, 1986), p. 117.

117 Happy optimists. William N. Dember and Judith Brooks, "A New Instrument for Measuring Optimism and Pessimism: Test-retest Reliability and

Relations with Happiness and Religious Commitment," *Bulletin of the Psychonomic Society* 27 (1989): 365–66.

117 Cultural attitude differences. Ronald Inglehart, *Culture Shift in Advanced Industrial Society* (Princeton: Princeton University Press, 1990), pp. 29–31.

117 Harvard graduates. Christopher Peterson, Martin E. P. Seligman, and George E. Vaillant, "Pessimistic Explanatory Style Is a Risk Factor for Physical Illness: A Thirty-five-Year Longitudinal Study," *Journal of Personality and Social Psychology* 55 (1988): 23–27.

117 Optimism, surgery, and health. Michael F. Scheier and Charles S. Carver, "Dispositional Optimism and Physical Well-being: The Influence of Generalized Outcome Expectancies on Health," *Journal of Personality* 55 (1987): 169–210; Michael F. Scheier and Charles S. Carver, "Dispositional Optimism and Recovery from Coronary Artery Bypass Surgery: The Beneficial Effects on Physical and Psychological Well-being," *Journal of Personality and Social Psychology* 57 (1987): 1024–40; and Michael F. Scheier and Charles S. Carver, "Effects of Optimism on Psychological and Physical Well-being."

117 Optimism and cancer recovery. Sandra Levy et al., "Survival Hazards Analysis in First Recurrent Breast Cancer Patients: Seven-year Follow-up," *Psychosomatic Medicine* 50 (1988): 520–28; and K. W. Pettingale et al., "Mental Attitudes to Cancer: An Additional Prognostic Factor," *Lancet*, March 30, 1985, p. 750.

117 Optimism and immune functioning. Leslie Kamen et al., "Pessimism and Cell-Mediated Immunity" (ms., University of Pennsylvania, 1988).

117 Life insurance sales representatives. Martin E. P. Seligman and Peter Schulman, "Explanatory Style as a Predictor of Productivity and Quitting Among Life Insurance Sales Agents," *Journal of Personality and Social Psychology* 50 (1986): 832–38.

117 Bob Dell. Reported in W. T. Buckley, "How to Cope with Crisis," *Reader's Digest*, July 1990, pp. 93–96.

118 "The good news is . . ." Robert Schuller, *The Be-Happy Attitudes: Eight Positive Attitudes That Can Transform Your Life!* (Waco, TX: Word Books, 1985).

118 College enrollment trends and projections. *Chronicle of Higher Education Almanac* (Washington, DC: Chronicle of Higher Education, Inc., 1990).

119 La Rochefoucauld. Quoted by Wladyslaw Tatarkiewicz, *Analysis of Happiness* (The Hague: Martinus Nijhoff, 1976), p. 226.

120 Extraversion-happiness link in universities. Robert A. Emmons and Ed

Diener, "Personality Correlates of Subjective Well-being," *Personality and Social Psychology Bulletin* 11 (1985): 89–97; Robert A. Emmons and Ed Diener, "An Interactional Approach to the Study of Personality and Emotion," *Journal of Personality* 54 (1986): 371–84; Robert A. Emmons and Ed Diener, "Influence of Impulsivity and Sociability on Subjective Well-being," *Journal of Personality and Social Psychology* 50 (1986): 1211–15; and William Pavot, Ed Diener, and Frank Fujita, "Extraversion and Happiness," *Personality and Individual Differences* 11, no. 12 (1990): 1299–1306.

120 As have Michael Argyle. Michael Argyle and Luo Lu, "The Happiness of Extraverts," *Personality and Individual Differences* 11 (1990): 1011–17; and Michael Argyle and Luo Lu, "Happiness and Social Skills," *Personality and Individual Differences* 11 (1990): 1255–61.

120 Extraversion-happiness link in Australians. Bruce Headey and Alex Wearing, "Personality, Life Events, and Subjective Well-being: Toward a Dynamic Equilibrium Model," *Journal of Personality and Social Psychology* 57 (1989): 731–39.

120 Extraversion-happiness link in older Americans. Paul T. Costa, Jr., and Robert R. McCrae, "Personality as a Lifelong Determinant of Well-being," in *Emotion in Adult Development*, ed. Carol Z. Malatesta and Carroll E. Izard (Newbury Park, CA: Sage, 1984).

120 "Extraverts are simply." Robert R. McCrae and Paul T. Costa, Jr., "Adding *Liebe und Arbeit:* The Full Five-Factor Model and Well-being" (Paper presented at the American Psychological Association Convention, New Orleans, August 1989).

120 Extraverts experience more positive events. Heady and Wearing, "Personality," pp. 731–39; and K. Magnus and Ed Diener, "A Longitudinal Analysis of Personality, Life Events, and Well-being" (Paper presented at the Midwestern Psychological Association Convention, Chicago, May 1991).

122 Behavior genetic studies of personality. Auke Tellegen et al., "Personality Similarity in Twins Reared Apart and Together," *Journal of Personality and Social Psychology* 54 (1988): 1031–39; B. Floderus-Myrhed, Nancy Pedersen, and I. Rasmuson, "Assessment of Heritability for Personality, Based on a Short-form of the Eysenck Personality Inventory: A Study of 13,898 Twin Pairs," *Behavior Genetics* 10 (1980): 153–62; John C. Loehlin, Lee Willerman, and Joseph M. Horn, "Personality Resemblance in Adoptive Families: A 10-year Follow-up," *Journal of Personality and Social Psychology* 53 (1987): 961–69; Robert Plomin and J. C. DeFries, *The Origins of Individual Differences in Infancy* (Orlando, FL: Academic

Press, 1985); Richard J. Rose et al., "Shared Genes, Shared Experiences, and Similarity in Personality: Data from 14,228 Adult Finnish Co-twins," *Journal of Personality and Social Psychology* 54 (1988): 161–71; and Sandra Scarr and Richard A. Weinberg, "The Minnesota Adoption Studies: Genetic Differences and Malleability," *Child Development* 54 (1983): 260–67.

122 Troubled children becoming competent adults. Jean Macfarlane, "Perspectives on Personality Consistency and Change from the Guidance Study," *Vita Humana* 7 (1964): 115–26; and study of 166 people from babyhood to age thirty. See also Alexander Thomas and Stella Chess, "The New Year Longitudinal Study: From Infancy to Early Adult Life," in *The Study of Temperament: Changes, Continuities, and Challenges*, ed. Robert Plomin and Judy Dunn (Hillsdale, NJ: Erlbaum, 1986).

122 Temper tantrums and risk of divorce. Avshalom Caspi and Daryl J. Bem, "Personality Continuity and Change Across the Life Course," in *Handbook of Personality: Theory and Research*, ed. L. A. Pervin (New York: Guilford Press, 1990).

122 Swedish study of boyhood aggression and adult crime. David Magnusson and Lars R. Bergman, "A Pattern Approach to the Study of Pathways from Childhood to Adulthood," in *Straight and Devious Pathways from Childhood to Adulthood*, ed. Lee N. Robins and Michael Rutter (Cambridge: Cambridge University Press, 1990).

122 Stability of adult personality traits. James J. Conley, "Longitudinal Stability of Personality Traits: A Multitrait-Multimethod-Multioccasion Analysis," *Journal of Personality and Social Psychology* 49 (1985): 1266–82; Paul T. Costa, Jr., and Robert R. McCrae, "Personality in Adulthood: A Six-Year Longitudinal Study of Self-reports and Spouse Ratings on the NEO Personality Inventory," *Journal of Personality and Social Psychology* 54 (1988): 853–63; and Stephen E. Finn, "Stability of Personality Self-ratings over 30 Years: Evidence for an Age/Cohort Interaction," *Journal of Personality and Social Psychology* 50 (1986): 813–18.

122 Optimism endures. Seligman, "Explanatory Style."

123 Obedience studies. Stanley Milgram, *Obedience of Authority* (New York: Harper & Row, 1974), p. 10.

123 Greek torturers. Mika Haritos-Fatouros, "The Official Torturer: A Learning Model for Obedience to the Authority of Violence," *Journal of Applied Social Psychology* 18 (1988): 1107–20; and Ervin Staub, *The Roots of Evil: The Psychological and Cultural Sources of Genocide* (New York: Cambridge University Press, 1989).

124 Pretending self-esteem increases self-esteem. Herbert L. Mirels and Robert W. McPeek, "Self-advocacy and Self-esteem," *Journal of Consulting and Clinical Psychology* 45 (1977): 1132–38; Edward Jones et al., "Effects of Strategic Self-presentation on Subsequent Self-esteem," *Journal of Personality and Social Psychology* 41 (1981): 407–21; and Frederick Rhodewalt and Sjofn Agustsdottir, "Effects of Self-presentation on the Phenomenal Self," *Journal of Personality and Social Psychology* 50 (1986): 47–55.

124 Mood manipulation statements. Emmett Velten, "A Laboratory Task for Induction of Mood States," *Behavior Research and Therapy* 6 (1968): 473–82.

124 Norman Vincent Peale's spirit lifters. From *Inspiring Messages for Dialing Living,* 1950.

125 Frowning vs. smiling. James D. Laird, "Self-attribution of Emotion: The Effects of Expressive Behavior on the Quality of Emotional Experience," *Journal of Personality and Social Psychology* 29 (1974): 475–86; James D. Laird, "The Real Role of Facial Response in the Experience of Emotion: A Reply to Tourangeau and Ellsworth, and Others," *Journal of Personality and Social Psychology* 47 (1984): 909–17; and Sandra E. Duclos et al., "Emotion-Specific Effects of Facial Expressions and Postures on Emotional Experience," *Journal of Personality and Social Psychology* 57 (1989): 100–108.

125 To find out. Joan Kellerman, James Lewis, and James D. Laird, "Looking and Loving: The Effects of Mutual Gaze on Feelings of Romantic Love," *Journal of Research in Personality* 23 (1989): 145–61.

125 Pen in teeth experiment. Fritz Strack, Leonard Martin, and Sabine Stepper, "Inhibiting and Facilitating Conditions of the Human Smile: A Nonobtrusive Test of the Facial Feedback Hypothesis," *Journal of Personality and Social Psychology* 54 (1988): 768–77.

125 Hearty smile, with cheeks. Paul Ekman, Richard J. Davidson, and Wallace V. Friesen, "The Duchenne Smile: Emotional Expression and Brain Physiology II," *Journal of Personality and Social Psychology* 58 (1990): 342–53.

125 Skidmore College students. Sara E. Snodgrass, J. G. Higgins, and L. Todisco, "The Effects of Walking Behavior on Mood" (Paper presented at the American Psychological Association Convention, Washington, DC, August 1986).

126 We synchronize. Elaine Hatfield, John T. Cacioppo, and Richard Rapson, "The Logic of Emotion: Emotional Contagion," in *Review of Per-*

sonality and Social Psychology, ed. M. S. Clark (Newbury Park, CA: Sage, 1992).

126 "If we wish." William James, "What Is an Emotion?" (1884).

Chapter 7: "Flow" in Work and Play

127 Creation curse. Excerpted from Genesis 3:17, 19 *(NRSV).*

127 Work as a search. Studs Terkel, *Working: People Talk About What They Do All Day and How They Feel About What They Do* (New York: Pantheon Books, 1972), p. xi.

129 Unhappy unemployed man: Quoted by Jonathan Freedman, *Happy People* (New York: Harcourt Brace Jovanovich, 1978), p. 156.

129 "When work is." Maksim Gorky, *The Lower Depths,* trans. Alexander Bakshy (1903; reprint, New York: Avon Books, 1974).

129 Work satisfaction and life satisfaction, especially among singles. Freedman, *Happy People;* Susan E. Crohan et al., "Job Characteristics and Well-being at Midlife," *Psychology of Women Quarterly* 13 (1989): 223–35; and Robert W. Rice et al., "Job Importance as a Moderator of the Relationship Between Job Satisfaction and Life Satisfaction," *Basic and Applied Social Psychology* 6 (1985): 297–316.

129 Work environment and mental health. Rena L. Repetti, "Individual and Common Components of the Social Environment at Work and Psychological Well-being," *Journal of Personality and Social Psychology* 52 (1987): 710–20.

129 Work spillover into family life. Richard H. Price, "Work and Community," *American Journal of Community Psychology* 13 (1985): 1–12.

129 Assembly team member. Ann C. Crouter, "Participative Work as an Influence on Human Development," *Journal of Applied Developmental Psychology* 5 (1984): 71–90.

129 Young unemployed woman. Freedman, *Happy People,* p. 155.

130 "No task, rightly done." Woodrow Wilson, address at Princeton University, November 1, 1902.

130 "The Chicago piano tuner." Terkel, *Working,* p. xi.

130 Would you continue working? In University of Michigan national surveys, three fourths say yes (Angus Campbell, *The Sense of Well-being in America* [New York: McGraw-Hill, 1981], p. 115). In National Opinion Research Center surveys, more than seven in ten say yes (Richard Gene

Niemi, John Mueller, and Tom W. Smith, *Trends in Public Opinion: A Compendium of Survey Data* [New York: Greenwood Press, 1989], p. 242).

130 Would you choose the same work again? Freedman, *Happy People.*

130 Increasing job satisfaction. Alex C. Michalos, "Job Satisfaction, Marital Satisfaction, and the Quality of Life: A Review and a Preview," in *Research on the Quality of Life,* ed. Frank M. Andrews (Ann Arbor: Survey Research Center, University of Michigan, 1986); and see Eric Sundstrom, Kenneth P. DeMeuse, and David Futrell, "Work Teams: Applications and Effectiveness," *American Psychologist* 45 (1990): 120–33.

130 Bakery director. Terkel, *Working.*

131 "Words such as 'love.' " Max DePree, *Leadership Is an Art* (Garden City, NY: Doubleday, 1989).

131 Employee well-being and bottom line. K. I. Howard, "Employers' Attitudes About Mental Health Are Affecting Their Bottom Lines," *Northwestern Perspectives,* Spring 1991, p. 48.

132 "Flow." Mihaly Csikszentmihalyi and Isabella S. Csikszentmihalyi, *Optimal Experience: Psychological Studies of Flow in Consciousness* (Cambridge: Cambridge University Press, 1988).

133 "In real play." Madeleine L'Engle, *A Circle of Quiet* (New York: Seabury, 1972), p. 10.

133 Beeper study. Mihaly Csikszentmihalyi and Judith LeFevre, "Optimal Experience in Work and Leisure," *Journal of Personality and Social Psychology* 56 (1989): 815–22.

133 Challenge and work satisfaction. Campbell, *Sense of Well-being,* p. 116; and Paula K. Adelmann, "Occupational Complexity, Control, and Personal Income: Their Relation to Psychological Well-being in Men and Women," *Journal of Applied Psychology* 72 (1987): 529–37.

133 Stone mason. Terkel, *Working,* p. xvi.

133 Abraham Maslow. Quoted by Anthony Storr, *Solitude: A Return to Self* (New York: Free Press, 1988), p. 201.

133 Dehumanization of labor. Karl Marx, *Das Kapital,* trans. S. L. Trask, vol. 2, p. 9.

133 Charles Reich. Quoted by Campbell, *Sense of Well-being,* p. 42.

134 Workers, 25 percent not working. Mihaly Csikszentmihalyi, *Flow: The Psychology of Optimal Experience* (New York: Harper & Row, 1990), p. 158.

134 Productivity and self-esteem. Mihaly Csikszentmihalyi, "The Future of Flow," in *Optimal Experience: Psychological Studies of Flow in Consciousness,* ed. Mihaly Csikszentmihalyi and Isabella S. Csikszentmihalyi (Cambridge: Cambridge University Press, 1988).

134 John F. Donnelly. Quoted by Eddie Malloy, Donnelly Inaugural Lecture, Notre Dame University, April 19, 1988.

135 Adversity into enjoyment. Csikszentmihalyi, *Flow:,* pp. 209–13.

136 "I am doing work." C. S. Lewis, "Good Work and Good Works," in *Screwtape Proposes a Toast* (Glasgow: William Collins, 1965), p. 114.

136 "The relative poverty." Csikszentmihalyi, "The Future of Flow," p. 378. A statistical digest of 107 studies confirms that "social activity is significantly related to subjective well-being"—Morris Okun et al., "The Social Activity/Subjective Well-being Relation: A Quantitative Synthesis," *Research on Aging* 6 (1984): 45–65.

137 Flow and apathy in leisure. Fausto Massimini and Massimo Carli, "The Systematic Assessment of Flow in Daily Experience," in *Optimal Experience: Psychological Studies of Flow in Consciousness,* ed. Mihaly Csikszentmihalyi and Isabella S. Csikszentmihalyi (Cambridge: Cambridge University Press, 1988), p. 99.

137 Sunday mornings. Csikszentmihalyi, *Flow,* p. 168.

137 Apathy and joylessness. M. Csikszentmihalyi, "The Future of Flow."

137 Active leisure in traditional societies. M. Csikszentmihalyi and LeFevre, "Optimal Experience," pp. 815–22.

138 "In every part." Robert Louis Stevenson, *Memories and portraits: Old mortality,* 1903.

138 Sleep deprivation and malaise. Mario Mikulincer et al., "The Effects of 72 Hours of Sleep Loss on Psychological Variables," *British Journal of Psychology* 80 (1989): 145–62.

138 Sleep and depression. T. Frederick, Ralph R. Frerichs, and Virginia A. Clark, "Personal Health Habits and Symptoms of Depression at the Community Level," *Preventive Medicine* 17 (1988): 173–82.

139 Carbohydrates and sleepiness. Bonnie Spring, "Foods, Brain and Behavior: New Links," *Harvard Medical School Mental Health Letter* 4, no. 7 (1988): 4–6.

139 National sleep debt. William Dement, in the PBS film, *Sleep Alert,* quoted by *Behavior Today,* March 12, 1990, p. 8.

139 REST. Peter Suedfeld, *Restricted Environmental Stimulation: Research and Clinical Applications* (New York: Wiley, 1980); and Peter Suedfeld,

"Aloneness as a Healing Experience," in *Loneliness: Sourcebook of Current Theory, Research, and Therapy,* ed. Letitia A. Peplau and Daniel Perlman (New York: Wiley, 1982).

140 Outward Bound. Herbert W. Marsh, Garry E. Richards, and Jennifer Barnes, "Multidimensional Self-concepts: The Effect of Participation in an Outward Bound Program," *Journal of Personality and Social Psychology* 50 (1986): 195–204.

140 "It is in silence." Thomas Merton, *The Silent Life,* 1957.

141 Meditative relaxation. Herbert Benson and Miriam Z. Klipper, *The Relaxation Response* (New York: Morrow, 1976); Herbert Benson and William Proctor, *Beyond the Relaxation Response: How to Harness the Healing Power of Your Personal Beliefs* (New York: Times Books, 1984); and Herbert Benson, *Your Maximum Mind* (New York: Times Books, 1987).

141 Relaxation and immune responses. Mary L. Jasnoski, Joachim Kugler, and David C. McClelland, "Power Imagery and Relaxation Affect Psychoneuroimmune Indices" (Paper presented at the American Psychological Association Convention, Washington, DC, August 1986).

141 Meditation and longevity. Charles Alexander et al., "Transcendental Meditation, Mindfulness, and Longevity: An Experimental Study with the Elderly," *Journal of Personality and Social Psychology* 57 (1989): 950–64.

Chapter 8: The Friendship Factor

142 Linda and Emily. Shelley E. Taylor, *Positive Illusions* (New York: Basic Books, 1989), pp. 139–42.

143 "Hell is others." Jean-Paul Sartre, *No Exit,* 1944, p. 5.

143 Family stress. Peter Warr and Roy Payne, "Experiences of Strain and Pleasure Among British Adults," *Social Science and Medicine* 16 (1982): 1691–97.

143 Social ties and health. Sheldon Cohen, "Psychosocial Models of the Role of Social Support in the Etiology of Physical Disease," *Health Psychology* 7 (1988): 269–97; and James S. House, Karl R. Landis, and Debra Umberson, "Social Relationships and Health," *Science* 241 (1988): 540–45.

144 Finnish study of widowhood and death risk. Jaakko Kaprio, Markku Koskenvuo, and Heli Rita, "Mortality After Bereavement: A Prospective

Study of 95,647 Widowed Persons," *American Journal of Public Health* 77 (1987): 283–87.

144 National Academy of Sciences on widowhood and disease. Bruce Dohren-wend et al., "Report on Stress and Life Events," in *Stress and Human Health: Analysis and Implications of Research,* ed. Glen R. Elliott and Carl Eisdorfer (New York: Springer-Verlag, 1982).

144 A friend is good medicine. Carolyn E. Cutrona, "Behavioral Manifesta-tions of Social Support: A Microanalytic Investigation," *Journal of Per-sonality and Social Psychology* 51 (1986): 201–8; and Karen S. Rook, "Social Support Versus Companionship: Effects on Life Stress, Loneli-ness, and Evaluations by Others," *Journal of Personality and Social Psy-chology* 52 (1987): 1132–47.

144 "Friendship is a sovereign." Seneca, "Seneca of a Happy Life," *Morals.*

144 Expression of grief and health. James W. Pennebaker, *The Psychology of Physical Symptoms* (New York: Springer-Verlag, 1982); James W. Pen-nebaker and S. Beall, "Cognitive, Emotional, and Physiological Compo-nents of Confiding: Behavioral Inhibition and Disease" (ms., Southern Methodist University, 1984); and James W. Pennebaker and Robin C. O'Heeron, "Confiding in Others and Illness Rate Among Spouses of Suicide and Accidental Death Victims," *Journal of Abnormal Psychology* 93 (1984): 473–76. For an excellent, nontechnical summary see James W. Pennebaker, *Opening Up: The Healing Power of Confiding in Others* (New York: Morrow, 1990).

145 Holocaust survivors. James W. Pennebaker, Steven D. Barger, and John Tiebout, "Disclosure of Traumas and Health Among Holocaust Survi-vors," *Psychosomatic Medicine* 51 (1989): 577–89.

145 Individualism and hopelessness. Martin E. P. Seligman, "Why Is There So Much Depression Today?" in *G. Stanley Hall Lectures,* ed. I. S. Cohen, vol. 9 (Washington, DC: American Psychological Association, 1988).

145 Individualist vs. communal identity. Harry C. Triandis et al., "Individual-ism and Collectivism: Cross-cultural Perspectives on Self-Ingroup Rela-tionships," *Journal of Personality and Social Psychology* 54 (1988): 323–38.

146 "Gestalt credo." Fritz Perls, "Gestalt Therapy (interview)," in *Inside Psychotherapy,* ed. Adelaide Bry (New York: Basic Books, 1972), p. 70.

146 "The only question." Quoted by Michael A. Wallach and Lise Wallach, "How Psychology Sanctions the Cult of the Self," *Washington Monthly,* February 1985, pp. 46–56.

147 Hong Kong students. Ladd Wheeler, Harry T. Reis, and Michael H.

Bond, "Collectivism-Individualism in Everyday Social Life: The Middle Kingdom and the Melting Pot," *Journal of Personality and Social Psychology* 57 (1989): 79–86.

147 Communal society interdependence. C. Harry Hui, "West Meets East: Individualism Versus Collectivism in North America and Asia" (Invited address, Hope College, November 1990).

147 Japanese/Chinese mother-infant closeness. Hazel Markus and Shinobu Kitayama, "Culture and the Self: Implications for Cognition, Emotion, and Motivation," *Psychological Review* 98 (1991): 224–53.

147 Pros and cons of individualism and collectivism. See Harry C. Triandis, "The Self and Social Behavior of Differing Cultural Contexts," *Psychological Review* 96 (1989): 506–20; Harry C. Triandis, "Cross-cultural Studies of Individualism and Collectivism," in *Nebraska Symposium on Motivation 1989*, ed. J. J. Berman, vol. 37 (Lincoln: University of Nebraska Press, 1989); Harry C. Triandis, Richard Brislin, and C. Harry Hui, "Cross-cultural Training Across the Individualism-Collectivism Divide," *International Journal of Intercultural Relations* 12 (1988): 269–89; and Karen K. Dion and Kenneth L. Dion, "Psychological Individualism and Romantic Love," *Journal of Social Behavior and Personality* 6 (1991): 17–33.

148 "Woe to him." Ecclesiastes 4:10b *(NRSV)*.

148 "Rampant individualism carries." Seligman, "Why Is There So Much Depression Today?"

148 Natural selection of group living. William D. Hamilton, "Innate Social Aptitudes of Man: An Approach from Evolutionary Genetics," in *Biosocial Anthropology*, ed. R. Fox (London: Malaby Press, 1975).

148 "Intimate attachments to other." John Bowlby, *Loss, Sadness and Depression*, vol. 3 of *Attachment and Loss* (London: Basic Books, 1980), p. 442.

149 "It redoubleth joys." Francis Bacon, "Of Friendship," *Essays*.

149 Number of intimates and happiness. Ronald S. Burt, *Strangers, Friends and Happiness*, GSS Technical Report No. 72 (Chicago: National Opinion Research Center, University of Chicago, 1986).

149 University students' love life. Robert Emmons et al., "Factors Predicting Satisfaction Judgments: A Comparative Examination" (Paper presented at the Midwestern Psychological Association Convention, Chicago, May 1983).

149 Close relationships and stress. Antonio Abbey and Frank M. Andrews, "Modeling the Psychological Determinants of Life Quality," *Social Indicators Research* 16 (1985): 1–34; and Daniel Perlman and Karen S.

Rook, "Social Support, Social Deficits, and the Family: Toward the Enhancement of Well-being," in *Family Processes and Problems: Social Psychological Aspects*, ed. Stuart Oskamp (Newbury Park, CA: Sage, 1987).

149 A-teams. Frederick J. Manning and Terrence D. Fullerton, "Health and Well-being in Highly Cohesive Units of the U.S. Army," *Journal of Applied Social Psychology* 18 (1988): 503–19.

149 Goal support and well-being. Barbara A. Israel and Toni C. Antonucci, "Social Network Characteristics and Psychological Well-being: A Replication and Extension," *Health Education Quarterly* 14 (1987): 461–81; and Linda S. Ruehlman and Sharlene A. Wolchik, "Personal Goals and Interpersonal Support and Hindrance as Factors in Psychological Distress and Well-being," *Journal of Personality and Social Psychology* 55 (1988): 293–301.

·149 Yuppie values. H. W. Perkins, "Religious Commitment, Yuppie Values, and Well-being in Post-collegiate Life," *Review of Religious Research* 32 (1991): 244–51.

150 Close relationships necessary for happiness. Ellen Berscheid, "Interpersonal Attraction," in *The Handbook of Social Psychology*, ed. Gardner Lindzey and Elliot Aronson (New York: Random House, 1985); and Ellen Berscheid and Letitia A. Peplau, "The Emerging Science of Relationships," in *Close Relationships*, ed. H. H. Kelly et al. (New York: Freeman, 1983).

150 "The sun looks." C. S. Lewis, "Membership," in *The Weight of Glory and Other Addresses* (New York: Macmillan, 1949).

150 Elizabeth Taylor. Lois Wyse, "The Way We Are," *Good Housekeeping*, April 1991, p. 254.

150 Single-parent families. U.S. Bureau of the Census, reported in *American Enterprise*, March/April, 1991, p. 93.

150 Trust vs. anxiety. John G. Holmes and John K. Rempel, "Trust in Close Relationships," in *Review of Personality and Social Psychology*, ed. Clyde Hendrick, vol. 10 (Newbury Park, CA: Sage, 1989).

150 Mood and self-disclosure. Michael R. Cunningham, "Does Happiness Mean Friendliness? Induced Mood and Heterosexual Self-disclosure," *Personality and Social Psychology Bulletin* 14 (1988): 283–97.

151 Masks and love. Sidney M. Jourard, *The Transparent Self* (Princeton: Van Nostrand, 1964).

151 Friendship and threats to self-image. William G. Swann, Jr., and Steven

C. Predmore, "Intimates as Agents of Social Support: Sources of Consolation or Despair?" *Journal of Personality and Social Psychology* 41 (1985): 1119–28.

151 Self-disclosure vs. loneliness. John Berg and Letitia A. Peplau, "Loneliness: The Relationship of Self-disclosure and Androgyny," *Personality and Social Psychology Bulletin* 8 (1982): 624–30; and Cecilia H. Solano, Phillip G. Batten, and Elizabeth A. Parish, "Loneliness and Patterns of Self-Disclosure," *Journal of Personality and Social Psychology* 43 (1982): 524–31.

151 "I lie awake." Psalm 102:7 *(NRSV).*

151 "Desert of our loneliness." Henri J. M. Nouwen, *Reaching Out: The Three Movements of the Spiritual Life* (Garden City, NY: Doubleday, 1975).

151 Disclosure reciprocity. John Berg, Responsiveness and Self-disclosure," in *Self-disclosure: Theory, Research, and Therapy,* ed. Valerian J. Derlega and John H. Berg (New York: Plenum, 1987; and Harry T. Reis and Phillip Shaver, "Intimacy as an Interpersonal Process," in *Handbook of Personal Relationships: Theory, Relationships and Interventions,* ed. Steve Duck (Chichester, England: Wiley, 1988).

151 Skilled openers. Lynn C. Miller, John H. Berg, and Richard L. Archer, "Openers: Individuals Who Elicit Intimate Self-disclosure," *Journal of Personality and Social Psychology* 44 (1983): 1234–44; and James A. Purvis, James M. Dabbs, and Charles H. Hopper, "The 'Opener': Skilled User of Facial Expression and Speech Pattern," *Personality and Social Psychology Bulletin* 10 (1984): 61–66.

151 "Growth-promoting" listeners. Carl R. Rogers, *A Way of Being* (Boston: Houghton Mifflin, 1980), p. 10.

151 Carl R. Rogers, "Reinhold Niebuhr's *The Self and the Dramas of History:* A Criticism," *Pastoral Psychology* 9 (1958): 15–17.

152 Rogers conversation. B. D. Meador and Carl R. Rogers, "Person-Centered Therapy," in *Current Psychotherapies,* ed. Raymond J. Corsini (Itasca, IL: Peacock, 1984), p. 167.

153 Benefits of psychotherapy. Mary Lee Smith and Gene V. Glass, "Meta-analysis of Psychotherapy Outcome Studies," *American Psychologist* 31 (1977): 752–60; and Mary Lee Smith and Gene V. Glass, *The Benefits of Psychotherapy* (Baltimore: Johns Hopkins University Press, 1980).

153 Psychotherapy effectiveness. Jerome D. Frank, "Therapeutic Components Shared by All Psychotherapies," in *Psychotherapy Research and*

Behavior Change, vol. 1 of *The Master Lecture Series* ed. John H. Harvey and Marjorie M. Parks (Washington, DC: American Psychological Association, 1982).

153 Psychotherapy effectiveness. Marvin R. Goldfried and Wendy Padawer, "Current Status and Future Directions in Psychotherapy," in *Converging Themes in Psychotherapy: Trends in Psychodynamic, Humanistic, and Behavioral Practice,* ed. Marvin R. Goldfried (New York: Springer-Verlag, 1982).

153 Psychotherapy effectiveness. Hans H. Strupp, "Psychotherapy: Research, Practice, and Public Policy (How to Avoid Dead Ends)," *American Psychologist* 41 (1986): 120–30.

153 Therapists vs. lay people. John A. Hattie, Christopher F. Sharpley, and H. Jane Rogers, "Comparative Effectiveness of Professional and Paraprofessional Helpers," *Psychological Bulletin* 95 (1984): 534–41; see also Jeffrey S. Berman and Nicholas C. Norton, "Does Professional Training Make a Therapist More Effective?" *Psychological Bulletin* 98 (1985): 401–7.

153 Social support reduced need for therapy. Jerome D. Frank, "Therapeutic Components Shared"; and Pat O'Connor and George W. Brown, "Supportive Relationships: Fact or Fancy?" *Journal of Social and Personal Relationships* 1 (1984): 159–75.

154 Not good to be alone. Genesis 2: 18a *(NRSV).*

Chapter 9: Love and Marriage

155 Love as missing element, and quotes. Jonathan Freedman, *Happy People* (New York: Harcourt Brace Jovanovich, 1978).

156 Marriage and happiness. For summary of West European surveys, see Ronald Inglehart, *Culture Shift in Advanced Industrial Society* (Princeton: Princeton University Press, 1990); see also Norval D. Glenn and Charles N. Weaver, "The Changing Relationship of Marital Status to Reported Happiness," *Journal of Marriage and the Family* 50 (1988): 317–24; and Walter R. Gove, Carolyn B. Style, and Michael Hughes, "The Effect of Marriage on the Well-being of Adults: A Theoretical Analysis," *Journal of Family Issues* 11 (1990): 4–35.

156 Statistical summary. Wendy Wood, Nancy Rhodes, and Melanie Whelan, "Sex Differences in Positive Well-being: A Consideration of Emotional Style and Marital Status," *Psychological Bulletin* 106 (1989): 249–64.

156 Marriage and psychological disorder. Robert H. Coombs, "Marital Status and Personal Well-being: A Literature Review," *Family Relations* 40 (January 1991): 97–102.

156 Marriage quality and happiness. Walter R. Gove, Michael Hughes, and Carolyn B. Style, "Does Marriage Have Positive Effects on the Psychological Well-being of the Individual?" *Journal of Health and Social Behavior* 24 (1983): 122–31; Jacqueline M. Golding, "Role Occupancy and Role-Specific Stress and Social Support as Predictors of Depression," *Basic and Applied Social Psychology* 10 (1989): 173–95; and Robert C. Smolen et al., "Examination of Marital Adjustment and Marital Assertion in Depressed and Nondepressed Women," *Journal of Social and Clinical Psychology* 7 (1988): 284–89.

156 Most people happy with their marriage. National Opinion Research Center survey, reported in *Public Opinion,* October/November 1984, p. 23. See also Andrew M. Greeley, *Faithful Attraction* (New York: Tor Books, 1991).

156 Spouse as best friend and would marry again. Greeley, *Faithful Attraction,* p. 238.

157 "Depressed persons induced." Stephen Strack and James C. Coyne, "Social Confirmation of Dysphoria: Shared and Private Reactions to Depression," *Journal of Personality and Social Psychology* 44 (1983): 798–806.

157 Male medical students. Coombs, "Marital Status," pp. 97–102.

157 Multiple roles. Faye J. Crosby, *Spouse, Parent, Worker: On Gender and Multiple Roles* (New Haven: Yale University Press, 1987).

158 95 percent marry by age forty. Bureau of the Census, *Statistical Abstract of the United States* (Washington, DC: Superintendent of Documents, Government Printing Office, 1987).

158 Overconfidence in lifelong romance. Darrin R. Lehman and Richard E. Nisbett, "Effects of Higher Education on Inductive Reasoning" (ms. University of Michigan, 1985).

158 U.S. and Canadian divorce data. T. R. Balakrishan et al., "A Hazard Model Analysis of the Covariates of Marriage Dissolution in Canada," *Demography* 24 (1987): 395–406.

158 Well-married person. Henry Ward Beecher, *Proverbs from Plymouth Pulpit,* 1887.

158 Happiness of those happily married or not. Norval D. Glenn, "The Social and Cultural Meaning of Contemporary Marriage," in *The Retreat from Marriage,* ed. Bryce Christensen (Rockford, IL: The Rockford Institute, 1990).

158 Glenn analyzed. Glenn, "Social and Cultural Meaning"; and Norval D. Glenn, "The Recent Trend in Marital Success in the United States," *Journal of Marriage and the Family* 53 (1991): 261–70. After studying the 1985 U.S. government population survey, Teresa Castro Martin and Larry L. Bumpass, "Recent Trends in Marital Disruption," *Demography* 26 (1989): 37–51, similarly estimate that two thirds of recent marriages are destined for divorce or separation.

159 Gallup report. Diane Colasanto and James Shriver, "Mirror of America: Middle-aged Face Marital Crisis," *Gallup Report*, no. 284, May 1989, pp. 34–38.

159 Marriage market. Glenn, "The Recent Trend in Marital Success," pp. 261–70.

159 Woman teacher. Digested from Freedman, *Happy People.*

159 "Marry, and with luck." Euripides, *Orestes*, trans. William Arrowsmith.

160 European divorce. Ronald Inglehart, *Culture Shift*, p. 203.

160 Hedonistic marriages. Glenn, "Social and Cultural Meaning."

160 Social forces and changing divorce norms. Inglehart, *Culture Shift*, p. 178.

160 Declining percent "very happy" among the still married. Glenn, "Social and Cultural Meaning."

160 Declining marital happiness gap. Ibid.

161 "Traditional families." Bureau of the Census, *Statistical Abstract of the United States* (Washington, DC: Superintendent of Documents, Government Printing Office, 1990).

161 Cohabitation trends. Neil G. Bennett, Ann K. Blanc, and David E. Bloom, "Commitment and the Modern Union: Assessing the Link Between Premarital Cohabitation and Subsequent Marital Stability," *American Sociological Review* 53 (1988): 127–38; and Larry L. Bumpass and James A. Sweet, "National Estimates of Cohabitation," *Demography* 26 (1989); 615–25; and Inglehart, *Culture Shifts.*

161 Marriage among eighteen- to fifty-four-year-olds. U.S. Census data reported in *American Enterprise*, May/June 1991, p. 101.

161 Living apart and divorce. Ronald R. Rindfuss and Elizabeth Hervey Stephen, "Marital Noncohabitation: Separation Does Not Make the Heart Grow Fonder," *Journal of Marriage and the Family* 52 (1990): 259–70.

162 Teen birth control and abortion. National Research Council, *Risking the Future: Adolescent Sexuality, Pregnancy, and Childbearing* (Washington, DC: National Academic Press, 1987), p. 1.

162 College survey regarding trial marriage. Alexander W. Astin, William S.

Korn, and E. R. Berz, *The American Freshman: National Norms for Fall 1989* (Los Angeles: Higher Education Research Institute, Graduate School of Education, UCLA, 1989).

162 Cohabitation and subsequent divorce. American data: Alan Booth and David Johnson, "Premarital Cohabitation and Marital Success," *Journal of Family Issues* 9 (1988): 255–72; E. Lowell Kelly and James J. Conley, "Personality and Compatibility: A Prospective Analysis of Marital Stability and Marital Satisfaction," *Journal of Personality and Social Psychology* 52 (1987): 27–40; and Michael D. Newcomb, "Cohabitation and Marriage: A Quest for Independence and Relatedness," in *Family Processes and Problems: Social Psychological Aspects,* ed. Stuart Oskamp (Newbury Park, CA: Sage, 1987). U.S. national data: Bumpass and Sweet, "National Estimates of Cohabitation," pp. 615–25. Canadian data: Balakrishan et al., "A Hazard Model Analysis," pp. 395–406; S. S. Halli and Z. Zimmer, "Common Law Union as a Differentiating Factor in the Failure of Marriage in Canada, 1984," *Social Indicators Research* 24 (1991): 329–45; and James M. White, "Reply to Comment by Professors Trussell and Rao: A Reanalysis of the Data," *Journal of Marriage and the Family* 51 (1989): 540–44. Swedish data: Bennett, Blanc, and Bloom, "Commitment and the Modern Union," pp. 127–38.

163 Premarital sex and marital unhappiness. Michael D. Newcomb and Peter M. Bentler, "Impact of Adolescent Drug Use and Social Support on Problems of Young Adults: A Longitudinal Study," *Journal of Abnormal Psychology* 97 (1988): 64–75.

163 Cohabitation and marital quality. Alfred DeMaris and Gerald R. Leslie, "Cohabitation with the Future Spouse: Its Influence upon Marital Satisfaction and Communication," *Journal of Marriage and the Family* 46 (1984): 77–84. Elizabeth Thomson and Ugo Colella, "Cohabitation and Marital Stability: Quality or Commitment," *Journal of Marriage and the Family,* in press.

163 Centers for Disease Control. Report summarized by the Associated Press, January 5, 1991.

164 "Teen promiscuity is known." Neil M. Malamuth et al., "Characteristics of Aggressors Against Women: Testing a Model Using a National Sample of College Students," *Journal of Consulting and Clinical Psychology* 59 (1991): 670–81; and Joan R. Kahn and Kathryn A. London, "Premarital Sex and the Risk of Divorce," *Journal of Marriage and the Family* 53 (1991): 845–55.

164 Soap operas. Dennis T. Lowry and David E. Towles, "Soap Opera Por-

trayals of Sex, Contraception, and Sexually Transmitted Diseases," *Journal of Communication* 39, no. 2 (1989): 76–83.

164 Sex disinformation. Planned Parenthood Federation of America, 1986; "10,000 do it"—from a 1986 Planned Parenthood ad, "Sex Education for Parents," *USA Today,* December 15, 1986, p. 11A.

164 "That intensely sexual material." Michael Medved, "Popular Culture and the War Against Standards," *Imprimis* 20, no. 2 (February 1991): 1–7.

164 "Our children will." Louis Sullivan, *Washington Post* quote from address to the March 12, 1991, National Health Forum, *Grand Rapids Press,* March 24, 1991, p. D7.

164 Footnote. One in four women have experienced rape or attempted rape. From surveys by Mary P. Koss, Christine A. Gidycz, and Nadine Wisniewski, "The Scope of Rape: Incidence and Prevalence of Sexual Aggression and Victimization in a National Sample of Higher Education Students," *Journal of Consulting and Clinical Psychology* 55 (1987): 162–70; Mary P. Koss and Barry R. Burkhart, "A Conceptual Analysis of Rape Victimization," *Psychology of Women Quarterly* 13 (1989): 27–40; Mary P. Koss, Paul Koss, and W. Joy Woodruff, "Relation of Criminal Victimization to Health Perceptions Among Women Medical Patients," *Journal of Consulting and Clinical Psychology* 58, no. 2 (1990): 147–52.

164 Footnote. Pornography research. See Ed Donnerstein, Daniel Linz, and Steven Penrod, *The Question of Pornography* (New York: Free Press, 1987); Neil M. Malamuth, "Sexually Violent Media, Thought Patterns, and Antisocial Behavior," in *Public Communication and Behavior,* ed. George Comstock, vol. 2 (San Diego: Academic Press, 1989); and Dolf Zillmann, "Effects of Prolonged Consumption of Pornography," in *Pornography: Research Advances and Policy Considerations,* ed. Dolf Zillmann and Jennings Bryant (Hillsdale, NJ: Erlbaum, 1989).

165 National surveys on children of divorce and of unhappily married parents. Norval D. Glenn and Kathryn B. Kramer, "The Psychological Well-being of Adult Children of Divorce," *Journal of Marriage and Family* 47 (1985): 905–12; and Alan Booth and John N. Edwards, "Transmission of Marital and Family Quality over the Generations: The Effect of Parental Divorce on Unhappiness," *Journal of Divorce* 12 (1989): 41–58.

165 "Children at increased risk." E. Mavis Hetherington, Margaret Stanley-Hagan, and Edward R. Anderson, "Marital Transitions: A Child's Perspective," *American Psychologist* 44 (1989): 303–12. Also see E. Mavis Hetherington and W. G. Clingempeel, "Coping with Marital Transi-

tions: A Family Systems Perspective," *Society for Research in Child Development Monographs*, in press; Paul R. Amato and Bruce Keith, "Parental Divorce and the Well-being of Children: A Meta-analysis, *Psychological Bulletin* 110 (1991): 26–46; and Paul R. Amato and Bruce Keith, "Parental Divorce and Adult Well-being," *Journal of Marriage and the Family* 53 (1991): 43–58.

165 British seven-year-olds. Andrew J. Cherlin et al., "Longitudinal Studies of Effects of Divorce on Children in Great Britain and the United States," *Science* 252 (1991): 1386–89.

165 Remarriage rates. Booth and Edwards, "Transmission of Marital and Family Quality," pp. 41–58.

165 First marriage satisfaction. Elizabeth Vemer et al., "Marital Satisfaction in Remarriage: A Meta-analysis," *Journal of Marriage and the Family* 51 (1989): 713–25.

165 25 percent greater risk of divorce in remarried. Martin and Bumpass, "Recent Trends," pp. 37–51.

165 Affairs. Joyce Brothers, "Why Wives Have Affairs," *Parade*, February 18, 1990, pp. 4–7.

166 Marital fidelity. Beliefs about fidelity and Gallup survey: Greeley, *Faithful Attraction*. British fidelity: British Market Research Limited, 1987. NORC: Tom W. Smith, "Adult Sexual Behavior in 1989: Number of Partners, Frequency, and Risk," General Social Survey Topic Report No. 18 (Chicago: National Opinion Research Center, University of Chicago, 1990).

166 "All is not well." Glenn, "Social and Cultural Meaning."

166 In a 1990 survey. American Psychological Association, *Survey of American Psychological Association Members* (Washington, DC: American Psychological Association, 1990).

166 Love in various close relationships. Keith E. Davis, "Near and Dear: Friendship and Love Compared," *Psychology Today*, February 1985, pp. 22–30; G. M. Maxwell, "Behavior of Lovers: Measuring the Closeness of Relationships," *Journal of Social and Personal Relationships* 2 (1985): 215–38; and Robert J. Sternberg and Susan Grajek, "The Nature of Love," *Journal of Personality and Social Psychology* 47 (1984): 312–29.

167 Eye-contact study. Zick Rubin, "Measurement of Romantic Love," *Journal of Personality and Social Psychology* 16 (1970): 265–73; and Zick Rubin, *Liking and Loving: An Invitation to Social Psychology* (New York: Holt, Rinehart and Winston, 1973).

167 "All the world." Anthony Storr, *Solitude: A Return to Self* (New York: Free Press, 1988).

167 Joyful woman in love. Quoted by Dorothy Tennov, *Love and Limerence: The Experience of Being in Love* (New York: Stein & Day, 1979), p. 22.

167 Bottled note. UPI news story reported in the *Milwaukee Journal,* August 27, 1981, p. 1.

168 Surprising sense of loss upon divorce or death. John G. Carlson and Elaine Hatfield, *Psychology of Emotion* (Belmont, CA: Wadsworth, 1989).

168 Romantic high to disappointment. Greeley, *Faithful Attraction,* p. 50.

168 Passionate and romantic love. Ellen Berscheid, Steven W. Gangestad, and D. Kulakowski, "Emotion in Close Relationship Counseling," in *Handbook of Counseling Psychology,* ed. Steven D. Brown and Robert W. Lent (New York: Wiley, 1984).

168 "The sharp rise in the divorce rate." Jeffry A. Simpson, Bruce Campbell, and Ellen Berscheid, "The Association Between Romantic Love and Marriage: Kephart (1967) Twice Revisited," *Personality and Social Psychology Bulletin* 12 (1986): 363–72.

168 Asians' attachments. Karen K. Dion and Kenneth L. Dion, "Personality, Gender, and the Phenomenology of Romantic Love," in *Review of Personality and Social Psychology,* ed. Phillip R. Shaver, vol. 6 (Newbury Park, CA: Sage, 1985).

168 Waning passion aids children's survival. Douglas T. Kenrick and Melanie R. Trost, "A Biosocial Theory of Heterosexual Relationships," in *Females, Males, and Sexuality,* ed. Kathryn Kelly (Albany: SUNY Press, 1987).

168 Well-being before, during, and after child-rearing. C. Walker, "Some Variations in Marital Satisfaction," in *Equalities and Inequalities in Family Life,* ed. Robert Chester and John Peel (London: Academic Press, 1977); Andrew M. Greeley, "The State of the Nation's Happiness," *Psychology Today,* January 1981, pp. 14–15; Sara McLanahan and Julia Adams, "Parenthood and Psychological Well-being," *Annual Review of Sociology* 13 (1987): 237–57; and Sara McLanahan and Julia Adams, "The Effects of Children on Adults' Psychological Well-being: 1957–1976," *Social Forces* 68 (1989): 124–46.

169 Sensitization to children. Philip Cowan and Susan Cowan, as reported by Carin Rubenstein, "The Baby Bomb," *New York Times/Good Health Magazine,* October 8, 1989, pp. 34–41.

169 "No man or woman." Mark Twain, *Notebook,* 1935.

169 Predictors of marital success. Balakrishan et al., "A Hazard Model Analysis," pp. 395–406. See also Colasanto and Shriver, "Mirror of America," pp. 34–38; and Tim B. Heaton and E. L. Pratt, "The Effects of Religious

Homogamy on Marital Satisfaction and Stability," *Journal of Family Issues* 11 (1990): 191–207.

170 Similarity and marital success. Donn Byrne, *The Attraction Paradigm* (New York: Academic Press, 1971).

170 India couples. Usha Gupta and Pushpa Singh, "Exploratory Study of Love and Liking and Type of Marriages," *Indian Journal of Applied Psychology* 19 (1982): 92–97.

171 *Reader's Digest.* S. Jacoby, "When Opposites Attract," *Reader's Digest,* December 1986, pp. 95–98.

171 "Can two walk." Amos 3:3 *(KJV)*.

172 Sex, arguments, and marital happiness. J. W. Howard and Robyn M. Dawes, "Linear Prediction of Marital Happiness," *Personality and Social Psychology Bulletin* 2 (1976): 478–80; and Tom W. Smith, "Adult Sexual Behavior in 1989: Number of Partners, Frequency, and Risk." General Social Survey Topic Report No. 18, National Opinion Research Center, University of Chicago, 1990, pp. 18–30.

172 Sex therapy and marital happiness. Lorne M. Hartman, "Effects of Sex and Marital Therapy on Sexual Interaction and Marital Happiness," *Journal of Sex and Marital Therapy* 9 (1983) 137–51.

172 Finnish sex holidays. Associated Press story reported in *Grand Rapids Press,* February 25, 1989, p. A9.

172 "Forced against a brick wall." Ellen Berscheid, "Some Comments on Love's Anatomy: Or Whatever Happened to Old-fashioned Lust?" In *The Psychology of Love,* ed. R. J. Sternberg and M. L. Barnes (New Haven: Yale University Press, 1988).

173 Sex quantity, sex quality, and marital happiness. See Freedman, *Happy People,* pp. 56–58.

173 "People cannot fully." Bertrand Russell, *Marriage and Morals,* 1929.

173 "If two lie together." Ecclesiastes 4:11 *(NRSV)*.

173 Prayer and marital happiness. Greeley, *Faithful Attraction,* pp. 189–90.

174 Marital equity. Irving Sarnoff and Suzanne Sarnoff, *Love-Centered Marriage in a Self-Centered World* (New York: Hemisphere, 1989), p. 20.

174 Equity. Bernedette Gray-Little, and Nancy Burks, "Power and Satisfaction in Marriage: A Review and Critique," *Psychological Bulletin* 93 (1983): 513–38; Elaine Hatfield et al., "Equity and Intimate Relations: Recent Research," in *Compatible and Incompatible Relationships,* ed. William Ickes (New York: Springer-Verlag, 1985); Susan E. Crohan and Joel Veroff, "Dimensions of Marital Well-being Among White and Black Newlyweds," *Journal of Marriage and the Family* 51 (1989): 373–83; and Bartolomeo J. Palisi, "Marriage Companionship and Marriage Well-

being: A Comparison of Metropolitan Areas in Three Countries," *Journal of Comparative Family Studies* 15 (1984): 43–57.

174 Distress in inequitable marriage. Robert B. Schafer and Pat M. Keith, "Equity and Depression Among Married Couples," *Social Psychology Quarterly* 43 (1980): 430–35.

174 Actress. Carol Tavris and Carole Wade, *The Longest War: Sex Differences in Perspective* (New York: Harcourt Brace Jovanovich, 1984), p. 366.

175 Unhappy and happy couples. Patricia Noller and Mary Anne Fitzpatrick, "Marital Communication in the Eighties," *Journal of Marriage and the Family* 52 (1990): 832–43.

175 " 'Living happily ever after.' " Robert J. Sternberg, "Triangulating Love," in *The Psychology of Love,* ed. Robert J. Sternberg and Michael L. Barnes (New Haven: Yale University Press, 1988).

175 Velveteen rabbit. Margaret Williams, *The Velveteen Rabbit: Or How Toys Become Real* (Garden City, NY: Doubleday, 1926).

Chapter 10: Faith, Hope, and Joy

178 Lee Atwater with Todd Brewster, "Lee Atwater's Last Campaign," *Life,* February 1991, p. 67.

178 Jeff (not his actual name). Quoted by Jonathan Freedman, *Happy People* (New York: Harcourt Brace Jovanovich, 1978), pp. 195–96.

179 Decline in materialism. Ronald Inglehart, *Culture Shift in Advanced Industrial Society* (Princeton: Princeton University Press, 1990), p. 180.

179 Chris Evert. Christopher Whipple, "Chrissie," *Life,* June 1986, pp. 64–72.

181 "My people have." Jeremiah 2:13 *(NRSV).*

181 Human religion. Donald Bloesch, *Essentials of Evangelical Theology,* vol. 1 (San Francisco: Harper & Row, 1978), p. 98.

182 Religious existence. Langdon Gilkey, *The Shantung Compound: The Story of Men and Women Under Pressure* (New York: Harper & Row, 1966), p. 223.

182 American religious census: Telephone survey of 113,000 adults conducted by ICR Research Group for the City University of New York Graduate School. Reported by George W. Cornell "Melting-pot Image Still Applies to Religion in U.S., Survey Shows," *Grand Rapids Press,* June 22, 1991, p. B4. The Gallup Organization reports that two tenths of 1 percent of 30,233 Americans they interviewed during 1990 claimed the

Muslim or Islamic faith. Hindus numbered three tenths of 1 percent (from the Princeton Religion Research Center's newsletter, *Emerging Trends* 13 [September 1991]: 4–5).

182 Jesus. John 15:11 *(NRSV)*.

182 "Obsessional neurosis." Sigmund Freud, *The Future of an Illusion* (Garden City, NY: Doubleday, 1964), p. 71.

183 Spiritual commitment. George Gallup, Jr., "Commentary on the State of Religion in the U.S. Today," *Religion in America: The Gallup Report*, no. 222, March 1984, pp. 1–20.

183 Surveys of religion and well-being. Robert A. Witter et al., "Religion and Subjective Well-being in Adulthood: A Quantitative Synthesis," *Review of Religious Research* 26 (1985): 332–42; C. Kirk Hadaway, "Life Satisfaction and Religion: A Reanalysis," *Social Forces* 57 (1978): 636–43; C. Kirk Hadaway and Wade C. Roof, "Religious Commitment and the Quality of Life in American Society," *Review of Religious Research* 19 (1978): 295–307; Margaret M. Poloma and Brian F. Pendleton, "Religious Domains and General Well-being," *Social Indicators Research* 22 (1990): 255–76; Melvin Pollner, "Divine Relations, Social Relations, and Well-being," *Journal of Health and Social Behavior* 30 (1989): 92–104; and F. K. Willits and D. M. Crider, "Religion and Well-being: Men and Women in the Middle Years," *Review of Religious Research* 29 (1988): 281–94.

183 Atheist and religious Europeans. Inglehart, *Culture Shift*, p. 447.

183 Church attendance and life satisfaction. Inglehart, *Culture Shift*, p. 229. This sample was slightly reduced from the sixteen-nation study reported earlier because data from Spain and Portugal were unavailable.

183 Elderly well-being and religiousness. Morris A. Okun and William A. Stock, "Correlates and Components of Subjective Well-being Among the Elderly," *Journal of Applied Gerontology* 6 (1987): 95–112. See also William A. Stock et al., "Age and Subjective Well-being: A Meta-analysis," in *Evaluation Studies: Review Annual*, ed. Richard J. Light, vol. 8 (Beverly Hills: Sage, 1983); Bruce Hunsberger, "Religion, Age, Life Satisfaction, and Perceived Sources of Religiousness: A Study of Older Persons," *Journal of Gerontology* 40 (1985): 615–30; Harold G. Koenig, James N. Kvale, and Carolyn Ferrel, "Religion and Well-being in Later Life," *The Gerontologist* 28 (1988): 18–28; Jeffrey S. Levin and Kyriakos S. Markides, "Religious Attendance and Psychological Well-being in Middle-aged and Older Mexican Americans," *Sociological Analysis* 49 (1988): 66–72; Kyriakos S. Markides, Jeffrey S. Levin, and Laura A. Ray, "Religion, Aging, and Life Satisfaction: An Eight-Year, Three-Wave

Longitudinal Study," *The Gerontologist* 27 (1987): 660–65; and Poloma and Pendleton, "Religious Domains and General Well-being," pp. 255–76.

184 Religion and coping with stress and crisis. Crystal Park, Lawrence H. Cohen, and Lisa Herb, "Intrinsic Religiousness and Religious Coping as Life Stress Moderators for Catholics Versus Protestants," *Journal of Personality and Social Psychology* 59 (1990): 562–74.

184 Religiously active widows and widowers. Thomas H. McGloshen and Shirley L. O'Bryant, "The Psychological Well-being of Older, Recent Widows," *Psychology of Women Quarterly* 12 (1988): 99–116; Carol D. Harvey, Gordon E. Barnes, and Leonard Greenwood, "Correlates of Morale Among Canadian Widowed Persons," *Social Psychiatry* 22 (1987): 65–72; and Judith M. Siegel and David H. Kuykendall, "Loss, Widowhood, and Psychological Distress Among the Elderly," *Journal of Consulting and Clinical Psychology* 58 (1990): 519–24.

184 Religion and coping with retardation. William N. Friedrich, Donna S. Cohen, and Lorna T. Wilturner, "Specific Beliefs as Moderator Variables in Maternal Coping with Mental Retardation," *Children's Health Care* 17 (1988): 40–44.

184 Faith and trauma. Christopher G. Ellison, "Religious Involvement and Subjective Well-being," *Journal of Health and Social Behavior* 32 (1991): 80–99.

185 Religion, delinquency, drugs, divorce, and suicide. For reviews, see C. Daniel Batson and W. Larry Ventis, *The Religious Experience: A Social-Psychological Perspective* (New York: Oxford University Press, 1982); Bernard Spilka, Ralph W. Hood, Jr., and Richard L. Gorsuch, *The Psychology of Religion: An Empirical Approach* (Englewood Cliffs, NJ: Prentice-Hall, 1985); John Gartner et al., "Religious Commitment and Psychopathology: A Review of the Empirical Literature," *Journal of Psychology and Theology* 19 (1991): 6–25; and Diane Colasanto and James Shriver, "Mirror of America: Middle-aged Face Marital Crisis," *Gallup Report*, no. 284, May 1989, pp. 34–38.

185 Religion and physical health and mortality. Jeffrey S. Levin and Preston L. Schiller, "Is There a Religious Factor in Health?" *Journal of Religion and Health* 26 (1987): 9–36; Gartner et al., "Religious Commitment"; Harold G. Koenig, Mona Smiley, and Jo Ann P. Gonzales, *Religion, Health, and Aging: A Review and Theoretical Integration* (Westport, CT: Greenwood Press, 1988); D. McIntosh and Bernard B. Spilka, "Religion and Physical Health: The Role of Personal Faith and Control Beliefs," in *Research in the Social Scientific Study of Religion*, ed. Monty L. Lynn

and David O. Moberg, vol. 2 (Greenwich, CT: JAI Press, 1990); and Jeffrey W. Dwyer, Leslie L. Clarke, and Michael K. Miller, "The Effect of Religious Concentration and Affiliation on County Cancer Mortality Rates," *Journal of Health and Social Behavior* 31 (1990): 185–202.

185 Religion and sense of fate control. Batson and Ventis, *The Religious Experience.*

185 Religion, depression, and disorder. Ibid.; Gartner et al., "Religious Commitment," pp. 6–25; Jerome Kroll and William Sheehan, "Religious Beliefs and Practices Among 52 Psychiatric Inpatients in Minnesota," *American Journal of Psychiatry* 146 (1989): 67–72; Koenig, Smiley, and Gonzales, *Religion, Health, and Aging;* and I. R. Payne et al., "Review of Religion and Mental Health: Prevention and the Enhancement of Psychosocial Functioning," *Prevention in Human Services,* in press.

186 Special protection. Reinhold Niebuhr, *Beyond Tragedy* (New York: Scribner's, 1937), p. 97.

186 Individualism. Martin E. P. Seligman, "Boomer Blues," *Psychology Today,* October 1988, pp. 50–55.

187 Puritans. John Winthrop's 1630 remarks appear as "A Model of Christian Charity," in *Puritan Political Ideas, 1558–1794,* ed. Edmund S. Morgan (Indianapolis: Bobbs-Merrill, 1965), p. 92.

187 Modern individualism. Robert Bellah et al., *Habits of the Heart* (Berkeley: University of California Press, 1985).

188 Amish depression. Janice A. Egeland and Abram M. Hostetter, "Amish Study I: Affective Disorders Among the Amish, 1976–1980," *American Journal of Psychiatry* 140 (1983): 56–61; and Janice A. Egeland, Abram M. Hostetter, and S. Kendrick Eshleman, "Amish Study III: The Impact of Cultural Factors on Diagnosis of Bipolar Illness," *American Journal of Psychiatry* 140 (1983): 67–71.

188 294,000 congregations. From a Gallup/Independent Sector study of giving and volunteering, summarized by Virginia A. Hodgkinson, Murray S. Weitzman, and A. D. Kirsch, "From Commitment to Action: How Religious Involvement Affects Giving and Volunteering," in *Faith and Philanthropy in America: Exploring the Role of Religion in America's Voluntary Sector,* ed. Robert Wuthnow, Virginia A. Hodgkinson, and Associates (San Francisco: Jossey-Bass, 1990).

188 Spiritual well-being and loneliness. Ray F. Paloutzian and Craig W. Ellison, "Loneliness, Spiritual Well-being, and the Quality of Life," in *Loneliness: A Sourcebook of Current Theory, Research, and Therapy,* ed. Letitia A. Peplau and Daniel Perlman (New York: Wiley, 1982).

188 Controlling for social activity. Craig W. Ellison, David A. Gay, and

Thomas A. Glass, "Does Religious Commitment Contribute to Individual Life Satisfaction?" *Social Forces* 68 (1989): 100–23; Ellison, "Religious Involvement," pp. 80–99.

188 Cyprian Norwid, 1850. Wladyslaw Tatarkiewicz, *Analysis of Happiness* (The Hague: Martinus Nijhoff, 1976), p. 176.

189 Meaning and well-being. See, for example, Sheryl Zika and Kerry Chamberlain, "Relation of Hassles and Personality to Subjective Well-being," *Journal of Personality and Social Psychology* 53 (1987): 155–62.

189 Meaning and depression. Seligman, "Boomer Blues," pp. 50–55.

189 "My religious faith." Harold Kushner, "You've Got to Believe in Something," *Redbook,* December 1987, pp. 92–94.

189 Psychiatrist Viktor Frankl. Viktor E. Frankl, *Man's Search for Meaning: An Introduction to Logotherapy* (Boston: Beacon Press, 1962).

189 Devout Jews in concentration camps. Paul Marcus and Alan Rosenberg, "The Holocaust Survivor's Faith and Religious Behavior: Implications for Treatment," in *Healing Their Wounds: Psychotherapy with Holocaust Survivors and Their Families,* ed. Paul Marcus and Alan Rosenberg (New York: Praeger, 1989).

189 Well-being from goal. Mihaly Csikszentmihalyi, *Flow: The Psychology of Optimal Experience* (New York: Harper & Row, 1990).

189 Hillel. Quoted by Martin Buber, *The Way of Man* (New York: Citadel Press, 1963), p. 63.

190 Terrorism from group polarization. Clark R. McCauley and Mary E. Segal, "Social Psychology in Terrorist Groups," in *Group Processes and Intergroup Relations,* ed. Clyde Hendrick (Beverly Hills: Sage, 1987).

190 Religious individualists. Robert Wuthnow, "Evangelicals, Liberals, and the Perils of Individualism," *Perspectives,* May 1991, pp. 10–13.

191 Jesus. Matthew 5:3 *(TEV).*

191 "No one has ever." Mignon McLaughlin, source unknown.

191 "Unspeakable comfort." C. S. Lewis, *Mere Christianity* (New York: Macmillan, 1960), p. 25. "Christian religion is, in the long run, a thing of unspeakable comfort. But it does not begin in comfort; it begins in [dismay], and it is no use at all to try to go on to that comfort without first going through that dismay."

191 Pretensions. William James, *The Principles of Psychology* (New York: Holt, 1890).

192 "Lord, I have." Psalm 131:1a, 2a *(TEV).*

192 God-concept and marriage. Andrew M. Greeley, *Faithful Attraction* (New York: Tor Books, 1991), p. 193.

193 Spiritual disciplines. Ellison, "Religious Involvement," pp. 80–99.

193 Prayer. Margaret M. Poloma and George Gallup, Jr., *The Varieties of Prayer* (Philadelphia: Trinity Press, 1991), summarized by R. Bezilla, "Review Essay: The Varieties of Prayer," *Emerging Trends* 13, no. 5 (May 1991): 4.

193 Footnote. World Day of Prayer for Peace. P. A. Crow, Jr., "Assisi's Day of Prayer for Peace," *Christian Century*, December 3, 1986, pp. 1084–85; and Roberto Suro, "Twelve Faiths Join Pope to Pray for Peace," *New York Times*, October 28, 1986.

194 "Everybody longs to be." Fred Rogers, A PBS special, "Our Neighbor," March 18, 1990.

194 Jesus on losing self. Matthew 10:37–39, 16:25–26; March 8:35; Luke 9:24–25; John 12:25 *(NRSV)*.

194 Catholic personal fulfillment. Richard Rohr and Joseph Martos, "Eight Good Reasons for Being Catholic," *Catholic Update*, no. CU 0888 (1990).

194 Muggeridge and Mother Teresa. Robert Schuller, *The Be-Happy Attitudes: Eight Positive Attitudes That Can Transform Your Life!* (Waco, TX: Word Books, 1985), p. 137.

194 Happiness from unselfishness. Bernard B. Rimland, "The Altruism Paradox," *The Southern Psychologist* 2, no. 1 (1982): 8–9.

195 "Christians have given." Madeleine L'Engle, *Walking on Water: Reflections on Faith and Art* (Wheaton, IL: Harold Shaw, 1980), p. 59.

195 Prejudice and religion. I review this research in David G. Myers, *Social Psychology*, 4th ed. (New York: McGraw-Hill, in press).

196 Intrinsic religiosity and mental health. Allen E. Bergin, Kevin S. Masters, and P. Scott Richards, "Religiousness and Mental Health Reconsidered: A Study of an Intrinsically Religious Sample," *Journal of Counseling Psychology* 34 (1987): 197–204; Kevin S. Masters et al., "Religious Lifestyles and Mental Health: Conclusions from an Intensive Three-Year Project" (Paper presented at the Midwestern Psychological Association Convention, Chicago, May 1990); W. Dixon, J. Alexander, and W. Anderson, "The Relationship Between Intrinsic and Extrinsic Religious Orientation and Obsessions and Compulsions" (Paper presented at the Midwestern Psychological Association Convention, Chicago, May 1990); and V. Genia and D. G. Shaw, "Religion, Intrinsic-Extrinsic Orientation and Depression," *Review of Religious Research* 32 (1991): 274–83.

196 "We have just enough." Jonathan Swift, *Thoughts on Various Subjects*, 1727.

197 Religion and altruism in emergencies. C. Daniel Batson, Patricia A. Schoenrade, and Virginia Pych, "Brotherly Love or Self-concern? Behav-

ioral Consequences of Religion," in *Advances in the Psychology of Religion*, ed. L. D. Brown (Oxford, England: Pergamon Press, 1985).

197 "When it comes." Sam Levenson, *You Don't Have to Be in Who's Who to Know What's What* (New York: Pocket Books, 1979), p. 188.

197 Gallup 1989 poll on altruism. Diane Colasanto, "Voluntarism: Americans Show Commitment to Helping Those in Need," *Gallup Report*, no. 290, November 1989, pp. 17–24.

197 Congregational giving. Gallup Organization, *From Belief to Commitment: The Activities and Finances of Religious Congregations in the United States* (Washington, DC: Independent Sector, 1988).

197 1987 Gallup survey. Robert Wuthnow, Virginia A. Hodgkinson, and Associates, "From Commitment to Action: How Religious Involvement Affects Giving and Volunteering," in *Faith and Philanthropy in America* (San Francisco: Jossey-Bass, 1990).

197 Follow-up 1989 Gallup survey. Virginia A. Hodgkinson and Murray S. Weitzman, *Giving and Volunteering in the United States: Findings from a National Survey* (Washington, DC: Independent Sector, 1990).

198 Priority of care. Paul G. Schervish, "Wealth and the Spiritual Secret of Money," in *Faith and Philanthropy in America: Exploring the Role of Religion in America's Voluntary Sector*, ed. Robert Wuthnow, Virginia A. Hodgkinson, and Associates (San Francisco: Jossey-Bass, 1990).

198 Religious roots of community organizations. Bill Berkowitz, *Local Heroes* (Lexington, MA: Heath, 1987), pp. 317–18.

198 Mother of philanthropy. Frank Emerson Andrews, *Attitudes Toward Giving* (New York: Bureau of Social Research, 1953), p. 85.

198 College professors. Robert H. Frank, Thomas Gilovich, and Dennis T. Regan, "Is the Self-interest Model a Corrupting Force?" (ms., Cornell University, 1991).

199 Gallup on volunteerism. George Gallup, Jr., "Commentary on the State of Religion," *Religion in America: Gallup Report No. 222*, March 1984, pp. 1–20. See also Peter Benson et al., "Intrapersonal Correlates of Nonspontaneous Helping Behavior," *Journal of Social Psychology* 110 (1980): 87–95.

199 Eric Liddell story. Assembled from a biography by Sally Magnusson, *The Flying Scotsman* (London: Quartet Books, 1981); D. J. Michell, "I Remember Eric Liddell," in *The Disciplines of the Christian Life*, ed. Eric Liddell (London: Triangle, 1985); and Gilkey, *The Shantung Compound*, pp. 224–26.

200 "Those who wait." Isaiah 40:31 *(NRSV)*.

201 Samuel Johnson. Quoted in Boswell's *Life of Samuel Johnson*, 1791.

201 Young Germans on hope. Tatarkiewicz, *Happiness*.

201 Isaiah 51:6 *(NRSV)*.

201 John of Patmos. Revelation 21:1, 3b, 4 *(NRSV)*.

202 British veteran. Quoted by William Barclay, *Through the Year with William Barclay*, ed. D. Duncan (London: Arthur James, 1971), p. 67.

202 Worldviews for coping. Sheldon Solomon, Jeffery Greenberg, and Tom Pyszczynski, "A Terror Management Theory of Social Behavior: The Psychological Functions of Self-esteem and Cultural Worldviews," *Advances in Experimental Social Psychology* 24 (1991): 93–159.

202 Betty. Quoted by John Powell, *Happiness Is an Inside Job* (Valencia, CA: Tabor, 1989), p. 125.

203 "I have a dream." Martin Luther King, *New York Times*, June 6, 1964, p. 10.

203 Ignacio Martin-Baro, as reported by Arthur Aron, "A Tribute to Ignacio Martin-Baro (1942–1989)," *SPSSI Newsletter* (April 1990): 4.

203 Laszlo Tokes, as reported by Jill Schaeffer, "Romania: The Eighth Circle of Hell," *Perspectives*, May 1990, pp. 4–6.

203 "Hope is hearing." Reubem Alves, *Tomorrow's Child: Imagination, Creativity, and the Rebirth of Culture* (New York: Harper & Row, 1972), p. 195.

204 "Believe in God." C. S. Lewis, *Christian Reflections* (Glasgow: Collins [Fount Paperbacks], 1981), p. 61.

Bibliography

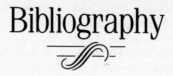

Abbey, Antonio, and Frank M. Andrews. "Modeling the Psychological Determinants of Life Quality." *Social Indicators Research* 16 (1985): 1–34.

Ackroyd, Peter. *T. S. Eliot: A Life.* New York: Simon & Schuster, 1984.

Adelmann, Paula K. "Occupational Complexity, Control, and Personal Income: Their Relation to Psychological Well-being in Men and Women." *Journal of Applied Psychology* 72 (1987): 529–37.

———. "Work and Well-being in Women: A Meta-analysis." Manuscript, University of Michigan, 1988.

——— et al. "Empty Nest, Cohort, and Employment in the Well-being of Midlife Women." *Sex Roles* 20 (1989): 173–89.

Adler, Tina. "Judd Leaves NIMH, Returns to Old Job." *APA Monitor* (December 1990): 6.

Advertising Age. February 10, 1958.

Ahearn, Marie Lucy. "Firewalking: From Sacred to Secular." *Journal of Popular Culture* 21 (1987): 11–18.

Alexander, Charles N. et al. "Transcendental Meditation, Mindfulness, and Longevity: An Experimental Study with the Elderly." *Journal of Personality and Social Psychology* 57 (1989): 950–64.

Allman, A. L. "Subjective Well-being of Students With and Without Disabilities." Paper presented at the Midwestern Psychological Association Convention, Chicago, May 1989.

———, and Ed Diener. "Measurement Issues and the Subjective Well-being of People with Disabilities." Manuscript, University of Illinois, 1990.

Alves, Rubem. *Tomorrow's Child: Imagination, Creativity, and the Rebirth of Culture.* New York: Harper & Row, 1972.

Amabile, Teresa M., and Ann H. Glazebrook. "A Negativity Bias in Interpersonal Evaluation." *Journal of Experimental Social Psychology* 18 (1982): 1–22.

Amato, Paul R., and Bruce Keith. "Parental Divorce and Adult Well-being." *Journal of Marriage and the Family* 53 (1991): 43–58.

———. "Parental Divorce and the Well-being of Children: A Meta-analysis." *Psychological Bulletin* 110 (1991): 26–46.

American Institutes for Research. *Women and their Health in Massachusetts.* Cambridge, MA: Cambridge Research Center, 1986.

American Psychological Association. *Survey of American Psychological Association Members.* Washington, DC: American Psychological Association, 1990.

Anderson, Barbara L., Barrie Anderson, and Charles deProsse. "Controlled Prospective Longitudinal Study of Women with Cancer: II. Psychological Outcomes." *Journal of Consulting and Clinical Psychology* 57 (1989): 692–97.

Anderson, D. R., and W. S. Jose. "Employee Lifestyle and the Bottom Line: Results from the Stay Well Evaluation." *Fitness in Business,* December 1987, pp. 86–91.

Andrews, Frank Emerson. *Attitudes Toward Giving.* New York: Bureau of Social Research, 1953.

Andrews, Frank M. "Stability and Change in Levels and Structure of Subjective Well-being: USA 1972 and 1988." *Social Indicators Research* 25 (1991): 1–30.

———, and Stephen B. Withey. *Social Indicators of Well-being: Americans' Perceptions of Life Quality.* New York: Plenum, 1976.

Argyle, Michael. *The Psychology of Happiness.* London: Methuen, 1986.

————, and Luo Lu. "Happiness and Social Skills." *Personality and Individual Differences* 11 (1990): 1255–61.

————. "The Happiness of Extraverts." *Personality and Individual Differences* 11 (1990): 1011–17.

Aron, Arthur. "A Tribute to Ignacio Martin-Baro (1942–1989)." *SPSSI Newsletter* (April 1990): 4.

Astin, Alexander W. "This Year's College Freshmen: Attitudes and Characteristics." *The Chronicle of Higher Education*, January 30, 1991, pp. A30–31.

————, Kenneth C. Green, and William S. Korn. *The American Freshman: Twenty Year Trends* (a report of the Cooperative Institutional Research Program sponsored by the American Council on Education). Los Angeles: Higher Education Research Institute, Graduate School of Education, UCLA, 1987.

Astin, Alexander W., William S. Korn, and E. R. Berz. *The American Freshman: National Norms for Fall 1989* (a report of the Cooperative Institutional Research Program sponsored by the American Council on Education). Los Angeles: Higher Education Research Institute, Graduate School of Education, UCLA, 1989.

Atwater, Lee, with Todd Brewster. "Lee Atwater's Last Campaign." *Life*, February 1991, pp. 58–67.

Auday, Brian C., J. L. Mellett, and P. M. Williams. "Self-improvement Using Subliminal Self-help Audiotapes: Consumer Benefit or Consumer Fraud?" Manuscript, Gordon College, 1990.

Bach, Richard. *Illusions: Adventures of a Reluctant Messiah.* New York: Delacorte Press, 1977.

Bachman, Jerald, and Patrick O'Malley. "Yea-saying, Nay-saying, and Going to Extremes: Black-White Differences in Response Styles." *Public Opinion Quarterly* 48 (1984): 491–509.

Baker, Elgan L. "The State of the Art of Clinical Hypnosis." *International Journal of Clinical and Experimental Hypnosis* 35 (1987): 203–14.

Balakrishan, T. R. et al. "A Hazard Model Analysis of the Covariates of Marriage Dissolution in Canada." *Demography* 24 (1987): 395–406.

Balatsky, Galina, and Ed Diener. "Subjective Well-being Among Soviet Students." Manuscript, University of Illinois, 1991.

Baldassare, Mark, Sarah Rosenfield, and Karen S. Rook. "The Types of Social Relations Predicting Elderly Well-being." *Research on Aging* 6 (1984): 549–59.

Barclay, William. *Through the Year with William Barclay.* Edited by D. Duncan. London: Arthur James, 1971.

Baron, Robert A. "Interviewer's Mood and Reaction to Job Applicants: The Influence of Affective States on Applied Social Judgments." *Journal of Applied Social Psychology* 17 (1987): 911–26.

Baruch, Grace K., and Rosaline Barnett. "Role Quality, Multiple Role Involvement, and Psychological Well-being in Midlife Women." *Journal of Personality and Social Psychology* 51 (1986): 578–85.

Batson, C. Daniel, Patricia A. Schoenrade, and Virginia Pych. "Brotherly Love or Self-concern? Behavioral Consequences of Religion." In *Advances in the Psychology of Religion*, edited by L. D. Brown. Oxford, England: Pergamon Press, 1985.

Batson, C. Daniel, and W. Larry Ventis. *The Religious Experience: A Social-Psychological Perspective.* New York: Oxford University Press, 1982.

Baucom, Donald H., and Pamela Danker-Brown. "Sex Role Identity and Sex-stereotyped Tasks in the Development of Learned Helplessness in Women." *Journal of Personality and Social Psychology* 46 (1984): 422–30.

Baumeister, Roy F., Diane M. Tice, and Debra G. Hutton. "Self-presentational Motivations and Personality Differences in Self-esteem. *Journal of Personality* 57 (1989): 547–79.

Beaman, Arthur L., and Bonnel Klentz. "The Supposed Physical Attractiveness Bias Against Supporters of the Women's Movement: A Meta-analysis." *Personality and Social Psychology Bulletin* 9 (1983): 544–50.

Belck, Jack, ed. *The Faith of Helen Keller.* Kansas City: Hallmark Cards, 1967.

Bellah, Robert et al. *Habits of the Heart.* Berkeley: University of California Press, 1985.

Bennett, Neil G., Ann K. Blanc, and David E. Bloom. "Commitment and the Modern Union: Assessing the Link Between Premarital Cohabitation and Subsequent Marital Stability." *American Sociological Review* 53 (1988): 127–38.

Benson, Herbert. *Your Maximum Mind.* New York: Times Books, 1987.

———, and Miriam Z. Klipper. *The Relaxation Response.* New York: Morrow, 1976.

Benson, Herbert, and William Proctor. *Beyond the Relaxation Response: How to Harness the Healing Power of Your Personal Beliefs.* New York: Times Books, 1984.

Benson, Peter et al. "Intrapersonal Correlates of Nonspontaneous Helping Behavior." *Journal of Social Psychology* 110 (1980): 87–95.

Berg, John. "Responsiveness and Self-disclosure." In *Self-disclosure: Theory, Research, and Therapy,* edited by Valerian J. Derlega and John H. Berg. New York: Plenum, 1987.

————, and Letitia A. Peplau. "Loneliness: The Relationship of Self-disclosure and Androgyny." *Personality and Social Psychology Bulletin* 8 (1982): 624–30.

Bergin, Allen E., Kevin S. Masters, and P. Scott Richards. "Religiousness and Mental Health Reconsidered: A Study of an Intrinsically Religious Sample." *Journal of Counseling Psychology* 34 (1987): 197–204.

Berkowitz, Bill. *Local Heroes.* Lexington, MA: Heath, 1987.

Berman, Jeffrey S., and Nicholas C. Norton. "Does Professional Training Make a Therapist More Effective?" *Psychological Bulletin* 98 (1985): 401–7

Berscheid, Ellen. "Interpersonal Attraction." In *The Handbook of Social Psychology,* edited by Gardner Lindzey and Elliot Aronson. New York: Random House, 1985.

————. "Some Comments on Love's Anatomy: Or Whatever Happened to Old-fashioned Lust?" In *The Psychology of Love,* edited by R. J. Sternberg and M. L. Barnes. New Haven: Yale University Press, 1988.

————, Steven W. Gangestad, and D. Kulakowski. "Emotion in Close Relationships: Implications for Relationship Counseling." In *Handbook of Counseling Psychology,* edited by Steven D. Brown and Robert W. Lent. New York: Wiley, 1984.

Berscheid, Ellen, and Letitia A. Peplau. "The Emerging Science of Relationships." In *Close Relationships,* edited by H. H. Kelly et al. New York: Freeman, 1983.

Bezilla, R. "Review Essay: The Varieties of Prayer." *Emerging Trends* 13, no. 5 (May 1991): 4.

Block, Jack. "Some Enduring and Consequential Structures of Personality." In *Further Explorations in Personality,* edited by A. I. Rabin. New York: Wiley, 1981.

Bloesch, Donald. *Essentials of Evangelical Theology.* Vol. 1. San Francisco: Harper & Row, 1978.

Bolger, Niall et al. "Effects of Daily Stress on Negative Mood." *Journal of Personality and Social Psychology* 57 (1989): 808–18.

Booth, Alan, and John N. Edwards. "Transmission of Marital and Family Quality over the Generations: The Effect of Parental Divorce on Unhappiness." *Journal of Divorce* 12 (1989): 41–58.

273

Booth, Alan, and David Johnson. "Premarital Cohabitation and Marital Success." *Journal of Family Issues* 9 (1988): 255–72.

Bornstein, Robert F. et al. "The Temporal Stability of Ratings of Parents: Test-retest Reliability and Influence of Parental Contact." *Journal of Social Behavior and Personality* 6 (1991): 641–49.

Bostick, R. M. "Quality of Life Survey Among a Severely Handicapped Population." Ph.D. diss., University of Houston, 1977.

Bower, Gordon H. "Mood Congruity of Social Judgments." In *Emotional and Social Judgments,* edited by Joseph P. Forgas. Oxford, England: Pergamon Press, 1991.

Bowers, Kenneth S. "Hypnosis." In *Personality and Behavioral Disorders,* edited by Norman Endler and J. McVicker Hunt. 2d ed. New York: Wiley, 1984.

———. Personal correspondence, July 1987.

———, and Samuel LeBaron. "Hypnosis and Hypnotizability: Implications for Clinical Intervention." *Hospital and Community Psychiatry* 37 (1986): 456–67.

Bowlby, John. *Loss, Sadness and Depression.* Vol. 3 of *Attachment and Loss.* London: Basic Books, 1980.

Bradburn, Norman M. *The Structure of Psychological Well-being.* Chicago: Aldine, 1969.

Brickman, Philip, and Donald T. Campbell. "Hedonic Relativism and Planning the Good Society." In *Adaptation-level Theory,* edited by M. H. Appley. New York: Academic Press, 1971.

Brickman, Philip, Dan Coates, and Ronnie J. Janoff-Bulman. "Lottery Winners and Accident Victims: Is Happiness Relative?" *Journal of Personality and Social Psychology* 36 (1978): 917–27.

Briggs, David. "Poll: Americans Want to Be Rich." Associated Press article, *Holland Sentinel,* November 1, 1991, p. B6.

Brockner, Joel, and A. J. Blethyn Hulton. "How to Reverse the Vicious Cycle of Low Self-esteem: The Importance of Attentional Focus." *Journal of Experimental Social Psychology* 14 (1978): 564–78.

Brothers, Joyce. "Why Wives Have Affairs." *Parade,* February 18, 1990, pp. 4–7.

Brown, Jonathon D. "Accuracy and Bias in Self-knowledge. Can Knowing the Truth Be Hazardous to Your Health?" In *Handbook of Social and Clinical Psychology: The Health Perspective,* edited by C. R. Snyder and D. F. Forsyth. New York: Pergamon Press, 1991.

Buber, Martin. *The Way of Man.* New York: Citadel Press, 1963.

Buckley, W. T. "How to Cope with Crisis." *Reader's Digest,* July 1990, pp. 93–96.

Bulka, Reuben P. "Religion in Contemporary Times: For Denial or for Pleasure." *Psychologists Interested in Religious Issues Newsletter* 15, no. 1 (1990): 1–4.

Bumpass, Larry L., and James A. Sweet. "National Estimates of Cohabitation." *Demography* 26 (1989): 615–25.

Bureau of the Census. *Statistical Abstract of the United States.* Washington, DC: Superintendent of Documents, Government Printing Office, 1987.

———. *Statistical Abstract of the United States.* Washington, DC: Superintendent of Documents, Government Printing Office, 1989.

———. *Statistical Abstract of the United States.* Washington, DC: Superintendent of Documents, Government Printing Office, 1990.

Burns, David D. *Feeling Good: The New Mood Therapy.* New York: Signet, 1980.

Burt, Ronald S. "Strangers, Friends and Happiness." GSS Technical Report No. 72. Chicago: National Opinion Research Center, University of Chicago, 1986.

Byrne, Donn. *The Attraction Paradigm.* New York: Academic Press, 1971.

Campbell, Angus. *The Sense of Well-being in America.* New York: McGraw-Hill, 1981.

———, Phillip E. Converse, and Willard L. Rodgers. *The Quality of American Life: Perceptions, Evaluations and Satisfactions.* New York: Sage, 1976.

Carlson, John G., and Elaine Hatfield. *Psychology of Emotion.* Belmont, CA: Wadsworth, 1989.

Carlson, Shawn. "A Double-blind Test of Astrology." *Nature* 318 (1985): 419–25.

Carnegie Council on Adolescent Development. *Turning Points: Preparing American Youth for the 21st Century.* New York: Task Force on Education of Young Adolescents, 1989.

Carr, Thomas H., A. Kontowicz, and Dale Dagenbach. "Subthreshold Priming and the Cognitive Unconscious." Invited paper presented to the Midwestern Psychological Association Convention, Chicago, May 1987.

Caspi, Avshalom, and Daryl J. Bem. "Personality Continuity and Change Across the Life Course." In *Handbook of Personality: Theory and Research,* edited by L. A. Pervin. New York: Guilford Press, 1990.

Castro, Janice. "How's Your Pay?" *Time*, April 15, 1991, pp. 40–41.

Centers for Disease Control Vietnam Experience Study, "Health Status of Vietnam Veterans." *Journal of the American Medical Association* 259 (1988): 2701–9.

Cherlin, Andrew J. et al. "Longitudinal Studies of Effects of Divorce on Children in Great Britain and the United States." *Science* 252 (1991): 1386–89.

Chronicle of Higher Education Almanac (projections of college enrollment, 1990–2000, p. 14, and administrator's views of enrollment changes in the next five years, p. 28). Washington DC: Chronicle of Higher Education, Inc., 1990.

Chwalisz, Kathleen, Ed Diener, and Dennis Gallagher. "Autonomic Arousal Feedback and Emotional Experience: Evidence from the Spinal Cord Injured." *Journal of Personality and Social Psychology* 54 (1988): 820–28.

Cialdini, Robert B., and Kenneth D. Richardson. "Two Indirect Tactics of Image Management: Basking and Blasting." *Journal of Personality and Social Psychology* 39 (1980): 406–15.

Clancy, Frank, and Heidi Yorkshire. "The Bandler Method." *Mother Jones*, February/March 1989, pp. 24–28, 63–64.

Clark, Lee A., and David Watson. "Mood and the Mundane: Relations Between Daily Life Events and Self-reported Mood." *Journal of Personality and Social Psychology* 54 (1988): 296–308.

Cohen, Lawrence H., Lynn C. Towbes, and Regina Flocco. "Effects of Induced Mood on Self-reported Life Events and Perceived and Received Social Support." *Journal of Personality and Social Psychology* 55 (1988): 669–74.

Cohen, Sheldon. "Psychological Models of the Role of Social Support in the Etiology of Physical Disease." *Health Psychology* 7 (1988): 269–97.

———, and Gail M. Williamson. "Perceived Stress in a Probability Sample of the United States." In *The Social Psychology of Health*, edited by Shirlynn Spacapan and Stuart Oskamp. Newbury Park, CA: Sage, 1988.

Colasanto, Diane. "Voluntarism: Americans Show Commitment to Helping Those in Need." *Gallup Report*, no. 290, November 1989, pp. 17–24.

———, and James Shriver. "Mirror of America: Middle-aged Face Marital Crisis." *Gallup Report*, no. 284, May 1989, pp. 34–38.

Coles, Robert. *Privileged Ones: The Well-off and the Rich in America*. Boston: Atlantic Monthly Press, 1977.

Collins, Rebecca L., Shelley E. Taylor, and Laurie A. Skokan. "A Better World or a Shattered Vision? Changes in Life Perspectives Following Victimization." *Social Cognition* 8 (1990): 263–85.

Conley, James J. "Longitudinal Stability of Personality Traits: A Multitrait-Multi-Method-Multioccasion Analysis." *Journal of Personality and Social Psychology* 49 (1985): 1266–82.

Coombs, Robert H. "Marital Status and Personal Well-being: A Literature Review." *Family Relations* 40 (January 1991): 97–102.

Cooper, Kenneth. *The New Aerobics.* New York: Bantam, 1970.

Cornell, George W. "Melting-pot Image Still Applies to Religion in U.S., Survey Shows." *Grand Rapids Press,* June 22, 1991, p. B4.

Costa, Paul T., Jr., and Robert R. McCrae. "Still Stable After All These Years: Personality as a Key to Some Issues in Adulthood and Old Age." In *Life-Span Development and Behavior,* edited by Paul B. Baltes and O. Brim, Jr. Vol. 3. New York: Academic Press, 1980.

———. "Personality as a Lifelong Determinant of Well-being." In *Emotion in Adult Development,* edited by Carol Z. Malatesta and Carroll E. Izard. Newbury Park, CA: Sage, 1984.

———. "Personality in Adulthood: A Six-Year Longitudinal Study of Self-report and Spouse Ratings on the NEO Personality Inventory." *Journal of Personality and Social Psychology* 54 (1988): 853–63.

———, and Alan B. Zonderman. "Environmental and Dispositional Influences on Well-being: Longitudinal Follow-up of an American National Sample." *British Journal of Psychology* 78 (1987): 299–306.

Cousins, Norman. *Head First: The Biology of Hope.* New York: E. P. Dutton, 1989.

Coyne, James C., Sue A. L. Burchill, and William B. Stiles. "An Interactional Perspective on Depression." In *Handbook of Social and Clinical Psychology: The Health Perspective,* edited by C. R. Snyder and D. O. Forsyth. New York: Pergamon Press, 1991.

Crider, Donald M., Fern K. Willits, and C. L. Kanagy. "Rurality and Well-being During the Middle Years of Life." *Social Indicators* 24 (1991): 253–68.

Crocker, Jennifer, and Lisa Gallo. "The Self-enhancing Effect of Downward Comparison." Paper presented at the American Psychological Association Convention, Los Angeles, August 1985.

Crocker, Jennifer, and Brenda Major. "Social Stigma and Self-esteem: The Self-protective Properties of Stigma." *Psychological Review* 96 (1989): 608–30.

Crocker, Jennifer et al. "Downward Comparison, Prejudice, and Evaluation of Others: Effects of Self-esteem and Threat." *Journal of Personality and Social Psychology* 52 (1987): 907–16.

Crohan, Susan E., and Joel Veroff. "Dimensions of Marital Well-being

Among White and Black Newlyweds." *Journal of Marriage and the Family* 51 (1989): 373–83.

Crohan, Susan E. et al. "Job Characteristics and Well-being at Midlife." *Psychology of Women Quarterly* 13 (1989): 223–35.

Crosby, Faye J. *Spouse, Parent, Worker: On Gender and Multiple Roles.* New Haven: Yale University Press, 1987.

———. "Divorce and Work Life Among Women Managers." *The Experience and Meaning of Work in Women's Lives,* edited by H. Y. Grossman and N. L. Chester. Hillsdale, NJ: Erlbaum, 1990.

———. "Combining Work and Home." In *Male and Female,* edited by A. Campbell. Oxford, England: Andromede Press, in press.

Crouter, Ann C. "Participative Work as an Influence on Human Development." *Journal of Applied Developmental Psychology* 5 (1984): 71–90.

Crow, P. A., Jr. "Assisi's Day of Prayer for Peace." *Christian Century,* December 3, 1986, pp. 1084–85.

Csikszentmihalyi, Mihaly. "The Future of Flow." In *Optimal Experience: Psychological Studies of Flow in Consciousness,* edited by Mihaly Csikszentmihalyi and Isabella S. Csikszentmihalyi. Cambridge: Cambridge University Press, 1988.

———. *Flow: The Psychology of Optimal Experience.* New York: Harper & Row, 1990.

———, and Isabella S. Csikszentmihalyi. *Optimal Experience: Psychological Studies of Flow in Consciousness.* Cambridge: Cambridge University Press, 1988.

Csikszentmihalyi, Mihaly, and Randy Larson. *Being Adolescent: Conflict and Growth in the Teenage Years.* New York: Basic Books, 1984.

Csikszentmihalyi, Mihaly, and Judith LeFevre. "Optimal Experience in Work and Leisure." *Journal of Personality and Social Psychology* 56 (1989): 815–22.

Cunningham, Michael R. "Does Happiness Mean Friendliness? Induced Mood and Heterosexual Self-disclosure." *Personality and Social Psychology Bulletin* 14 (1988): 283–97.

Cutrona, Carolyn E. "Behavioral Manifestations of Social Support: A Microanalytic Investigation." *Journal of Personality and Social Psychology* 51 (1986): 201–8.

Danzig, F. "Subliminal Advertising—Today It's Just Historic Flashback for Researcher Vicary." *Advertising Age,* September 17, 1962, pp. 73–74.

Davis, Earl E., and Margaret Fine-Davis. "Social Indicators of Living Conditions in Ireland with European Comparisons." *Social Indicators Research* 25 (1991): 103–365.

Davis, Keith E. "Near and Dear: Friendship and Love Compared." *Psychology Today*, February 1985, pp. 22–30.

Davis-Van Atta, David et al., eds. *Educating America's Scientists: The Role of the Research Colleges*. Oberlin: Oberlin College Press, 1985.

Decker, Susan D., and Richard Schulz. "Correlates of Life Satisfaction and Depression in Middle-aged and Elderly Spinal Cord–Injured Persons." *American Journal of Occupational Therapy* 39 (1985): 740–45.

DeMaris, Alfred, and Gerald R. Leslie. "Cohabitation with the Future Spouse: Its Influence upon Marital Satisfaction and Communication." *Journal of Marriage and the Family*, February 1984, pp. 77–84.

Dember, William N. and Judith Brooks. "A New Instrument for Measuring Optimism and Pessimism: Test-retest Reliability and Relations with Happiness and Religious Commitment." *Bulletin of the Psychonomic Society* 27 (1989): 365–66.

Dement, William. In the PBS film, *Sleep Alert*. Quoted by *Behavior Today*, March 12, 1990, p. 8.

Dennett, Michael R. "Firewalking: Reality or Illusion?" *Skeptical Inquirer* 10 (Fall 1985): 36–40.

D'Eon, Joyce L. "Hypnosis in the Control of Labor Pain." In *Hypnosis: The Cognitive-Behavioral Perspective*, edited by Nicholas P. Spanos and John F. Chaves. Buffalo, NY: Prometheus Books, 1989.

DePree, Max. *Leadership Is an Art*. Garden City, NY: Doubleday, 1989.

Dermer, Marshall et al. "Evaluative Judgments of Aspects of Life as a Function of Vicarious Exposure to Hedonic Extremes." *Journal of Personality and Social Psychology* 37 (1979): 247–60.

Diener, Ed. "Subjective Well-being." *Psychological Bulletin* 93 (1984): 542–75.

———— et al. "The Costs of Intense Positive Emotions." *Journal of Personality and Social Psychology*, 61 (1991): 492–503.

Diener, Ed, Robert A. Emmons, and Ed Sandvik. "The Dual Nature of Happiness: Independence of Positive and Negative Moods." Manuscript, University of Illinois, 1986.

Diener, Ed, J. Horwitz, and Robert A. Emmons. "Happiness of the Very Wealthy." *Social Indicators* 16 (1985): 263–74.

Diener, Ed, Ed Sandvik, and William Pavot. "Happiness Is the Frequency, Not the Intensity, of Positive Versus Negative Affect." In *The Social Psychology of Subjective Well-being*, edited by Fritz Strack, Michael Argyle, and Norbert Schwarz. Oxford, England: Pergamon Press, 1990.

————, and Dennis Gallagher. "Response Artifacts in the Measurement of Subjective Well-being." *Social Indicators Research* 24 (1991): 35–56.

Dion, Karen K., and Kenneth L. Dion. "Personality, Gender, and the Phenomenology of Romantic Love." In *Review of Personality and Social Psychology,* edited by Phillip R. Shaver. Vol. 6. Newbury Park, CA: Sage, 1985.

———. "Psychological Individualism and Romantic Love." *Journal of Social Behavior and Personality* 6 (1991): 17–33.

DiStefano, Linda. "Pressures of Modern Life Bring Increased Importance to Friendship." *Gallup Poll Monthly,* no. 294, March 1990, pp. 24–33.

Dixon, W., J. Alexander, and W. Anderson. "The Relationship Between Intrinsic and Extrinsic Religious Orientation and Obsessions and Compulsions." Paper presented at the Midwestern Psychological Association Convention, Chicago, May 1990.

Dohrenwend, Bruce et al. "Report on Stress and Life Events." In *Stress and Human Health: Analysis and Implications of Research,* edited by Glen R. Elliot and Carl Eisdorfer (a study by the Institute of Medicine, National Academy of Sciences). New York: Springer-Verlag, 1982.

Donnerstein, Ed., Daniel Linz, and Steven Penrod. *The Question of Pornography.* New York: Free Press, 1987.

Doyle, Daniel, and Marilyn J. Forehand. "Life Satisfaction and Old Age: A Reexamination." *Research on Aging* 6 (1984): 432–48.

Druckman, Daniel, and John A. Swets, eds. *Enhancing Human Performance: Issues, Theories, and Techniques.* Washington, DC: National Academy Press, 1988.

Duclos, Sandra E. et al. "Emotion-Specific Effects of Facial Expressions and Postures on Emotional Experience." *Journal of Personality and Social Psychology* 57 (1989): 100–8.

Dumont, Matthew P. "An Unfolding Memoir of Community Mental Health." *Readings: A Journal of Reviews and Commentary in Mental Health* (September 1989): 4–7.

Dwyer, Jeffrey W., Leslie L. Clarke, and Michael K. Miller. "The Effect of Religious Concentration and Affiliation on County Cancer Mortality Rates." *Journal of Health and Social Behavior* 31 (1990): 185–202.

Dywan, Jane, and Kenneth S. Bowers. "The Use of Hypnosis to Enhance Recall." *Science* 222 (1983): 184–85.

Easterlin, Richard A. "Does Money Buy Happiness?" *Public Interest* 30 (1973): 3–10.

Egeland, Janice A., and Abram M. Hostetter. "Amish Study I: Affective Disorders Among the Amish, 1976–1980." *American Journal of Psychiatry* 140 (1983): 56–61.

———, and S. Kendrick Eshleman. "Amish Study III: The Impact of Cultural Factors on Diagnosis of Bipolar Illness." *American Journal of Psychiatry* 140 (1983): 67–71.

Eisenberg, Nancy, and Randy Lennon. "Sex Differences in Empathy and Related Capacities." *Psychological Bulletin* 94 (1983): 100–31.

Ekman, Paul, Richard J. Davidson, and Wallace V. Friesen. "The Duchenne Smile: Emotional Expression and Brain Physiology II." *Journal of Personality and Social Psychology* 58 (1990): 342–53.

Ellison, Christopher G. "Religious Involvement and Subjective Well-being." *Journal of Health and Social Behavior* 32 (1991): 80–99.

———, David A. Gay, and Thomas A. Glass. "Does Religious Commitment Contribute to Individual Life Satisfaction?" *Social Forces* 68 (1989): 100–23.

Emmons, Robert A., and Ed Diener. "Personality Correlates of Subjective Well-being." *Personality and Social Psychology Bulletin* 11 (1985): 89–97.

———. "Influence of Impulsivity and Sociability on Subjective Well-being." *Journal of Personality and Social Psychology* 50 (1986): 1211–15.

———. "An Interactional Approach to the Study of Personality and Emotion." *Journal of Personality* 54 (1986): 371–84.

Emmons, Robert A. et al. "Factors Predicting Satisfaction Judgments: A Comparative Examination." Paper presented at the Midwestern Psychological Association Convention, Chicago, May 1983.

Endler, Norman. *Holiday of Darkness*. New York: Wiley, 1982.

Falbo, Toni, and Dudley Polit. "Quantitative Review of the Only Child Literature: Research Evidence and Theory Development." *Psychological Bulletin* 100 (1986): 179–89.

Ferree, Myra M. "Class, Housework, and Happiness: Women's Work and Life Satisfaction." *Sex Roles* 11 (1984): 1057–74.

Fiedler, K., and Joseph P. Forgas. *Affect, Cognition, and Social Behavior*. Toronto: Hogrefe, 1988.

Fincham, Frank D., Steven R. Beach, and Donald H. Baucom. "Attribution Processes in Distressed and Nondistressed Couples: 4. Self-partner Attribution Differences." *Journal of Personality and Social Psychology* 52 (1987): 739–48.

Findley, Maureen J., and Harris M. Cooper. "Locus of Control and Academic Achievement: A Literature Review." *Journal of Personality and Social Psychology* 33 (1983): 419–27.

Finn, Stephen E. "Stability of Personality Self-ratings over 30 Years: Evidence for an Age/Cohort Interaction." *Journal of Personality and Social Psychology* 50 (1986): 813–18.

Floderus-Myrhed, B., Nancy Pedersen, and I. Rasmuson. "Assessment of Heritability for Personality, Based on a Short-form of the Eysenck Personality Inventory: A Study of 12,898 Twin Pairs." *Behavior Genetics* 10 (1980): 153–62.

Fordyce, Michael W. "The Psychology of Happiness: The Book Version of the Fourteen Fundamentals." Manuscript, Edison Community College, 1978.

———. "The PSYCHAP INVENTORY: A Multi-Scale Test to Measure Happiness and Its Concomitants." *Social Indicators Research* 18 (1985): 1–33.

Forer, Bertram R. "The Fallacy of Personal Validation: A Classroom Demonstration of Gullibility." *Journal of Abnormal and Social Psychology* 44 (1949): 118–23.

Forgas, Joseph P. "Mood and the Perception of Atypical People: Affect and Prototypicality in Person Memory and Impressions." *Journal of Personality and Social Psychology,* in press.

Fowler, Carol A. et al. "Lexical Access with and Without Awareness." *Journal of Experimental Psychology: General* 110 (1981): 341–62.

Frank, Jerome D. "Therapeutic Components Shared by All Psychotherapies." In *Psychotherapy Research and Behavior Change.* Vol. 1 of *The Master Lecture Series,* edited by John H. Harvey and Marjorie M. Parks. Washington, DC: American Psychological Association, 1982.

Frank, Robert H., Thomas Gilovich, and Dennis T. Regan. "Is the Self-interest Model a Corrupting Force?" Manuscript, Cornell University, 1991.

Frank, Susan J., Patricia A. Towell, and Margaret Huyck. "The Effects of Sex-Role Traits on Three Aspects of Psychological Well-being Is a Sample of Middle-aged Women." *Sex Roles* 12 (1985): 1073–87.

Frankl, Viktor E. *Man's Search for Meaning: An Introduction to Logotherapy.* Boston: Beacon Press, 1962.

Frazier, Kenneth. "Gallup Poll of Beliefs: Astrology Up, ESP down." *Skeptical Inquirer* 13 (1989): 244–45.

———. "Astrology in the White House: Nancy Reagan's View." *Skeptical Inquirer* 14 (1990): 228–30.

Frederick, T., Ralph R. Frerichs, and Virginia A. Clark. "Personal Health Habits and Symptoms of Depression at the Community Level." *Preventive Medicine* 17 (1988): 173–82.

Freedman, Jonathan. *Happy People.* New York: Harcourt Brace Jovanovich, 1978.

Freud, Sigmund. *A General Introduction to Psychoanalysis.* 1935. Reprint. New York: Washington Square Press, 1960.

———. *The Future of an Illusion.* Garden City, NY: Doubleday, 1964.

Freund, Michael. "Toward a Critical Theory of Happiness: Philosophical Background and Methodological Significance." *New Ideas in Psychology* 3 (1985): 3–12.

Friedman, Meyer, and Diane Ulmer. *Treating Type A Behavior—and Your Heart.* New York: Knopf, 1984.

Friedman, Myra. *Buried Alive: The Biography of Janis Joplin.* New York: Morrow, 1973.

Friedrich, William N., Donna S. Cohen, and Lorna T. Wilturner. "Specific Beliefs as Moderator Variables in Maternal Coping with Mental Retardation." *Children's Health Care* 17 (1988): 40–44.

Frijda, Nico H. "The Laws of Emotion." *American Psychologist* 43 (1988): 349–58.

Fuchs, Victor, and Diane Reklis. "America's Children: Economic Perspectives and Policy Options." *Science* 255 (1992): 41–46.

Fujita, Frank, Ed Diener, and Ed Sandvik. "Gender Differences in Negative Affect and Well-being: The Case for Emotional Intensity." *Journal of Personality and Social Psychology* 61 (1991): 427–34.

Gallup, George, Jr. "Commentary on the State of Religion in the U.S. Today." *Religion in America: The Gallup Report,* no. 222, March 1984, pp. 1–20.

———, and F. Newport. "Americans Widely Disagree on What Constitutes 'Rich.'" *Gallup Poll Monthly,* July 1990, pp. 28–36.

Gallup Organization. *Survey of the Public's Recollection of 1981 Charitable Donations.* Princeton: Independent Sector, 1982.

———. *From Belief to Commitment: The Activities and Finances of Religious Congregations in the United States.* Washington, DC: Independent Sector, 1988.

Gallup Report. "Importance of Social Values." Report nos. 282/283, March/April 1989, p. 42.

Gartner, John et al. "Religious Commitment and Psychopathology: A Review of the Empirical Literature." *Journal of Psychology and Theology* 19 (1991): 6–25.

Genia, V., and D. G. Shaw. "Religion, Intrinsic-Extrinsic Orientation and Depression." *Review of Religious Research* 32 (1991): 274–83.

Gibbons, Frederick X. "Social Comparison and Depression: Company's Effect on Misery." *Journal of Personality and Social Psychology* 51 (1986): 140–48.

——, and Meg Gerard. "Effects of Upward and Downward Social Comparison on Mood States." *Journal of Social and Clinical Psychology* 8 (1989): 14–31.

Gilkey, Langdon. *The Shantung Compound: The Story of Men and Women Under Pressure.* New York: Harper & Row, 1966.

Glatzer, W. "Quality of Life in Advanced Industrialized Countries: The Case of West Germany." In *Subjective Well-being: An Interdisciplinary Perspective,* edited by Fritz Strack, Michael Argyle, and Norbert Schwarz. Oxford, England: Pergamon Press, 1990.

Glenn, Norval D. "Psychological Well-being in the Postparental Stage: Some Evidence from National Surveys." *Journal of Marriage and the Family* 37 (1975): 105–10.

——. "The Social and Cultural Meaning of Contemporary Marriage." In *The Retreat from Marriage,* edited by Bryce Christensen. Rockford, IL: The Rockford Institute, 1990.

——. "The Recent Trend in Marital Success in the United States." *Journal of Marriage and the Family* 53 (1991): 261–70.

——, and Sue K. Hoppe. "Only Children as Adults: Psychological Well-being." *Journal of Family Issues* 5 (1984): 363–82.

Glenn, Norval D., and Kathryn B. Kramer. "The Psychological Well-being of Adult Children of Divorce." *Journal of Marriage and Family* 47 (1985): 905–12.

Glenn, Norval D., and Charles N. Weaver. "The Changing Relationship of Marital Status to Reported Happiness." *Journal of Marriage and the Family* 50 (1988): 317–24.

Goldfried, Marvin R., and Wendy Padawer. "Current Status and Future Directions in Psychotherapy." In *Converging Themes in Psychotherapy: Trends in Psychodynamic, Humanistic, and Behavioral Practice,* edited by Marvin R. Goldfried. New York: Springer-Verlag, 1982.

Golding, Jacqueline M. "Role Occupancy and Role-Specific Stress and Social Support as Predictors of Depression." *Basic and Applied Social Psychology* 10 (1989): 173–95.

Goodchilds, Jacqueline. Quoted by Carol Tavris, "Old Age Is Not What It Used to Be." *New York Times/Good Health Magazine,* September 27, 1987, pp. 24–25, 91–92.

Gorky, Maksim. *The Lower Depths.* Translated by Alexander Bakshy. 1903. Reprint. New York: Avon Books, 1974.

Gove, Walter R., Michael Hughes, and Carolyn B. Style. "Does Marriage

Have Positive Effects on the Psychological Well-being of the Individual?" *Journal of Health and Social Behavior* 24 (1983): 122–31.

———. "The Effect of Marriage on the Well-being of Adults: A Theoretical Analysis." *Journal of Family Issues* 11 (1990): 4–35.

Gray-Little, Bernedette, and Nancy Burks. "Power and Satisfaction in Marriage: A Review and Critique." *Psychological Bulletin* 93 (1983): 513–38.

Greeley, Andrew M. "The State of the Nation's Happiness." *Psychology Today*, January 1981, pp. 14–15.

———. *Faithful Attraction.* New York: Tor Books, 1991.

Greenwald, Anthony G., and Anthony R. Pratkanis. "The Self." In *Handbook of Social Cognition*, edited by Robert S. Wyer and Thomas K. Srull. Hillsdale, NJ: Erlbaum, 1984.

Greenwald, Anthony et al. "Double-blind Tests of Subliminal Self-help Audiotapes." *Psychological Science* 2 (1991): 119–22.

Greenwald, John. "Taking Away His Credit Cards." *Time*, July 9, 1990, p. 51.

Gross, Alan E., and C. Crofton. "What Is Good Is Beautiful." *Sociometry* 40 (1977): 85–90.

Gruder, Charles L. "Choice of Comparison Persons in Evaluating Oneself." In *Social Comparison Processes*, edited by Jerry M. Suls and R. L. Miller. New York: Hemisphere, 1977.

Guinness, A. E. *ABC's of the Human Mind: A Family Answer Book.* Pleasantville, NY: Reader's Digest, 1990.

Gupta, Usha, and Pushpa Singh. "Exploratory Study of Love and Liking and Type of Marriages." *Indian Journal of Applied Psychology* 19 (1982): 92–97.

Gutierrez, Gustavo. *We Drink from Our Own Wells: The Spiritual Journey of a People.* Maryknoll, NY: Orbis Books, 1985.

Hadaway, C. Kirk. "Life Satisfaction and Religion: A Reanalysis." *Social Forces* 57 (1978): 636–43.

———, and Wade C. Roof. "Religious Commitment and the Quality of Life in American Society." *Review of Religious Research* 19 (1978): 295–307.

Haemmerlie, Frances M., and Robert L. Montgomery. "Psychological State and the Menstrual Cycle." *Journal of Social Behavior and Personality* 2 (1987): 233–42.

Haes, J. C. J. M. de, and F. C. E. Van Knippenberg. "The Quality of Life of Cancer Patients: A Review of the Literature." *Social Science and Medicine* 10 (1985): 809–17.

Hall, Judith A. *Nonverbal Sex Differences: Communication Accuracy and Expressive Style.* Baltimore: Johns Hopkins University Press, 1984.

Halli, S. S., and Z. Zimmer. "Common Law Union as a Differentiating Factor in the Failure of Marriage in Canada, 1984." *Social Indicators Research* 24 (1991): 329–45.

Hamilton, William D. "Innate Social Aptitudes of Man: An Approach from Evolutionary Genetics." In *Biosocial Anthropology*, edited by R. Fox. London: Malaby Press, 1975.

Hare-Mustin, Rachel T. "The Impossible Pursuit of Perfection." In *Every Woman's Emotional Well-being*, edited by Carol Tavris. New York: Prentice-Hall, 1986.

Haring, Marilyn J., William A. Stock, and Morris A. Okun. "A Research Synthesis of Gender and Social Class as Correlates of Subjective Well-being." *Human Relations* 37 (1984): 645–57.

Haritos-Fatouros, Mika. "The Official Torturer: A Learning Model for Obedience to the Authority of Violence." *Journal of Applied Social Psychology* 18 (1988): 1107–20.

Hart, Archibald D. *15 Principles for Achieving Happiness*. Dallas: Word, 1988.

Hartman, Lorne M. "Effects of Sex and Marital Therapy on Sexual Interaction and Marital Happiness." *Journal of Sex and Marital Therapy* 9 (1983) 137–51.

Harvey, Carol D., Gordon E. Barnes, and Leonard Greenwood. "Correlates of Morale Among Canadian Widowed Persons." *Social Psychiatry* 22 (1987): 65–72.

Hatfield, Elaine, John T. Cacioppo, and Richard Rapson. "The Logic of Emotion: Emotional Contagion." In *Review of Personality and Social Psychology*, edited by M. S. Clark. Newbury Park, CA: Sage, 1992.

Hatfield, Elaine, and Susan Sprecher. *Mirror, Mirror: The Importance of Looks in Everyday Life*. Albany, NY: SUNY Press, 1986.

Hatfield, Elaine et al. "Equity and Intimate Relations: Recent Research." In *Compatible and Incompatible Relationships*, edited by William Ickes. New York: Springer-Verlag, 1985.

Hattie, John A., Christopher F. Sharpley, and H. Jane Rogers. "Comparative Effectiveness of Professional and Paraprofessional Helpers." *Psychological Bulletin* 95 (1984): 534–41.

Headey, Bruce, and Alex Wearing. "The Sense of Relative Superiority— Central to Well-being." *Social Indicators Research* 20 (1988): 497–516.

———. "Personality, Life Events, and Subjective Well-being: Toward a Dynamic Equilibrium Model." *Journal of Personality and Social Psychology* 57 (1989): 731–39.

———. "Subjective Well-being: A Stocks and Flows Framework." In *Subjec-*

tive Well-being: An Interdisciplinary Perspective, edited by Fritz Strack, Michael Argyle, and Norbert Schwarz. Oxford, England: Pergamon Press, 1990.

Heaton, Tim B., and E. L. Pratt. "The Effects of Religious Homogamy on Marital Satisfaction and Stability." *Journal of Family Issues* 11 (1990): 191–207.

Helson, Ravenna, Teresa Elliot, and Janet Leigh. "Number and Quality of Roles." *Psychology of Women Quarterly* 14 (1990): 83–101.

Hennigan, Karen et al. "Impact of the Introduction of Television on Crime in the United States: Empirical Findings and Theoretical Implications." *Journal of Personality and Social Psychology* 42 (1982): 461–77.

Herzog, A. Regula, and Willard L. Rogers. "Satisfaction Among Older Adults." In *Research on the Quality of Life,* edited by Frank M. Andrews. Ann Arbor: Survey Research Center, University of Michigan, 1986.

———, and Joseph Woodworth. *Subjective Well-being Among Different Age Groups.* Ann Arbor: Survey Research Center, University of Michigan, 1982.

Hessing, Dick J., Henk Elffers, and Russell H. Weigel. "Exploring the Limits of Self-reports and Reasoned Action: An Investigation of the Psychology of Tax Evasion Behavior." *Journal of Personality and Social Psychology* 54 (1988): 405–13.

Hetherington, E. Mavis, and W. G. Clingempeel. "Coping with Marital Transitions: A Family Systems Perspective." *Society for Research in Child Development Monographs,* in press.

Hetherington, E. Mavis, Margaret Stanley-Hagan, and Edward R. Anderson. "Marital Transitions: A Child's Perspective." *American Psychologist* 44 (1989): 303–12.

Hilgard, Ernest R. *Divided Consciousness: Multiple Controls in Human Thought and Action.* New York: Wiley, 1986.

Hinkle, J. Scott. "Psychological Benefits of Aerobic Running: Implications for Mental Health Counselors." *Journal of Mental Health Counseling* 10 (1988): 245–51.

Hirst, William, Ulric Neisser, and Elizabeth Spelke. "Divided Attention." *Human Nature,* June 1978, pp. 54–61.

Hodgkinson, Virginia A., and Murray S. Weitzman. *Giving and Volunteering in the United States: Findings from a National Survey.* Washington, DC: Independent Sector, 1990.

———, and A. D. Kirsch. "From Commitment to Action: How Religious Involvement Affects Giving and Volunteering." In *Faith and Philan-*

thropy in America: Exploring the Role of Religion in America's Voluntary Sector, edited by Robert Wuthnow, Virginia A. Hodgkinson, and Associates. San Francisco: Jossey-Bass, 1990.

Hogan, Joyce. "Personality Correlates of Physical Fitness." *Journal of Personality and Social Psychology* 56 (1989): 284–88.

Holahan, Carole K. "Relation of Life Goals at Age 70 to Activity Participation and Health and Psychological Well-being Among Terman's Gifted Men and Women." *Psychology and Aging* 3 (1988): 286–91.

Holmes, John G., and John K. Rempel. "Trust in Close Relationships." In *Review of Personality and Social Psychology*, edited by Clyde Hendrick. Vol. 10. Newbury Park, CA: Sage, 1989.

House, James S., Karl R. Landis, and Debra Umberson. "Social Relationships and Health." *Science* 241 (1988): 540–45.

Howard, J. W., and Robyn M. Dawes. "Linear Prediction of Marital Happiness." *Personality and Social Psychology Bulletin* 2 (1976): 478–80.

Howard, K. I. "Employers' Attitudes About Mental Health Are Affecting Their Bottom Lines." *Northwestern Perspective*, Spring 1991, p. 48.

Hui, C. Harry. "West Meets East: Individualism Versus Collectivism in North America and Asia." Invited address, Hope College, November 1990.

Hunsberger, Bruce. "Religion, Age, Life Satisfaction, and Perceived Sources of Religiousness: A Study of Older Persons." *Journal of Gerontology* 40 (1985): 615–30.

Hunter, Ski, and Martin Sundel, eds. *Midlife Myths: Issues, Findings, and Practice Implications*. Newbury Park, CA: Sage, 1989.

Inglehart, Ronald. *Culture Shift in Advanced Industrial Society*. Princeton: Princeton University Press, 1990.

Institute of Medicine, National Academy of Sciences. *Research Briefing: Behavioral Influences on the Endocrine and Immune Systems*. Washington, DC: National Academy Press, 1989.

Isen, Alice M. "The Influence of Positive and Negative Affect on Cognitive Organization: Some Implications for Development." In *Psychological and Biological Approaches to Emotion*, edited by Nancy Stein, Bennett Leventhal, and Tom Trabasso. Hillsdale, NJ: Erlbaum, 1990.

———, Kimberly A. Daubman, and Gary P. Nowicki. "Positive Affect Facilitates Creative Problem Solving." *Journal of Personality and Social Psychology* 52 (1987): 1122–31.

Isen, Alice et al. "Affect, Accessibility of Material in Memory, and Behavior: A Cognitive Loop?" *Journal of Personality and Social Psychology* 36 (1978): 1–12.

Israel, Barbara A., and Toni C. Antonucci. "Social Network Characteristics and Psychological Well-being: A Replication and Extension." *Health Education Quarterly* 14 (1987): 461–81.

Jacoby, S. "When Opposites Attract." *Reader's Digest,* December 1986, pp. 95–98.

James, William. *The Principles of Psychology.* New York: Holt, 1890.

———. *Varieties of Religious Experience.* 1902. Reprint. New York: Mentor Books, 1958.

Jasnoski, Mary L., Joachim Kugler, and David C. McClelland. "Power Imagery and Relaxation Affect Psychoneuroimmune Indices." Paper presented at the American Psychological Association Convention, Washington, DC, August 1986.

Jones, Edward et al. "Effects of Strategic Self-presentation on Subsequent Self-esteem." *Journal of Personality and Social Psychology* 41 (1981): 407–21.

Jourard, Sidney M. *The Transparent Self.* Princeton: Van Nostrand, 1964.

Kahn, Joan R., and Kathryn A. London. "Premarital Sex and the Risk of Divorce." *Journal of Marriage and the Family* 53 (1991): 845–55.

Kamen, Leslie et al. "Pessimism and Cell-Mediated Immunity." Manuscript, University of Pennsylvania, 1988.

Kammann, Richard. "Objective Circumstances, Life Satisfactions, and Sense of Well-being: Consistencies Across Time and Place." *New Zealand Journal of Psychology* 12 (1983): 14–22.

———, Carey Martin, and Malcolm McQueen. "Low Accuracy in Judgments of Others' Psychological Well-being as Seen from a Phenomenological Perspective." *Journal of Personality* 52 (1984): 107–23.

Kaprio, Jaakko, Markku Koskenvuo, and Heli Rita. "Mortality After Bereavement: A Prospective Study of 95,647 Widowed Persons." *American Journal of Public Health* 77 (1987): 283–87.

Kato, Pamela, S., and Diane N. Ruble. "Toward an Understanding of Women's Experience of Menstrual Cycle Symptoms." In *Psychological Perspectives on Women's Health,* edited by V. Adesso, D. Reddy, and R. Fleming. Washington, DC: Hemisphere, 1992.

Kaylor, Jeffrey A., Daniel W. King, and Lynda A. King. "Psychological Effects of Military Service in Vietnam: A Meta-analysis." *Psychological Bulletin* 102 (1987): 431–45.

Kellerman, Joan, James Lewis, and James D. Laird. "Looking and Loving: The Effects of Mutual Gaze on Feelings of Romantic Love." *Journal of Research in Personality* 23 (1989): 145–61.

Kelly, E. Lowell, and James J. Conley. "Personality and Compatibility: A

Prospective Analysis of Marital Stability and Marital Satisfaction." *Journal of Personality and Social Psychology* 52 (1987): 27–40.

Kenrick, Douglas T., and Sara E. Gutierres. "Contrast Effects and Judgments of Physical Attractiveness: When Beauty Becomes a Social Problem." *Journal of Personality and Social Psychology* 38 (1980): 131–40.

————, and Laurie L. Goldberg. "Influence of Popular Erotica on Judgments of Strangers and Mates." *Journal of Experimental Social Psychology* 25 (1989): 159–67.

Kenrick, Douglas T., and Melanie R. Trost. "A Biosocial Theory of Heterosexual Relationships." In *Females, Males, and Sexuality,* edited by Kathryn Kelley. Albany: SUNY Press, 1987.

Kihlstrom, John F. "Hypnosis." *Annual Review of Psychology* 36 (1985): 385–418.

King, Martin Luther, Jr. *New York Times,* June 6, 1964, p. 10.

King, Peter. "Bawl Players." *Sports Illustrated,* March 18, 1991, pp. 14–17.

Kitson, Gay C., and Marvin B. Sussman. "Marital Complaints, Demographic Characteristics, and Symptoms of Mental Distress in Divorce." *Journal of Marriage and the Family* 44 (1982): 87–101.

Klerman, Gerald L., and Myrna M. Weissman. "Increasing Rates of Depression." *Journal of the American Medical Association* 261 (1989): 2229–35.

Koenig, Harold G., James N. Kvale, and Carolyn Ferrel. "Religion and Well-being in Later Life." *The Gerontologist* 28 (1988): 18–28.

Koenig, Harold G., Mona Smiley, and Jo Ann P. Gonzales. *Religion, Health, and Aging: A Review and Theoretical Integration.* Westport, CT: Greenwood Press, 1988.

Koss, Mary P., and Barry R. Burkhart. "A Conceptual Analysis of Rape Victimization." *Psychology of Women Quarterly* 13 (1989): 27–40.

Koss, Mary P., Christine A. Gidycz, and Nadine Wisniewski. "The Scope of Rape: Incidence and Prevalence of Sexual Aggression and Victimization in a National Sample of Higher Education Students." *Journal of Consulting and Clinical Psychology* 55 (1987): 162–70.

Koss, Mary P., Paul Koss, and W. Joy Woodruff. "Relation of Criminal Victimization to Health Perceptions Among Women Medical Patients." *Journal of Consulting and Clinical Psychology* 58, no. 2 (1990): 147–52.

Kroll, Jerome, and William Sheehan. "Religious Beliefs and Practices Among 52 Psychiatric Inpatients in Minnesota." *American Journal of Psychiatry* 146 (1989): 67–72.

Kunst-Wilson, William R., and Robert B. Zajonc. "Affective Discrimination of Stimuli That Cannot Be Recognized." *Science* 207 (1980): 557–58.

Kurtz, Paul. "Stars, Planets, and People." *Skeptical Inquirer* (Spring 1983): 65–69.

Kushner, Harold. "You've Got to Believe in Something." *Redbook*, December 1987, pp. 92–94.

Laird, James D. "Self-attribution of Emotion: The Effects of Expressive Behavior on the Quality of Emotional Experience." *Journal of Personality and Social Psychology* 29 (1974): 475–86.

———. "The Real Role of Facial Response in the Experience of Emotion: A Reply to Tourangeau and Ellsworth, and Others." *Journal of Personality and Social Psychology* 47 (1984): 909–17.

Langer, Ellen J. *The Psychology of Control.* Beverly Hills: Sage, 1983.

Larsen, Randy J., and Margaret Kasimatis. "Individual Differences in Entrainment of Mood to the Weekly Calendar." *Journal of Personality and Social Psychology* 58 (1990): 164–71.

Larson, Randy. "Is Feeling 'In Control' Related to Happiness in Daily Life?" *Psychological Reports* 64 (1989): 775–84.

Latten, J. J. "Life-course and Satisfaction, Equal for Every-one?" *Social Indicators Research* 21 (1989): 599–610.

Laurence, Jean-Roch, and Campbell Perry. "Hypnotically Created Memory Among Highly Hypnotizable Subjects." *Science* 222 (1983): 523–24.

Lefcourt, Herbert M. *Locus of Control: Current Trends in Theory and Research.* Hillsdale, NJ: Erlbaum, 1982.

———, and Rod A. Martin. *Humor and Life Stress.* New York: Springer-Verlag, 1986.

Lehman, Darrin R., and Richard E. Nisbett. "Effects of Higher Education on Inductive Reasoning." Manuscript, University of Michigan, 1985.

Leikind, Bernard J., and William J. McCarthy. "An Investigation of Firewalking." *Skeptical Inquirer* 10 (1985): 23–34.

———. "Firewalking." *Experientia* 44 (1988): 310–15.

Lemly, B. "The Man Who Won't Be Defeated." *Parade*, November 26, 1989, pp. 12–13.

L'Engle, Madeleine. *A Circle of Quiet.* New York: Seabury, 1972.

———. *Walking on Water: Reflections on Faith and Art.* Wheaton, IL: Harold Shaw, 1980.

Lenz, S. "The Effect of Subliminal Auditory Stimuli on Academic Learning and Motor Skills Performance Among Police Recruits." Ph.D. diss., California School of Professional Psychology, 1989.

Levenson, Sam. *You Don't Have to Be in Who's Who to Know What's What.* New York: Pocket Books, 1979.

Levin, Jeffrey S., and Kyriakos S. Markides. "Religious Attendance and Psychological Well-being in Middle-aged and Older Mexican Americans." *Sociological Analysis* 49 (1988): 66–72.

Levin, Jeffrey S., and Preston L. Schiller. "Is There a Religious Factor in Health?" *Journal of Religion and Health* 26 (1987): 9–36.

Levinson, Daniel J. *The Seasons of a Man's Life.* New York: Knopf, 1979.

Levitt, Eugene E. "Coercion, Voluntariness, Compliance and Resistance: The Essence of Hypnosis Twenty-seven Years After Orne." Address to the American Psychological Association Convention, Washington, DC, August 1986.

Levy, Sandra et al. "Survival Hazards Analysis in First Recurrent Breast Cancer Patients: Seven-year Follow-up." *Psychosomatic Medicine* 50 (1988): 520–28.

Lewinsohn, Peter M., J. E. Redner, and J. R. Seeley. "The Relationship Between Life Satisfaction and Psychosocial Variables: New Perspectives." In *Subjective Well-being: An Interdisciplinary Perspective,* edited by Fritz Strack, Michael Argyle, and Norbert Schwarz. Oxford, England: Pergamon Press, 1990.

Lewinsohn, Peter M., and Michael Rosenbaum. "Recall of Parental Behavior by Acute Depressives, Remitted Depressives, and Nondepressives." *Journal of Personality and Social Psychology* 52 (1987): 611–19.

Lewis, C. S. "Membership." In *The Weight of Glory and Other Addresses.* New York: Macmillan, 1949.

———. *Mere Christianity.* New York: Macmillan, 1960.

———. "Good Work and Good Works." In *Screwtape Proposes a Toast.* Glasgow: William Collins, 1965.

———. *The Last Battle.* New York: Collier Books, 1974, p. 184.

———. *Christian Reflections.* Glasgow: Collins (Fount Paperbacks), 1981.

Lichtenstein, R. "Subliminal Messages Sell Tapes." *The Times,* December 14, 1989, pp. B1, B2.

Linville, Patricia W. "Self-complexity as a Cognitive Buffer Against Stress-related Illness and Depression." *Journal of Personality and Social Psychology* 52 (1987): 663–76.

Loehlin, John C., Lee Willerman, and Joseph M. Horn. "Personality Resemblance in Adoptive Families: A 10-year Follow-up." *Journal of Personality and Social Psychology* 53 (1987): 961–69.

Lowry, Dennis T., and David E. Towles. "Soap Opera Portrayals of Sex, Contraception, and Sexually Transmitted Diseases." *Journal of Communication* 39, no. 2 (1989): 76–83.

Luce, Clare Boothe. "A Doll's House." *Life,* October 16, 1970, pp. 54–67.

Lynn, Steven J., and Judith W. Rhue. "The Fantasy-prone Person: Hypnosis,

Imagination, and Creativity." *Journal of Personality and Social Psychology* 51 (1986): 404–8.

McCann, I. Lisa, and David S. Holmes. "Influence of Aerobic Exercise on Depression." *Journal of Personality and Social Psychology* 46 (1984): 1142–47.

McCauley, Clark R., and Mary E. Segal. "Social Psychology in Terrorist Groups." In *Group Processes and Intergroup Relations,* edited by Clyde Hendrick. Beverly Hills: Sage, 1987.

McCrae, Robert R., and Paul T. Costa, Jr. "Adding *Liebe und Arbeit:* The Full Five-Factor Model and Well-being." Paper presented at the American Psychological Association Convention, New Orleans, August 1989.

———. *Personality in Adulthood.* New York: Guilford Press, 1990.

McFarland, Cathy, Michael Ross, and Nancy DeCourville. "Women's Theories of Menstruation and Biases in Recall of Menstrual Symptoms." *Journal of Personality and Social Psychology* 57 (1989): 522–31.

Macfarlane, Jean W. "Perspectives on Personality Consistency and Change from the Guidance Study." *Vita Humana* 7 (1964): 115–26.

McGloshen, Thomas H., and Shirley L. O'Bryant. "The Psychological Well-being of Older, Recent Widows." *Psychology of Women Quarterly* 12 (1988): 99–116.

McIntosh, Daniel N. "Religion as Schema: Implications for the Relation Between Religion and Coping." Paper presented to the American Psychological Association Convention, San Francisco. August 1991.

———, and Bernard B. Spilka. "Religion and Physical Health: The Role of Personal Faith and Control Beliefs." In *Research in the Social Scientific Study of Religion,* edited by Monty L. Lynn and David O. Moberg. Vol. 2. Greenwich, CT: JAI Press, 1990.

MacKay, James L. "Selfhood: Comment on Brewster Smith." *American Psychologist* 35 (1980): 106–7.

McKenzie, Brad, and James Campbell. "Race, Socioeconomic Status, and the Subjective Well-being of Older Americans." *International Journal of Aging and Human Development* 25 (1987): 43–61.

McKinlay, John B., Sonja M. McKinlay, and Donald Brambilla. "Health Status and Utilization Behavior Associated with Menopause." *American Journal of Epidemiology* 125 (1987): 110–21.

———. "The Relative Contributions of Endocrine Changes and Social Circumstances to Depression in Mid-aged Women." *Journal of Health and Social Behavior* 28 (1987): 345–63.

McLanahan, Sara, and Julia Adams. "Parenthood and Psychological Well-being." *Annual Review of Sociology* 13 (1987): 237–57.

———. "The Effects of Children on Adults' Psychological Well-being: 1957–1976." *Social Forces* 68 (1989): 124–46.

McMillan, Marcia J., and R. O. Pihl. "Premenstrual Depression: A Distinct Entity." *Journal of Abnormal Psychology* 96 (1987): 149–54.

Magnus, K., and Ed Diener. "A Longitudinal Analysis of Personality, Life Events, and Well-being." Paper presented at the Midwestern Psychological Association Convention, Chicago, May 1991.

Magnusson, David, and Lars R. Bergman. "A Pattern Approach to the Study of Pathways from Childhood to Adulthood." In *Straight and Devious Pathways from Childhood to Adulthood,* edited by Lee N. Robins and Michael Rutter. Cambridge: Cambridge University Press, 1990.

Magnusson, Sally. *The Flying Scotsman.* London: Quartet Books, 1981.

Malamuth, Neil M. "Sexually Violent Media, Thought Patterns, and Antisocial Behavior." In *Public Communication and Behavior,* edited by George Comstock. Vol. 2. San Diego: Academic Press, 1989.

——— et al. "Characteristics of Aggressors Against Women: Testing a Model Using a National Sample of College Students." *Journal of Consulting and Clinical Psychology* 59 (1991): 670–81.

Manning, Frederick J., and Terrence D. Fullerton. "Health and Well-being in Highly Cohesive Units of the U.S. Army." *Journal of Applied Social Psychology* 18 (1988): 503–19.

Marcel, Anthony. "Conscious and Unconscious Perception: Experiments on Visual Masking and Word Recognition." *Cognitive Psychology* 15 (1983): 197–237.

Marcus, Paul, and Alan Rosenberg. "The Holocaust Survivor's Faith and Religious Behavior: Implications for Treatment." In *Healing Their Wounds: Psychotherapy with Holocaust Survivors and Their Families,* edited by Paul Marcus and Alan Rosenberg. New York: Praeger, 1989.

Markides, Kyriakos S., Jeffrey S. Levin, and Laura A. Ray. "Religion, Aging, and Life Satisfaction: An Eight-Year, Three-Wave Longitudinal Study." *The Gerontologist* 27 (1987): 660–65.

Markus, Hazel, and Shinobu Kitayama. "Culture and the Self: Implications for Cognition, Emotion, and Motivation." *Psychological Review* 98 (1991): 224–53.

Marsh, Herbert W., and John W. Parker. "Determinants of Student Self-concept: Is It Better to Be a Relatively Large Fish in a Small Pond Even If You Don't Learn to Swim as Well?" *Journal of Personality and Social Psychology* 47 (1984): 213–31.

Marsh, Herbert W., Garry E. Richards, and Jennifer Barnes. "Multidimensional Self-concepts: The Effect of Participation in an Outward

Bound Program." *Journal of Personality and Social Psychology* 50 (1986): 195–204.

Martin, Teresa Castro, and Larry L. Bumpass. "Recent Trends in Marital Disruption." *Demography* 26 (1989): 37–51.

Martinsen, Egil W. "The Role of Aerobic Exercise in the Treatment of Depression." *Stress Medicine* 3 (1987): 93–100.

Maslow, Bertha G. *Abraham H. Maslow: A Memorial Volume.* Monterey, CA: Brooks/Cole, 1972.

Massimini, Fausto, and Massimo Carli. "The Systematic Assessment of Flow in Daily Experience." In *Optimal Experience: Psychological Studies of Flow in Consciousness,* edited by Mihaly Csikszentmihalyi and Isabella S. Csikszentimihalyi. Cambridge: Cambridge University Press, 1988.

Masters, Kevin S. et al. "Religious Life-styles and Mental Health: Conclusions from an Intensive Three-Year Project." Paper presented to the Midwestern Psychological Association Convention, Chicago, May 1990.

Matlin, Margaret W., and David J. Stang. *The Pollyanna Principle: Selectivity in Language, Memory, and Thought.* Cambridge, MA: Schenkman, 1978.

Maxwell, G. M. "Behaviour of Lovers: Measuring the Closeness of Relationships." *Journal of Social and Personal Relationships* 2 (1985): 215–38.

Meador, B. D., and Carl R. Rogers. "Person-Centered Therapy." In *Current Psychotherapies,* edited by Raymond J. Corsini. Itasca, IL: Peacock, 1984.

Mecca, Andrew M., Neil J. Smelser, and John Vasconcellos, eds. *The Social Importance of Self-esteem.* Berkeley: University of California Press, 1989.

Medved, Michael. "Popular Culture and the War Against Standards." *Imprimis* 20, no. 2 (February 1991): 1–7.

Meindl, James R., and Melvin J. Lerner. "Exacerbation of Extreme Responses to an Out-group." *Journal of Personality and Social Psychology* 47 (1984): 71–84.

Merikle, Phillip M. "Subliminal Auditory Messages: An Evaluation." *Psychology and Marketing* 5 (1988): 355–72.

———. Unpublished manuscript regarding subliminal tapes and weight loss, University of Waterloo, 1991.

Meyer, Donald. *The Positive Thinkers: Religion as Pop Psychology from Mary Baker Eddy to Oral Roberts.* New York: Pantheon Books, 1980.

Michalos, Alex C. "Job Satisfaction, Marital Satisfaction, and the Quality of Life: A Review and a Preview." In *Research on the Quality of Life,* edited by Frank M. Andrews. Ann Arbor: Survey Research Center, University of Michigan, 1986.

————. *Life Satisfaction and Happiness.* Vol. 1 of *Global Report on Student Well-being.* New York: Springer-Verlag, 1991.

Michell, D. J. "I Remember Eric Liddell." In *The Disciplines of the Christian Life,* edited by Eric Liddell. London: Triangle, 1985.

Mikulincer, Mario et al. "The Effects of 72 Hours of Sleep Loss on Psychological Variables." *British Journal of Psychology* 80 (1989): 145–62.

Milberg, Sandra, and Margaret S. Clark. "Moods and Compliance." *British Journal of Social Psychology* 27 (1988): 79–90.

Milgram, Stanley. *Obedience to Authority.* New York: Harper & Row, 1974.

Mill, John Stuart. *Utilitarianism.* Ch. 2. 1863. Reprint. Oxford: Blackwell, 1949.

Miller, Katherine I., and Peter R. Monge. "Participation, Satisfaction, and Productivity: A Meta-analytic Review." *Academy of Management Journal* 29 (1986): 727–53.

Miller, Lynn C., John H. Berg, and Richard L. Archer. "Openers: Individuals Who Elicit Intimate Self-disclosure." *Journal of Personality and Social Psychology* 44 (1983): 1234–44.

Miller, Philip C. et al. "Marital Locus of Control and Marital Problem Solving." *Journal of Personality and Social Psychology* 51 (1986): 161–69.

Mirels, Herbert L., and Robert W. McPeek. "Self-advocacy and Self-esteem." *Journal of Consulting and Clinical Psychology* 45 (1977): 1132–38.

Montagu, Ashley. *Growing Young.* 2d ed. New York: Bergin & Garvey, 1989. (Abridged in *Utne Reader,* January/February 1990, p. 91.)

Moore, Timothy E. "The Case Against Subliminal Manipulation." *Psychology and Marketing* 5 (1988): 297–316.

————. "Discussion of: Subliminal Perception: Are There Any Practical Applications?" Symposium at the American Psychological Association Convention, Boston, August 1990.

Myers, David G. *Social Psychology.* 2d ed. New York: McGraw-Hill, 1987.

————. *Social Psychology.* 3d ed. New York: McGraw-Hill, 1990.

————. *Psychology.* 3d ed. New York: Worth Publishers, 1992.

Nadon, Robert et al. "Absorption and Hypnotizability: Context Effects Reexamined." *Journal of Personality and Social Psychology* 60 (1991): 144–53.

Nash, Michael. "What, If Anything, Is Regressed About Hypnotic Age Regression? A Review of the Empirical Literature." *Psychological Bulletin* 102 (1987): 42–52.

National Center for Education Statistics. *Digest of Education Statistics.* 25th ed. Washington, DC: Superintendent of Documents, Government Printing Office, 1989.

National Center for Health Statistics. *Natality.* Vol. 1 of *Vital Statistics of the United States, 1987.* DHHS Pub. No. (PHS) 89–1100. Washington, DC: Superintendent of Documents, Government Printing Office, 1989.

————. *Mortality, Part A.* Vol. 2 of *Vital Statistics of the United States, 1987.* Washington, DC: Superintendent of Documents, Government Printing Office, 1990.

National Council on the Aging. *The Myth and Reality of Aging in America.* Washington, DC: National Council on Aging, 1976.

National Research Council. *Risking the Future: Adolescent Sexuality, Pregnancy, and Childbearing.* Washington, DC: National Academic Press, 1987.

Naylor, Thomas H. "Redefining Corporate Motivation, Swedish Style." *Christian Century* 107 (1990): 566–70.

Neugarten, Bernice L. "The Roles We Play." In *Quality of Life: The Middle Years,* edited by American Medical Association. Action, MA: Publishing Sciences Group, 1974.

———— et al. "Women's Attitudes Towards the Menopause." *Vita Humana* 6 (1963): 140–51.

Newcomb, Michael D. "Cohabitation and Marriage: A Quest for Independence and Relatedness." In *Family Processes and Problems: Social Psychological Aspects,* edited by Stuart Oskamp. Newbury Park, CA: Sage, 1987.

————, and Peter M. Bentler. "Impact of Adolescent Drug Use and Social Support on Problems of Young Adults: A Longitudinal Study." *Journal of Abnormal Psychology* 97 (1988): 64–75.

————. "Marital Breakdown." In *Personal Relationships in Disorder.* Vol. 3 of *Personal Relationships,* edited by S. Duck and R. Gilmour. London: Academic Press, 1981.

Nezu, Arthur M., Christine M. Nezu, and Sonia E. Blissett. "Sense of Humor as a Moderator of the Relation Between Stressful Events and Psychological Distress: A Prospective Analysis." *Journal of Personality and Social Psychology* 54 (1988): 520–25.

Niebuhr, Reinhold. *Beyond Tragedy.* New York: Scribner's, 1937.

Niemi, Richard Gene, John Mueller, and Tom W. Smith. *Trends in Public Opinion: A Compendium of Survey Data.* New York: Greenwood Press, 1989.

Nisbett, Richard, and Lee Ross. *The Person and the Situation.* New York: McGraw-Hill, 1991.

Noller, Patricia, and Mary Anne Fitzpatrick. "Marital Communication in the Eighties." *Journal of Marriage and the Family* 52 (1990): 832–43.

Nouwen, Henri J. M. *Reaching Out: The Three Movements of the Spiritual Life.* Garden City, NY: Doubleday, 1975.

————. *Lifesigns: Intimacy, Fecundity, and Ecstasy in Christian Perspective.* Garden City, NY: Doubleday, 1986.

Oatley, Keith, and Winifred Bolton. "A Social-Cognitive Theory of Depression in Reaction to Life Events." *Psychological Review* 92 (1985): 372–88.

O'Connor, Pat, and George W. Brown. "Supportive Relationships: Fact or Fancy?" *Journal of Social and Personal Relationships* 1 (1984): 159–75.

Oettingen, Gabriele, and Martin E. P. Seligman. "Pessimism and Behavioural Signs of Depression in East Versus West Berlin." *European Journal of Social Psychology* 20 (1990): 207–20.

Okun, Morris A. "Subjective Well-being." *Encyclopedia on Aging,* in press.

Okun, Morris A., Robert W. Olding, and Catherine M. G. Cohn. "A Meta-analysis of Subjective Well-being Interventions Among Elders." *Psychological Bulletin* 108 (1990): 257–66.

Okun, Morris A., and William A. Stock. "The Construct Validity of Subjective Well-being Measures: An Assessment via Quantitative Research Syntheses." *Journal of Community Psychology* 15 (1987): 481–92.

————. "Correlates and Components of Subjective Well-being Among the Elderly." *Journal of Applied Gerontology* 6 (1987): 95–112.

Okun, Morris A. et al. "Health and Subjective Well-being: A Meta-analysis." *International Journal of Aging and Human Development* 19 (1984): 111–32.

————. "The Social Activity/Subjective Well-being Relation: A Quantitative Synthesis." *Research on Aging* 6 (1984): 45–65.

Oleckno, William A., and Michael J. Blacconiere. "Relationship of Religiosity to Wellness and Other Health-Related Behaviors and Outcomes." *Psychological Reports* 68 (1991): 819–26.

Olson, James M., C. Peter Herman, and Mark P. Zanna, eds. *Relative Deprivation and Social Comparison. The Ontario Symposium.* Vol. 4. Hillsdale, NJ: Erlbaum, 1986.

Orne, Martin T., and Frederick J. Evans. "Social Control in the Psychological Experiment: Antisocial Behavior and Hypnosis." *Journal of Personality and Social Psychology* 1 (1965): 189–200.

Orne, Martin. T. et al. "Hypnotically Induced Testimony." In *Eyewitness Testimony: Psychological Perspectives,* edited by Gary L. Wells and Elizabeth F. Loftus. New York: Cambridge University Press, 1984.

Paffenbarger, Ralph S., Jr., et al. "Physical Activity, All-Cause Mortality, and Longevity of College Alumni." *New England Journal of Medicine* 314 (1986): 605–12.

Palisi, Bartolomeo J. "Marriage Companionship and Marriage Well-being: A Comparison of Metropolitan Areas in Three Countries." *Journal of Comparative Family Studies* 15 (1984): 43–57.

Paloma, Margaret M., and Brian F. Pendleton. "The Effects of Prayer and Prayer Experiences on Measures of General Well-being." *Journal of Psychology and Theology* 19 (1991): 71–83.

Paloutzian, Ray F., and Craig W. Ellison. "Loneliness, Spiritual Well-being, and the Quality of Life." In *Loneliness: A Sourcebook of Current Theory, Research, and Therapy,* edited by Letitia A. Peplau and Daniel Perlman. New York: Wiley, 1982.

Parducci, Allen. "Value Judgments: Toward a *Relational* Theory of Happiness." In *Attitudinal Judgment,* edited by J. Richard Eiser. New York: Springer-Verlag, 1984.

Park, Crystal, Lawrence H. Cohen, and Lisa Herb. "Intrinsic Religiousness and Religious Coping as Life Stress Moderators for Catholics Versus Protestants." *Journal of Personality and Social Psychology* 59 (1990): 562–74.

Patterson, James, and Peter Kim. *The Day America Told the Truth: What People Really Believe About Everything That Matters.* Englewood Cliffs, NJ: Prentice-Hall, 1991.

Pavot, William et al. "Further Validation of the Satisfaction with Life Scale: Evidence for the Cross-Method Convergence of Well-being Measures." *Journal of Personality Assessment* 57 (1991): 149–61.

Pavot, William, Ed Diener, and Frank Fujita. "Extraversion and Happiness." *Personality and Individual Differences* 11, no. 12 (1990): 1299–1306.

Payne, I. R. et al. "Review of Religion and Mental Health: Prevention and the Enhancement of Psychosocial Functioning." *Prevention in Human Services,* in press.

Peale, Norman Vincent. *The Power of Positive Thinking.* Englewood Cliffs, NJ: Prentice-Hall, 1952.

———, and Smiley Blanton. *The Art of Real Happiness.* Englewood Cliffs, NJ: Prentice-Hall, 1950.

Pennebaker, James W. *The Psychology of Physical Symptoms.* New York: Springer-Verlag, 1982.

———. *Opening Up: The Healing Power of Confiding in Others.* New York: Morrow, 1990.

————, and S. Beall. "Cognitive, Emotional, and Physiological Components of Confiding: Behavioral Inhibition and Disease." Manuscript, Southern Methodist University, 1984.

Pennebaker, James W., and Robin C. O'Heeron. "Confiding in Others and Illness Rate Among Spouses of Suicide and Accidental Death Victims." *Journal of Abnormal Psychology* 93 (1984): 473–76.

Pennebaker, James W., Steven D. Barger, and John Tiebout. "Disclosure of Traumas and Health Among Holocaust Survivors." *Psychosomatic Medicine* 51 (1989): 577–89.

Peplau, Letitia A., and Daniel Perlman. *Loneliness: A Sourcebook of Current Theory, Research, and Therapy.* New York: Wiley, 1982.

Perkins, H. W. "Religious Commitment, Yuppie Values, and Well-being in Post-collegiate Life." *Review of Religious Research* 32 (1991): 244–51.

Perkins, Kenneth A. et al. "Cardiovascular Reactivity to Psychological Stress in Aerobically Trained Versus Untrained Mild Hypertensives and Normotensives." *Health Psychology* 5 (1986): 407–21.

Perlman, Daniel, and Karen S. Rook. "Social Support, Social Deficits, and the Family: Toward the Enhancement of Well-being." In *Family Processes and Problems: Social Psychological Aspects*, edited by Stuart Oskamp. Newbury Park, CA: Sage, 1987.

Perls, Fritz. "Gestalt Therapy (interview)." In *Inside Psychotherapy*, edited by Adelaide Bry. New York: Basic Books, 1972.

Peterson, Christopher, Martin E. P. Seligman, and George E. Vaillant. "Pessimistic Explanatory Style Is a Risk Factor for Physical Illness: A 35-Year Longitudinal Study." *Journal of Personality and Social Psychology* 55 (1988): 23–27.

Pettingale, K. W. et al. "Mental Attitudes to Cancer: An Additional Prognostic Factor." *Lancet*, March 30, 1985, p. 750.

Planned Parenthood Federation of America. "Sex Education for Parents." *USA Today*, December 15, 1986, p. 11A.

Plomin, Robert, and J. C. DeFries. *The Origins of Individual Differences in Infancy.* Orlando, FL: Academic Press, 1985.

Pollner, Melvin. "Divine Relations, Social Relations, and Well-being." *Journal of Health and Social Behavior* 30 (1989): 92–104.

Poloma, Margaret M., and George Gallup, Jr. *The Varieties of Prayer.* Philadelphia: Trinity Press, 1991.

Poloma, Margaret M., and Brian F. Pendleton. "Religious Domains and General Well-being." *Social Indicators Research* 22 (1990): 255–76.

Powell, John. *Happiness Is an Inside Job.* Valencia, CA: Tabor, 1989.

Powell, K. E. et al. "Physical Activity and the Incidence of Coronary Heart Disease." *Annual Review of Public Health* 8 (1987): 253–87.

Price, Richard H. "Work and Community." *American Journal of Community Psychology* 13 (1985): 1–12.

Purvis, James A., James M. Dabbs, and Charles H. Hopper. "The 'Opener': Skilled User of Facial Expression and Speech Pattern." *Personality and Social Psychology Bulletin* 10 (1984): 61–66.

Rae, S. "Brain Waves: Subliminal Self-help Messages While You Sleep?" *Elle,* April 1991, pp. 118–19.

Raskin, Robert, Jill Novacek, and Robert Hogan. "Narcissim, Self-esteem, and Defensive Self-enhancement." *Journal of Personality* 59 (1991): 19–38.

Reed, Kimberly. "Strength of Religious Affiliation and Life Satisfaction." *Sociological Analysis* 52 (1991): 205–10.

Reich, John W. et al. "Demands, Desires, and Well-being: An Assessment of Events, Responses, and Outcomes." *Journal of Community Psychology* 16 (1988): 392–402.

Reid, J. "Report of Subliminal M.A. Thesis Study Participants." Colorado State University, 1990.

Reis, H. T., and Phillip Shaver. "Intimacy as an Interpersonal Process." In *Handbook of Personal Relationships: Theory, Relationships and Interventions,* edited by Steve Duck. Chichester, England: Wiley, 1988.

Repetti, Rena L. "Individual and Common Components of the Social Environment at Work and Psychological Well-being." *Journal of Personality and Social Psychology* 52 (1987): 710–20.

———, and Faye Crosby. "Gender and Depression: Exploring the Adult-Role Explanation." *Journal of Social and Clinical Psychology* 2 (1984): 57–70.

Repetti, Rena L., Karen A. Matthews, and Ingrid Waldron. "Employment and Women's Health: Effects of Paid Employment on Women's Mental and Physical Health." *American Psychologist* 44 (1989): 1394–1401.

Reveen, Peter J. "Fantasizing Under Hypnosis: Some Experimental Evidence." *Skeptical Inquirer* 12 (1987–88): 181–83.

Rhodewalt, Frederick, and Sjofn Agustsdottir. "Effects of Self-presentation on the Phenomenal Self." *Journal of Personality and Social Psychology* 50 (1986): 47–55.

Rice, Robert W. et al. "Job Importance as a Moderator of the Relationship Between Job Satisfaction and Life Satisfaction." *Basic and Applied Social Psychology* 6 (1985): 297–316.

Richardson, John T. E. "Questionnaire Studies of Paramenstrual Symptoms." *Psychology of Women Quarterly* 14 (1990) 15–42.

Riddick, Carol C. "Life Satisfaction Determinants of Older Males and Females." *Leisure Sciences* 7 (1985): 47–63.

Rimland, Bernard B. "The Altruism Paradox." *The Southern Psychologist* 2, no. 1 (1982): 8–9.

Rindfuss, Ronald R., and Elizabeth Hervey Stephen. "Marital Noncohabitation: Separation Does Not Make the Heart Grow Fonder." *Journal of Marriage and the Family* 52 (1990): 259–70.

Robins, Lee N., and Daniel A. Reigier. *Psychiatric Disorders in America.* New York: Free Press, 1991.

Robinson, John P. "Who's Doing the Housework?" *American Demographics,* December 1988, pp. 24–28, 63.

Robinson, Vera M. "Humor and Health." In *Handbook of Humor Research,* edited by Paul E. McGhee and Jeffrey H. Goldstein. New York: Springer-Verlag, 1983.

Rodin, Judith. "Aging and Health: Effects of the Sense of Control." *Science* 233 (1986): 1271–76.

Rogers, Carl R. "Reinhold Niebuhr's *The Self and the Dramas of History:* A Criticism." *Pastoral Psychology* 9 (1958): 15–17.

———. *A Way of Being.* Boston: Houghton Mifflin, 1980.

Rogers, Fred. A PBS special, "Our Neighbor," March 18, 1990.

Rohr, Richard, and Joseph Martos. "Eight Good Reasons for Being Catholic." *Catholic Update,* no. CU 0888, 1990.

Rook, Karen S. "Social Support Versus Companionship: Effects on Life Stress, Loneliness, and Evaluations by Others." *Journal of Personality and Social Psychology* 52 (1987): 1132–47.

Rose, Richard J. et al. "Shared Genes, Shared Experiences, and Similarity in Personality: Data from 14,228 Adult Finnish Co-twins." *Journal of Personality and Social Psychology* 54 (1988): 161–71.

Roviaro, Susan, David S. Holmes, and R. David Holmsten. "Influence of a Cardiac Rehabilitation Program on the Cardiovascular, Psychological, and Social Functioning of Cardiac Patients." *Journal of Behavioral Medicine* 7 (1984): 61–81.

Rowlison, Richard T., and Robert D. Felner. "Major Life Events, Hassles, and Adaptation in Adolescence: Confounding in the Conceptualization and Measurement of Life Stress and Adjustment Revisited." *Journal of Personality and Social Psychology* 55 (1988): 432–44.

Ruback, R. Barry, Timothy S. Carr, and Charles H. Hopper. "Perceived Control in Prison: Its Relation to Reported Crowding, Stress, and Symptoms." *Journal of Applied Social Psychology* 16 (1986): 375–86.

Rubenstein, Carin. "The Baby Bomb." *New York Times/Good Health Magazine,* October 8, 1989, pp. 34–41.

Rubin, Lillian B. *Just Friends: The Role of Friendship in Our Lives.* New York: Harper & Row, 1985.

Rubin, Zick. "Measurement of Romantic Love." *Journal of Personality and Social Psychology* 16 (1970): 265–73.

———. *Liking and Loving: An Invitation to Social Psychology.* New York: Holt, Rinehart and Winston, 1973.

Ruehlman, Linda S., and Sharlene A. Wolchik. "Personal Goals and Interpersonal Support and Hindrance as Factors in Psychological Distress and Well-being." *Journal of Personality and Social Psychology* 55 (1988): 293–301.

Russell, Bertrand. *The Conquest of Happiness.* 1930. Reprint. London: Unwin Paperbacks, 1985.

Russell, T. G., W. Rowe, and A. D. Smouse. "Subliminal Self-help Tapes and Academic Achievement: An Evaluation." *Journal of Counseling and Development* 69 (1991): 359–62.

Salovey, Peter, and Deborah Birnbaum. "Influence of Mood on Health-Relevant Cognitions." *Journal of Personality and Social Psychology* 57 (1989): 539–51.

Sandvik, Edward, Ed Diener, and L. Seidlitz. "The Assessment of Well-being: A Comparison of Self-Report and Nonself-Report Strategies." Manuscript, University of Illinois, 1990.

Sapadin, Linda A. "Friendship and Gender: Perspectives of Professional Men and Women." *Journal of Social and Personal Relationships* 5 (1988): 387–403.

Sarnoff, Irving, and Suzanne Sarnoff. *Love-Centered Marriage in a Self-Centered World.* New York: Hemisphere, 1989.

Scanlan, C. "Weight-Loss Industry Diagnosed as Unhealthy." *Detroit Free Press,* March 27, 1990, pp. 1A, 8A.

Scanzoni, Letha D., and John Scanzoni. *Men, Women, and Change: A Sociology of Marriage and Family.* New York: McGraw-Hill, 1981.

Scarr, Sandra, Deborah Phillips, and Kathleen McCartney. "Working Mothers and Their Families." *American Psychologist* 44 (1989): 1402–9.

Scarr, Sandra, and Richard A. Weinberg. "The Minnesota Adoption Studies:

Genetic Differences and Malleability." *Child Development* 54 (1983): 260–67.

Schaeffer, Jill. "Romania: The Eighth Circle of Hell." *Perspectives,* May 1990, pp. 4–6.

Schafer, Robert B., and Pat M. Keith. "Equity and Depression Among Married Couples." *Social Psychology Quarterly* 43 (1980): 430–35.

Schaie, K. Warner, and James Geiwitz. *Adult Development and Aging.* Boston: Little, Brown, 1982.

Scheier, Michael F., and Charles S. Carver. "Dispositional Optimism and Physical Well-being: The Influence of Generalized Outcome Expectancies on Health." *Journal of Personality* 55 (1987): 169–210.

———. "Dispositional Optimism and Recovery from Coronary Artery Bypass Surgery: The Beneficial Effects on Physical and Psychological Well-being." *Journal of Personality and Social Psychology* 57 (1987): 1024–40.

———. "Effects of Optimism on Psychological and Physical Well-being: Theoretical Overview and Empirical Update." *Cognitive Therapy and Research,* in press.

Schervich, Paul G. "Wealth and the Spiritual Secret of Money." In *Faith and Philanthropy in America: Exploring the Role of Religion in America's Voluntary Sector,* edited by Robert Wuthnow, Virginia A. Hodgkinson, and Associates. San Francisco: Jossey-Bass, 1990.

Schuller, Robert. *The Be-Happy Attitudes: Eight Positive Attitudes That Can Transform Your Life!* Waco, TX: Word Books, 1985.

Schwarz, Norbert, and Gerald L. Clore. "Mood Misattribution, and Judgments of Well-being: Informative and Directive Functions of Affective States." *Journal of Personality and Social Psychology* 45 (1985): 513–23.

Schwarz, Norbert et al. "Soccer, Rooms and the Quality of Your Life: Mood Effects on Judgments of Satisfaction with Life in General and with Specific Domains." *European Journal of Social Psychology* 17 (1987): 69–79.

Schwarz, Norbert, and Fritz Strack. "Evaluating One's Life: A Judgment Model of Subjective Well-being." In *The Social Psychology of Well-being,* edited by Fritz Strack, Michael Argyle, and Norbert Schwarz. Oxford, England: Pergamon Press, 1990.

Scott, William A., and John Stumpf. "Personal Satisfaction and Role Performance: Subjective and Social Aspects of Adaptation." *Journal of Personality and Social Psychology* 47 (1984): 812–27.

Seligman, Martin E. P. *Helplessness: On Depression, Development and Death.* San Francisco: W. H. Freeman, 1975.

———. "Boomer Blues." *Psychology Today,* October 1988, pp. 50–55.

————. "Why Is There So Much Depression Today?" In *G. Stanley Hall Lectures*, edited by I. S. Cohen. Vol. 9. Washington, DC: American Psychological Association, 1988.

————. "Explanatory Style: Predicting Depression, Achievement, and Health." In *Brief Therapy Approaches to Treating Anxiety and Depression*, edited by Michael D. Yapko. New York: Brunner/Mazel, 1989.

————. *Learned Optimism*. New York: Random House, 1991.

————, and Peter Schulman. "Explanatory Style as a Predictor of Productivity and Quitting Among Life Insurance Sales Agents." *Journal of Personality and Social Psychology* 50 (1986): 832–38.

Siegel, Judith M., and David H. Kuykendall. "Loss, Widowhood, and Psychological Distress Among the Elderly." *Journal of Consulting and Clinical Psychology* 58 (1990): 519–24.

Silverman, Paul S., and Paul D. Retzlaff. "Cognitive Stage Regression Through Hypnosis: Are Earlier Cognitive Stages Retrievable?" *International Journal of Clinical and Experimental Hypnosis* 34 (1986): 192–204.

Simpson, Jeffry A., Bruce Campbell, and Ellen Berscheid. "The Association Between Romantic Love and Marriage: Kephart (1967) Twice Revisited." *Personality and Social Psychology Bulletin* 12 (1986): 363–72.

Smith, Marilyn C. "Hypnotic Memory Enhancement of Witnesses: Does It Work?" *Psychological Bulletin* 94 (1983): 387–407.

Smith, Mary Lee, and Gene V. Glass. "Meta-analysis of Psychotherapy Outcome Studies." *American Psychologist* 31 (1977): 752–60.

————, and Thomas I. Miller. *The Benefits of Psychotherapy*. Baltimore: Johns Hopkins University Press, 1980.

Smith, Richard H., Ed Diener, and Douglas H. Wedell. "Intrapersonal and Social Comparison Determinants of Happiness: A Range-Frequency Analysis." *Journal of Personality and Social Psychology* 56 (1989): 317–25.

Smith, Tom W. "Happiness: Time Trends, Seasonal Variations, Intersurvey Differences, and Other Mysteries." *Social Psychology Quarterly* 42 (1979): 18–30.

————. "Adult Sexual Behavior in 1989: Number of Partners, Frequency, and Risk." General Social Survey Topic Report No. 18, National Opinion Research Center, University of Chicago, 1990.

Smolen, Robert C. et al. "Examination of Marital Adjustment and Marital Assertion in Depressed and Nondepressed Women." *Journal of Social and Clinical Psychology* 7 (1988): 284–89.

Snodgrass, Sara E., J. G. Higgins, and L. Todisco. "The Effects of Walking

Behavior on Mood." Paper presented at the American Psychological Association Convention, Washington, DC, August 1986.

Snyder, C. R., and Raymond L. Higgins. "Excuses: Their Effective Role in the Negotiation of Reality." *Psychological Bulletin* 104 (1988): 23–35.

Solano, Cecilia H., Phillip G. Batten, and Elizabeth A. Parish. "Loneliness and Patterns of Self-Disclosure." *Journal of Personality and Social Psychology* 43 (1982): 524–31.

Solomon, Richard L. "The Opponent-Process Theory of Acquired Motivation: The Costs of Pleasure and the Benefits of Pain." *American Psychologist* 35 (1980): 691–712.

Solomon, Sheldon, Jeffery Greenberg, and Tom Pyszczynski. "A Terror Management Theory of Social Behavior: The Psychological Functions of Self-esteem and Cultural World-views." *Advances in Experimental Social Psychology* 24 (1991): 93–159.

Spanos, Nicholas P., and John F. Chaves. *Hypnosis: The Cognitive-Behavioral Perspective.* Buffalo, NY: Prometheus Books, 1989.

Spanos, Nicholas P., Robert J. Stenstrom, and Joseph C. Johnston. "Hypnosis, Placebo, and Suggestion in the Treatment of Warts." *Psychosomatic Medicine* 50 (1988): 245–60.

Spilka, Bernard, Ralph W. Hood, Jr., and Richard L. Gorsuch. *The Psychology of Religion: An Empirical Approach.* Englewood Cliffs, NJ: Prentice-Hall, 1985.

Spring, Bonnie. "Foods, Brain and Behavior: New Links." *Harvard Medical School Mental Health Letter* 4, no. 7 (1988): 4–6.

Staub, Ervin. *The Roots of Evil: The Psychological and Cultural Sources of Genocide.* New York: Cambridge University Press, 1989.

Stephens, T. "Physical Activity and Mental Health in the United States and Canada: Evidence from Four Population Surveys." *Preventive Medicine* 17 (1988): 35–47.

Sternberg, Robert J. "Triangulating Love." In *The Psychology of Love,* edited by Robert J. Sternberg and Michael L. Barnes. New Haven: Yale University Press, 1988.

———, and Susan Grajek. "The Nature of Love." *Journal of Personality and Social Psychology* 47 (1984): 312–29.

Stock, William A. et al. "Age and Subjective Well-being: A Meta-analysis." In *Evaluation Studies: Review Annual,* edited by Richard J. Light. Vol. 8. Beverly Hills: Sage, 1983.

———. "Race and Subjective Well-being in Adulthood." *Human Development* 28 (1985): 192–97.

Stone, Arthur A., and John M. Neale. "Effects of Severe Daily Events on

Mood." *Journal of Personality and Social Psychology* 46 (1984): 137–44.

Storr, Anthony. *Solitude: A Return to Self.* New York: Free Press, 1988.

Strack, Fritz, Leonard Martin, and Sabine Stepper. "Inhibiting and Facilitating Conditions of the Human Smile: A Nonobtrusive Test of the Facial Feedback Hypothesis." *Journal of Personality and Social Psychology* 54 (1988): 768–77.

Strack, Fritz, Norbert Schwarz, and Elisabeth Gschneidinger. "Happiness and Reminiscing: The Role of Time Perspective, Affect, and Mode of Thinking." *Journal of Personality and Social Psychology* 49 (1985): 1460–69.

Strack, Stephen, and James C. Coyne. "Social Confirmation of Dysphoria: Shared and Private Reactions to Depression." *Journal of Personality and Social Psychology* 44 (1983): 798–806.

Strumpel, Burkhard. "Economic Lifestyles, Values, and Subjective Welfare." In *Economic Means for Human Needs,* edited by Burkhard Strumpel. Ann Arbor: University of Michigan Survey Research Center, 1976.

Strupp, Hans H. "The Outcome Problem in Psychotherapy: Contemporary Perspectives." In *Psychotherapy Research and Behavior Change.* Vol. 1 of *The Master Lecture Series,* edited by John H. Harvey and Marjorie M. Parks. Washington, DC: American Psychological Association, 1982.

———. "Psychotherapy: Research, Practice, and Public Policy (How to Avoid Dead Ends)." *American Psychologist* 41 (1986): 120–30.

Suedfeld, Peter. *Restricted Environmental Stimulation: Research and Clinical Applications.* New York: Wiley, 1980.

———. "Aloneness as a Healing Experience." In *Loneliness: Sourcebook of Current Theory, Research, and Therapy,* edited by Letitia A. Peplau and Daniel Perlman. New York: Wiley, 1982.

Sullivan, Louis. *Washington Post* quote from address to the March 12, 1991, National Health Forum. *Grand Rapids Press,* March 24, 1991, p. D7.

Suls, Jerry M., and Frederick Tesch. "Students' Preferences for Information About Their Test Performance: A Social Comparison Study." *Journal of Applied Social Psychology* 8 (1978): 189–97.

Sundstrom, Eric, Kenneth P. DeMeuse, and David Futrell. "Work Teams: Applications and Effectiveness." *American Psychologist* 45 (1990): 120–33.

Suro, Robert. "Twelve Faiths Join Pope to Pray for Peace." *New York Times,* October 28, 1986.

Swann, William B., Jr., and Steven C. Predmore. "Intimates as Agents of Social Support: Sources of Consolation or Despair?" *Journal of Personality and Social Psychology* 41 (1985): 1119–28.

Sweet, L. L., and G. K. Murdock. "Subliminal Effect on Self-esteem." Senior thesis, Missouri Southern State College, 1990.

Tatarkiewicz, Wladyslaw. *Analysis of Happiness.* The Hague: Martinus Nijhoff, 1976.

Tavris, Carol. *The Mismeasure of Woman.* New York: Simon & Schuster, 1992.

———, and Carole Wade. *The Longest War: Sex Differences in Perspective.* New York: Harcourt Brace Jovanovich, 1984.

Taylor, Shelley E. "Adjustment to Threatening Events: A Theory of Cognitive Adaptation." *American Psychologist* 38 (1983): 1161–74.

———. *Positive Illusions.* New York: Basic Books, 1989.

Tellegen, Auke et al. "Personality Similarity in Twins Reared Apart and Together." *Journal of Personality and Social Psychology* 54 (1988): 1031–39.

Tennov, Dorothy. *Love and Limerence: The Experience of Being in Love.* New York: Stein & Day, 1979.

Terkel, Studs. *Working: People Talk About What They Do All Day and How They Feel About What They Do.* New York: Pantheon Books, 1972.

Thayer, Richard E. "Energy, Tiredness, and Tension Effects of a Sugar Snack Versus Moderate Exercise." *Journal of Personality and Social Psychology* 52 (1987): 119–25.

Thomas, Alexander, and Stella Chess. "The New York Longitudinal Study: From Infancy to Early Adult Life." In *The Study of Temperament: Changes, Continuities, and Challenges,* edited by Robert Plomin and Judy Dunn. Hillsdale, NJ: Erlbaum, 1986.

Thomson, Elizabeth, and Ugo Colella. "Cohabitation and Marital Stability: Quality or Commitment." *Journal of Marriage and the Family,* in press.

Tidball, M. Elizabeth, and Vera Kistiakowsky. "Baccalaureate Origins of American Scientists and Scholars." *Science* 193 (1976): 646–52.

Tierney, John. "The Perplexing Life of Erno Rubik." *Discover,* March 1986, pp. 81–88.

Tonkon, B. B. "A Social Psychological Perspective on Aging Patterns in Male Runners and Non-runners." *Dissertation Abstracts International* 45 (1985): 3591–92A.

Triandis, Harry C. "Cross-cultural Studies of Individualism and Collectivism." In *Nebraska Symposium on Motivation 1989,* edited by J. J. Berman. Vol. 37. Lincoln: University of Nebraska Press, 1989.

———. "The Self and Social Behavior in Differing Cultural Contexts." *Psychological Review* 96 (1989): 506–20.

——— et al. "Individualism and Collectivism: Cross-cultural Perspectives on

Self-Ingroup Relationships." *Journal of Personality and Social Psychology* 54 (1988): 323–38.

Triandis, Harry C., Richard Brislin, and C. Harry Hui. "Cross-cultural Training Across the Individualism-Collectivism Divide." *International Journal of Intercultural Relations* 12 (1988): 269–89.

Tucker, Larry A. "Physical Fitness and Psychological Distress." *International Journal of Sport Psychology* 21 (1990): 185–201.

Turner, J. et al. "The Effects of Subliminal Messages on Weight Loss." Manuscript, Aims Biofeedback Institute and University of Northern Colorado, 1989.

Uhlenberg, Peter, and David Eggebeen. "The Declining Well-being of Adolescents." *Public Interest* 82 (1986): 25–38.

Umberson, Debra, and Michael Hughes. "The Impact of Physical Attractiveness on Achievement and Psychological Well-being." *Social Psychological Quarterly* 50 (1987): 227–36.

Veenhoven, Ruut. "The Utility of Happiness." *Social Indicators Research* 20 (1988): 333–54.

———, ed. *How Harmful Is Happiness? Consequences of Enjoying Life or Not.* Gravenhage: Universitaire Pers Rotterdam, 1989.

———. "National Wealth and Individual Happiness." In *Understanding Economic Behaviour,* edited by Klaus G. Grunert and Folke Olander. Dordrecht: Kluwer Academic Publishers, 1989.

———. "Is Happiness Relative?" *Social Indicators Research* 24 (1991): 1–34.

———, and Piet Ouweneel. "Happiness as an Indicator of the Livability of Society." Paper presented at the International Conference on Social Reporting, Wissenschaftszentrum, Berlin, 1989.

Veenhoven, Ruut, and Maykel Verkuyten. "The Well-being of Only Children." *Adolescence* 14 (1989): 155–66.

Velten, Emmett. "A Laboratory Task for Induction of Mood States." *Behavior Research and Therapy* 6 (1968): 473–82.

Vemer, Elizabeth et al. "Marital Satisfaction in Remarriage: A Meta-analysis." *Journal of Marriage and the Family* 51 (1989): 713–25.

Venn, Jonathon. "Hypnosis and the Lamaze Method: A Reply to Wideman and Singer." *American Psychologist* 41 (1986): 475–76.

Viorst, Judith. *Necessary Losses.* New York: Ballantine/Fawcett, 1987.

Wachtel, Paul L. *The Poverty of Affluence: A Psychological Portrait of the American Way of Life.* Philadelphia: New Society Publishers, 1989.

Walker, C. "Some Variations in Marital Satisfaction." In *Equalities and Inequalities in Family Life,* edited by Robert Chester and John Peel. London: Academic Press, 1977.

Walker, Iain, and Leon Mann. "Unemployment, Relative Deprivation, and Social Protest." *Personality and Social Psychology Bulletin* 13 (1987): 275–83.

Wallach, Michael A., and Lise Wallach. "How Psychology Sanctions the Cult of the Self." *Washington Monthly,* February 1985, pp. 46–56.

Wallis, Claudia. "Back Off, Buddy: A New Hite Report Stirs Up a Furor over Sex and Love in the '80s." *Time,* October 12, 1987, pp. 68–73.

Warr, Peter, and Roy Payne. "Experiences of Strain and Pleasure Among British Adults." *Social Science and Medicine* 16 (1982): 1691–97.

Watson, David, and Lee A. Clark. "Self Versus Peer Ratings of Specific Emotional Traits: Evidence of Convergent and Discriminant Validity." *Journal of Personality and Social Psychology* 60 (1991): 927–40.

Weary, Gifford, Kerry L. Marsh, and Faith Gleicher. "Social-Cognitive Consequences of Depression." In *Control Motivation and Social Cognition,* edited by G. Weary, F. Gleicher, and K. L. Marsh. New York: Springer-Verlag, 1992.

Weaver, Charles N., and M. C. Matthews. *Personnel* 64 (September 1987): 62–65.

Weaver, James B., Jonathon L. Masland, and Dolf Zillmann. "Effect of Erotica on Young Men's Aesthetic Perceptions of Their Female Sexual Partners." *Perceptual and Motor Skills* 58 (1984): 929–30.

Weinstein, Neil D. "Unrealistic Optimism About Future Life Events." *Journal of Personality and Social Psychology* 39 (1980): 806–20.

———. "Unrealistic Optimism About Susceptibility to Health Problems." *Journal of Behavioral Medicine* 5 (1982): 441–60.

———. "Why It Won't Happen to Me: Perceptions of Risk Factors and Susceptibility." *Health Psychology* 3 (1984): 431–57.

Wener, Richard, William Frazier, and Jay Farbstein. "Building Better Jails." *Psychology Today,* June 1987, pp. 40–49.

Wheeler, Ladd, Harry T. Reis, and Michael H. Bond. "Collectivism-Individualism in Everyday Social Life: The Middle Kingdom and the Melting Pot." *Journal of Personality and Social Psychology* 57 (1989): 79–86.

Whipple, Christopher. "Chrissie." *Life,* June 1986, pp. 64–72.

White, James M. "Reply to Comment by Professors Trussel and Rao: A Reanalysis of the Data." *Journal of Marriage and the Family* 51 (1989): 540–44.

White, Lynn, and John N. Edwards. "Emptying the Nest and Parental Well-being: An Analysis of National Panel Data." *American Sociological Review* 55 (1990): 235–42.

Whitley, Bernard E., Jr. "Sex-Role Orientation and Psychological Well-being: Two Meta-analyses." *Sex Roles* 12 (1984): 207–25.

Wholey, Dennis. *Are You Happy?* Boston: Houghton Mifflin, 1986.

Wickless, Cynthia, and Irving Kirsch. "Effects of Verbal and Experiential Expectancy Manipulations on Hypnotic Susceptibility." *Journal of Personality and Social Psychology* 57 (1989): 762–68.

Will, George F. "The Seven Deadly Sins." In syndicated newspapers, July 8, 1978.

Williams, Margaret. *The Velveteen Rabbit: Or How Toys Become Real.* Garden City, NY: Doubleday, 1926.

Willits, Fern K., and D. M. Crider. "Religion and Well-being: Men and Women in the Middle Years." *Review of Religious Research* 29 (1988): 281–94.

Wing, Rena R., and Robert W. Jeffery. "Outpatient Treatments of Obesity: A Comparison of Methodology and Clinical Results." *International Journal of Obesity* 3 (1979): 261–79.

Winokur, Jon. *The Portable Curmudgeon.* New York: New American Library, 1987.

Winthrop, John. "A Model of Christian Charity." In *Puritan Political Ideas, 1558–1794,* edited by Edmund S. Morgan. Indianapolis: Bobbs-Merrill, 1965.

Witter, Robert A. et al. "Education and Subjective Well-being: A Meta-analysis." *Educational Evaluation and Policy Analysis* 6 (1984): 165–73.

———. "Religion and Subjective Well-being in Adulthood: A Quantitative Synthesis." *Review of Religious Research* 26 (1985): 332–42.

Wood, Joanne V., Judith A. Saltzberg, and Lloyd A. Goldsamt. "Does Affect Induce Self-Focused Attention?" *Journal of Personality and Social Psychology* 58 (1990): 899–908.

Wood, Wendy, Nancy Rhodes, and Melanie Whelan. "Sex Differences in Positive Well-being: A Consideration of Emotional Style and Marital Status." *Psychological Bulletin* 106 (1989): 249–64.

Wortman, Camille B., and Roxanne C. Silver. "Coping with Irrevocable Loss." In *Cataclysms, Crises, and Catastrophes: Psychology in Action,* edited by Gary R. VandenBos and Brenda K. Bryant. Washington, DC: American Psychological Association, 1987.

Wright, James D. "Are Working Women *Really* More Satisfied? Evidence from Several National Surveys." *Journal of Marriage and the Family* 40 (1978): 301–13.

Wuthnow, Robert. "Evangelicals, Liberals, and the Perils of Individualism." *Perspectives,* May 1991, pp. 10–13.

———, Virginia A. Hodgkinson, and Associates. *Faith and Philanthropy in America.* San Francisco: Jossey-Bass, 1990.

Wyche, James H., and Henry T. Frierson, Jr. "Minorities at Majority Institutions." *Science* 249 (1990): 989–91.

Wyse, Lois. "The Way We Are." *Good Housekeeping,* April 1991, p. 254.

Yardley, John K., and Robert W. Rice. "The Relationship Between Mood and Subjective Well-being." *Social Indicators Research* 24 (1991): 101–11.

Zika, Sheryl, and Kerry Chamberlain. "Relation of Hassles and Personality to Subjective Well-being." *Journal of Personality and Social Psychology* 53 (1987): 155–62.

Zillmann, Dolf. "Effects of Prolonged Consumption of Pornography." In *Pornography: Research Advances and Policy Considerations,* edited by Dolf Zillmann and Jennings Bryant. Hillsdale, NJ: Erlbaum, 1989.

Index

Page numbers, beginning with 209, refer to notes

A NOTE ABOUT THE AUTHOR

Social psychologist David G. Myers is an award-winning teacher (at Michigan's Hope College), an award-winning researcher, and the author of psychology's most widely studied text. With support from the National Science Foundation, he devoted the first decade of his career to studies of group influence, for which he received the Gordon Allport Prize. Since the late 1970s, his efforts have turned to translating psychological research for the lay public.